Assessment of Physical Fitness and Training Effect in Individual Sports

Assessment of Physical Fitness and Training Effect in Individual Sports

Editors

Tadeusz Ambrozy
Mariusz Ozimek
Andrzej Ostrowski
Henryk Duda
Michał Spieszny

MDPI • Basel • Beijing • Wuhan • Barcelona • Belgrade • Manchester • Tokyo • Cluj • Tianjin

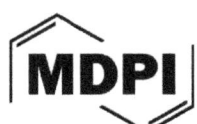

Editors

Tadeusz Ambrozy
University of Physical Education
Poland

Mariusz Ozimek
University of Physical Education
Poland

Andrzej Ostrowski
University of Physical Education
Poland

Henryk Duda
University of Physical Education
Poland

Michał Spieszny
University of Physical Education
Poland

Editorial Office
MDPI
St. Alban-Anlage 66
4052 Basel, Switzerland

This is a reprint of articles from the Special Issue published online in the open access journal *International Journal of Environmental Research and Public Health* (ISSN 1660-4601) (available at: https://www.mdpi.com/journal/ijerph/special_issues/Fitness_Training_Sports).

For citation purposes, cite each article independently as indicated on the article page online and as indicated below:

LastName, A.A.; LastName, B.B.; LastName, C.C. Article Title. *Journal Name* **Year**, *Volume Number*, Page Range.

ISBN 978-3-0365-6216-2 (Hbk)
ISBN 978-3-0365-6215-5 (PDF)

© 2023 by the authors. Articles in this book are Open Access and distributed under the Creative Commons Attribution (CC BY) license, which allows users to download, copy and build upon published articles, as long as the author and publisher are properly credited, which ensures maximum dissemination and a wider impact of our publications.

The book as a whole is distributed by MDPI under the terms and conditions of the Creative Commons license CC BY-NC-ND.

Contents

About the Editors vii

Preface to "Assessment of Physical Fitness and Training Effect in Individual Sports" ix

Jian Kim, Jooyeon Jin and Aeryung Hong
Creative Intercorporeality in Collaborative Work of Choreographers with and without Disabilities: A Grounded Theory Approach
Reprinted from: *Int. J. Environ. Res. Public Health* 2022, 19, 5548, doi:10.3390/ijerph19095548 . . . 1

Ruqayya Lockhart, Wiesław Błach, Manuela Angioi, Tadeusz Ambroży, Łukasz Rydzik and Nikos Malliaropoulos
A Systematic Review on the Biomechanics of Breakfall Technique (Ukemi) in Relation to Injury in Judo within the Adult Judoka Population
Reprinted from: *Int. J. Environ. Res. Public Health* 2022, 19, 4259, doi:10.3390/ijerph19074259 . . . 15

Szymon Price, Szczepan Wiecha, Igor Cieśliński, Daniel Śliż, Przemysław Seweryn Kasiak, Jacek Lach, Grzegorz Gruba, et al.
Differences between Treadmill and Cycle Ergometer Cardiopulmonary Exercise Testing Results in Triathletes and Their Association with Body Composition and Body Mass Index
Reprinted from: *Int. J. Environ. Res. Public Health* 2022, 19, 3557, doi:10.3390/ijerph19063557 . . . 33

Monika Kowalczyk, Małgorzata Zgorzalewicz-Stachowiak, Wiesław Błach and Maciej Kostrzewa
Principles of Judo Training as an Organised Form of Physical Activity for Children
Reprinted from: *Int. J. Environ. Res. Public Health* 2022, 19, 1929, doi:10.3390/ijerph19041929 . . . 49

Zepeng Lu, Limingfei Zhou, Wangcheng Gong, Samuel Chuang, Shixian Wang, Zhenxiang Guo, Dapeng Bao, et al.
The Effect of 6-Week Combined Balance and Plyometric Training on Dynamic Balance and Quickness Performance of Elite Badminton Players
Reprinted from: *Int. J. Environ. Res. Public Health* 2022, 19, 1605, doi:10.3390/ijerph19031605 . . . 59

Jarosław Jaszczur-Nowicki, Oscar Romero-Ramos, Łukasz Rydzik, Tadeusz Ambroży, Michał Biegajło, Marta Nogal, Waldemar Wiśniowski, et al.
Motor Learning of Complex Tasks with Augmented Feedback: Modality-Dependent Effectiveness
Reprinted from: *Int. J. Environ. Res. Public Health* 2021, 18, 12495, doi:10.3390/ijerph182312495 . 67

Tadeusz Ambroży, Łukasz Rydzik, Michał Spieszny, Wiesław Chwała, Jarosław Jaszczur-Nowicki, Małgorzata Jekiełek, Karol Görner, et al.
Evaluation of the Level of Technical and Tactical Skills and Its Relationships with Aerobic Capacity and Special Fitness in Elite Ju-Jitsu Athletes
Reprinted from: *Int. J. Environ. Res. Public Health* 2021, 18, 12286, doi:10.3390/ijerph182312286 . 75

Shiuan-Yu Tseng, Chung-Po Ko, Chin-Yen Tseng, Wei-Ching Huang, Chung-Liang Lai and Chun-Hou Wang
Is 20 Hz Whole-Body Vibration Training Better for Older Individuals than 40 Hz?
Reprinted from: *Int. J. Environ. Res. Public Health* 2021, 18, 11942, doi:10.3390/ijerph182211942 . 87

Jeong-Weon Kim and Sang-Seok Nam
Physical Characteristics and Physical Fitness Profiles of Korean Taekwondo Athletes: A Systematic Review
Reprinted from: *Int. J. Environ. Res. Public Health* 2021, 18, 9624, doi:10.3390/ijerph18189624 . . . 97

I-Lin Wang, Li-I Wang, Yang Liu, Yu Su, Shun Yao and Chun-Sheng Ho
Application of Real-Time Visual Feedback System in Balance Training of the Center of Pressure with Smart Wearable Devices
Reprinted from: *Int. J. Environ. Res. Public Health* **2021**, *18*, 9637, doi:10.3390/ijerph18189637 . . . 115

Karoly Dobos, Dario Novak and Petar Barbaros
Neuromuscular Fitness Is Associated with Success in Sport for Elite Female, but Not Male Tennis Players
Reprinted from: *Int. J. Environ. Res. Public Health* **2021**, *18*, 6512, doi:10.3390/ijerph18126512 . . . 125

Chin-Yi Gu, Xiang-Rui Li, Chien-Ting Lai, Jin-Jiang Gao, I-Lin Wang and Li-I Wang
Sex Disparity in Bilateral Asymmetry of Impact Forces during Height-Adjusted Drop Jumps
Reprinted from: *Int. J. Environ. Res. Public Health* **2021**, *18*, 5953, doi:10.3390/ijerph18115953 . . . 135

Wiesław Błach, Łukasz Rydzik, Łukasz Błach, Wojciech J. Cynarski, Maciej Kostrzewa and Tadeusz Ambroży
Characteristics of Technical and Tactical Preparation of Elite Judokas during the World Championships and Olympic Games
Reprinted from: *Int. J. Environ. Res. Public Health* **2021**, *18*, 5841, doi:10.3390/ijerph18115841 . . . 145

Wojciech J. Cynarski, Jan Słopecki, Bartosz Dziadek, Peter Böschen and Paweł Piepiora
Indicators of Targeted Physical Fitness in Judo and Jujutsu—Preliminary Results of Research
Reprinted from: *Int. J. Environ. Res. Public Health* **2021**, *18*, 4347, doi:10.3390/ijerph18084347 . . . 155

Alex Ojeda-Aravena, Tomás Herrera-Valenzuela, Pablo Valdés-Badilla, Jorge Cancino-López, José Zapata-Bastias and José Manuel García-García
Effects of 4 Weeks of a Technique-Specific Protocol with High-Intensity Intervals on General and Specific Physical Fitness in Taekwondo Athletes: An Inter-Individual Analysis
Reprinted from: *Int. J. Environ. Res. Public Health* **2021**, *18*, 3643, doi:10.3390/ijerph18073643 . . . 165

Rafel Cirer-Sastre, Francisco Corbi, Isaac López-Laval, Luis Enrique Carranza-García and Joaquín Reverter-Masià
Exercise-Induced Release of Cardiac Troponins in Adolescent vs. Adult Swimmers
Reprinted from: *Int. J. Environ. Res. Public Health* **2021**, *18*, 1285, doi:10.3390/ijerph18031285 . . . 183

Łukasz Rydzik, Tadeusz Ambroży, Zbigniew Obmiński, Wiesław Błach and Ibrahim Ouergui
Evaluation of the Body Composition and Selected Physiological Variables of the Skin Surface Depending on Technical and Tactical Skills of Kickboxing Athletes in K1 Style
Reprinted from: *Int. J. Environ. Res. Public Health* **2021**, *18*, 11625, doi:10.3390/ijerph182111625 . 189

Joanna M. Bukowska, Małgorzata Jekiełek, Dariusz Kruczkowski, Tadeusz Ambroży and Jarosław Jaszczur-Nowicki
Biomechanical Aspects of the Foot Arch, Body Balance and Body Weight Composition of Boys Training Football
Reprinted from: *Int. J. Environ. Res. Public Health* **2021**, *18*, 5017, doi:10.3390/ijerph18095017 . . . 205

Łukasz Rydzik and Tadeusz Ambroży
Physical Fitness and the Level of Technical and Tactical Training of Kickboxers
Reprinted from: *Int. J. Environ. Res. Public Health* **2021**, *18*, 3088, doi:10.3390/ijerph18063088 . . . 217

About the Editors

Tadeusz Ambrozy

Tadeusz Ambroży is a Full Professor of physical culture sciences, and is Director of the Institute of Sports Sciences of the University of Physical Education in Krakow. He has authored or co-authored over 300 scientific papers. He is a masterclass trainer in combat sports; a trainer of gymnastics, boxing, swimming, and bodybuilding; a personal trainer; sports manager; sailing, skiing, and water rescue instructor; and a yacht and motorboat captain.

Mariusz Ozimek

Mariusz Ozimek is a Professor of Physical Culture Sciences at the Institute of Sports Sciences of the University of Physical Education in Krakow. He has authored or co-authored many publications in the field of physical culture. He is also a masterclass trainer.

Andrzej Ostrowski

Andrzej Ostrowski is a Professor of Physical Culture Sciences at the Institute of Sports Sciences of the University of Physical Education in Krakow. He has authored or co-authored many publications in the field of physical culture. He is also a swimming coach and yacht and motorboat captain.

Henryk Duda

Henryk Duda is a Professor of Physical Culture Sciences at the Institute of Sports Sciences of the University of Physical Education in Krakow. He has authored or co-authored many publications in the field of physical culture. He is also a masterclass trainer.

Michał Spieszny

Michał Spieszny is a Professor of Physical Culture Sciences at the Institute of Sports Sciences of the University of Physical Education in Krakow. He has authored or co-authored many publications in the field of physical culture. He is also a masterclass trainer.

Preface to "Assessment of Physical Fitness and Training Effect in Individual Sports"

Physical fitness is the basis for the success of players in sports, and its monitoring makes it possible to assess the effectiveness of training and identify possible errors. During training, thanks to the use of control results, these activities are modified, which better prepares players for competition. This Special Issue, entitled "Assessment of Physical Fitness and the Effect of Training in Individual Sports" presents the results of coaching control and the results of monitoring progression in training, as well as an assessment of the physical fitness of athletes practicing individual sports.

Tadeusz Ambrozy, Mariusz Ozimek, Andrzej Ostrowski, Henryk Duda, and Michał Spieszny
Editors

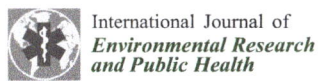

Article

Creative Intercorporeality in Collaborative Work of Choreographers with and without Disabilities: A Grounded Theory Approach

Jian Kim [1], Jooyeon Jin [2] and Aeryung Hong [3,*]

1 Department of Sports and Dance, Sangmyung University, Seoul 03016, Korea; artsedu@smu.ac.kr
2 Department of Sport Science, University of Seoul, Seoul 02504, Korea; jjin13@uos.ac.kr
3 Global Research Institute for Arts and Culture Education, Sangmyung University, Seoul 03016, Korea
* Correspondence: dphong@smu.ac.kr

Abstract: The purpose of this study was to present an academic discourse on a theoretical framework and acceptance process of 'creative intercorporeality' in the collaborative work of choreographers with and without disabilities. To this end, a grounded theory approach using a qualitative research method was employed to dancers who have participated in collaborative choreography. This study employed the perspective of social cognitive theory about the process in which dancers with and without disabilities form emotional empathy and trust relationships through continuous interactions for creative work. Physical, emotional, cognitive, and behavioral empathy and interactions in the collaborative work of choreographers with and without disabilities were discussed as a process of forming 'creative intercorporeality' that is defined as creative attitude and perspective consisting of harmony, concurrency, consistency, and balance.

Keywords: creative intercorporeality; collaborative work; choreographers with and without disabilities; social cognitive theory

1. Introduction

Choreography is an art that designs a series of human movements and the form is defined within movements [1,2]. Choreography is not just activity using body, but activity created through intellectual processes to express one's emotions and intentions using bodily movements [3]. It spans various fields of arts and sports such as dance, theater, musical, opera, gymnastics, figure skating, cheerleading, and artistic swimming. In particular, choreography created by two or more choreographers must contain dynamic exchange in intellectual capability, interact through bodily movements, and form creative solidarity. In this regard, well-developed collaborative choreography may include in-depth work and processes that harmonize methods of movement and expression by interacting cognitive, relational, aesthetic, and creative thinking skills among choreographers.

In the last two decades, collaborate work of choreographers with and without disabilities were actively attempted in different settings worldwide [4]. In addition, there have been recent scholarly activities dealing with topics such as experiences of children with disabilities in elementary school dance education [5–8], collaborative dance lessons in inclusive education environment [9], cooperative programs in traditional dance [10,11] and creative practice of dance artists [12,13]. These endeavors may guide, from the perspective of individuals with disabilities, how to overcome a lack of confidence and empowerment caused by disabilities, and from the perspective of individuals without disabilities, how to understand disabilities and develop an attitude away from prejudice. For these reasons, collaborative work of choreographers with and without disabilities is probably promising as it results in forming a positive attitude that recognizes and embraces the differences.

Meanwhile, most participation of people with disabilities in dance has been regarded as part of amateur or community dance rather than the area of "professional". The potential reason, regardless of the culture of the East and the West, might be that the audience has been only used to watching the dance performed by dancers with the best physical conditions at the best theater. In other words, prejudice that limits the artistic value of dance, centering on physical figures and dance movements of dancers without disabilities, has been socially prevalent for quite a long time. However, breaking away from this prejudice, over the past decade, the development of "adapted dance" and/or "physically integrated dance" has gradually been expanded from an inclusive perspective [4,14]. This is probably influenced by a disability paradigm shift to perceive the concept of disability as a social and non-categorical phenomenon rather than a medical and categorical phenomenon. This change may prompt an contextual extension of dance participation towards inclusive environment where dancers with and without disabilities perform together [15–18].

The goal of the inclusive perspective in dance is to break up the technical framework of people without disabilities in locomotion and balance, and to expand the language of dance movements in various ways, so that people with disabilities can enter the norm of choreography more actively [19]. For example, dancesport has been widely known as a representative genre of dance that shows inclusive and cooperative characteristics as at least one of the dancers is in a wheelchair. Even the team of dancers with and without disabilities perform all modern genres such as Tango, Waltz, and Quickstep, and Latin American dances such as Chacha, Samba, Pasodoble, Lumba, and Jive are called "Combi-dance". This collaborative choreography is not limited to the genre of dance in which the step routine is determined by certain criteria. The meaning of "creative integration" based on atypicality and possibility is important in that various creative elements must be drawn and new compositions must be created cooperatively. In the inclusive dance, directors and choreographers tend to focus on what dancers with disabilities can do in new and alternative ways, rather than focusing on what they cannot do. Due to the nature of inclusive environment, choreographers with disabilities may develop dance repertoire regardless of what disability conditions and degrees they have and collaborate through improvisation, and make new movements with their peers without disabilities.

However, there may be a dilemma in expressing "integrated" or "inclusive" dances through the performance of dancers with disabilities on a stage [4,20,21]. For example, it is necessary to take into account shortcomings such as blind access to infinite possibilities [22], directing dancers with disabilities treated as stage props, injuries and extreme damage caused by excessive technical attempts, and targeting audiences with disabilities rather than without disabilities. Nevertheless, it should be noted that the cooperative choreography is still as important as the serious creative process itself [23]. In inclusive dance process, one may have the following questions: "What movements can dancers with disabilities make?", "How do you communicate among dancers with and without disabilities," and "How do you solve the problem of movement for possible dance?" To answer those questions, cooperative choreography among dancers with and without disabilities aims for a more professional performance and presents a new vision for a "barrier-free society" [24].

The collaborative choreography goes through a cognitive process [25] that strives to empathize with each other and form a relationship for physical and emotional interactions; that is, bonding, intimacy, and trust, which soon shifts to movements as a dance language [26–29]. This process is explained by the concept of interaction that emphasizes the essential role of individuals with different abilities in the process of social understanding [30]. This notion is supported from the perspective of social cognitive theory, assuming that human behavior is a function of interactions of cognitive process and environment in a heterogeneous way, and the quality of human behavior is determined by experience in the particular environment [31–37].

With this core concept of the theory, Shogo Tanaka attempted to reexamine the concept of Merleau-Ponty's intercorporeality and specify it as a extended social cognitive theory [38,39]. He developed the concept of behavioral unity, primitive empathy, interactive synchronization, and a sense of mutual understanding. Based on the perspective of this cognitive science, intercorporeality is defined as a shared perception including emotions and thoughts of two independent individuals. This can be said to be the origin of empathy, arising from the connection of cognition and behavior among oneself and another self; that is, the interrelationship among one's body and another's body.

The purpose of this study was to clarify the meaning of the cooperative choreography process and experience of choreographers with and without disabilities in the context of "creative intercorporeality" and to re-examine the discourses related to the construct. To achieve the purpose, end, this study employed a grounded theory approach as a qualitative research method to build empirical knowledge and a theoretical framework for dancers who have participated in integrated dance, especially collaborative choreography.

2. Research Method

This study employs a grounded theory approach to examine the process by which choreographers with and without disabilities embrace creative intercorporeality for collaborative work. Based on the experiences of the choreographers, this study examined how adapted dance affects disability awareness in the context of creative intercorporeality, and how a choreographer's work embrace and transform a disability in the context of creative intercorporeality. The Grounded Theory, which was developed by sociologists Glaser and Strauss, was used for developing a theoretical model that explains interactions concerning systematic and comprehensive processes [40].

2.1. Research Participants

Ten participants who have experiences working with performers and/or choreographers with and without disabilities were conveniently recruited from an annual dance festival funded by Korean government. Demographic information of the participants are shown in Table 1. The approval (SMUIRB C-2020-017) from the Institutional Review Board (IRB) was obtained and the consent was collected from all research participants before data collection was initiated to ensure research ethics.

Table 1. Research participants.

No.	Name	Gender	Age	Occupation	Career
A	Kim, S.	Female	30+	Dancer, Arts instructor	16 years
B	Shin, J.	Female	30+	Dancer, Arts instructor	15 years
C	Kim, A.	Female	40+	Dancer, Arts instructor	17 years
D	Han, J.	Female	40+	Leader of dance company	26 years
E	Lee, Y.	Male	40+	Professor	25 years
F	Song, J.	Male	40+	Professor	23 years
G	Kim, Y.	Male	40+	Leader of dance project	15 years
H	Kim, E.	Female	50+	Artistic director	31 years
I	Kim, H.	Female	50+	Leader of dance company	35 years
J	Jung, S.	Male	50+	Artistic director	36 years

2.2. Data Collection and Analysis

Data were collected from November 2020 to January 2021 through in-depth interviews using a semi-structured questionnaire. For a research participant who is overseas and not available for in-depth interviews in person, the researchers collected data via emails. The semi-structured questionnaire covered four areas: introduction to disability art and the artist's portfolio, experience participating in disability art, difficulties in the collaborative work, and social recognition of disability and creative inter-corporeality. In order to collect data, an average of 1.5 in-depth interviews were conducted with the study participants for 1 hour 30 minutes to 2 hours, and the consent of the study participants was obtained and recorded. All interview contents were transcribed and coded and classified into upper and lower categories.

Data analysis was conducted according to the analytical methods of open coding, axial coding, and selective coding presented by Strauss and Corbin [41]. Through open coding, 190 significant concepts were classified among the interview contents, and 30 subcategories and 14 categories were categorized centering on similar concepts. Conditions, phenomenon, strategy, and sequences constituting the paradigm model were classified as axial coding. In the selective coding process, the core category and the entire story line are summarized. After analysis, the details of descriptions were confirmed by the researchers, and the names of the participants were changed to pseudonyms or initials.

3. Result (1) Concepts and Categories

To examine the process by which choreographers who have experiences working with ones with and without disabilities accept creative intercorporeality, 190 conceptual words were derived as a result of analyzing the data line by line. Those with similar meanings were gathered to derive 30 subcategories, from which those with similar meanings were placed into superordinate categories, deriving a total of 14 categories.

Among the experiences of choreographers with and without disabilities as a process of acceptance of creative intercorporeality was the "creative intercorporeality through integrated dance," which is a central phenomenon, as an interaction between causal conditions and contextual conditions; to overcome its difficulties, choreographers used action/interaction strategies. The process of reaching consequences as the impact of intervening conditions was determined. As a result of the analysis, the paradigm model on the collaborative choreography process was developed to demonstrate creative intercorporeality with subcategories.

3.1. Causal Conditions

Causal conditions indicate the conditions or events that lead a certain phenomenon to occur, lay the groundwork, or develop. The acceptance process of the collaborative work of choreographers with and without disabilities begins from new motivation in choreography; more specifically, choreographers pondered over the essence of dance and continuity in exploring the body and implemented work extended by a new perspective on dance. They attempted professional–nonprofessional movements in dance styles based on movements as the collaborative choreography began to contemplate the disability discourse in dance. The choreographers served as a link between works with artistic value and the public sector through adapted dance, conducting various activities in events hosted by the government and local governments. These activities are exposed to society due to these internal and external public events, and further opportunities bring more positive effects. As such, the awareness and consideration of the context of creative intercorporeality began at the same time that choreography work was born as an adapted dance. Therefore, elements of causal conditions could be categorized into personal situations such as 'new approach to the body' and 'motivation for new ideas'.

> We spent a few weeks getting to know each other, introducing and talking about performances of a dancer with a disability, watching performance videos, and moving our bodies together. As we experienced trial and error in experiencing new things, we started to change little by little. Remembering the elements of impromptu amusement that I learned from the Axis Dance Company, I applied the improvisation method to our class and witnessed the stages of transformation in our art. (Research participant B)

3.2. Contextual Conditions

Contextual conditions refer to the structural context that pertains to a certain phenomenon and the specific conditions for action and interaction. As a result of analysis, "mirroring others," "breaking the pattern of the body," and "shifting to a paradoxical way of thinking" were required as a "methodological agenda." It was necessary to break the stereotypes between choreographers for the collaborative work, and to communicate by determining the movements within the scope of potential capability. As such, the methodological agenda about diversity and integration accepts disabilities in the context of creative intercorporeality and provides the conditions of action and interaction regarding the process of integration required. Therefore, elements of context conditions could be categorized into personal situations such as 'acquiring mutually integrated choreography' and 'methodological agenda of support system'.

By showing the public the dance that engages our body most actively, it became a determining factor in breaking down the barrier between disability and art. (Research participant F)

3.3. Central Phenomenon

Central phenomenon is defined as how a certain phenomenon is handled or progressed, and experience or core issue commonly shared by the research participants, as well as a key event to which action and interaction are related. As a result of the analysis, awareness of creative intercorporeality in choreography was the core phenomenon and was more specifically classified into balanced exploration of disability related expressions, empathy from potential behavior, and acquiring mutually integrated choreography. This experience was became an important turning point for the research participants because they were able to develop a new perspective on disabilities, breaking their prejudice or bias after participation, claiming that they attempted to find the balance point in expression or lead the space through potential behavior. In particular, "creative intercorporeality through integrated dance" was the consequence of causal conditions and described by the participants as an important disability art experience in the context of creative intercorporeality; thus, it was presented as the central phenomenon.

With poliomyelitis, my body is in discomfort, and the center of gravity is different for me. In other words, my range of motion relying on a shifted center of gravity and the texture of my motion from different postures are completely different compared to others. However, I just take it as differences amongst performers and I think that can be the point of attraction. Would you say there is any difference between a student with a curved pelvis lifting a leg versus a person with a completely distorted center of gravity lifting a leg? When it comes to the performance of lifting a leg, there must be wholesome respect for the body. (Research participant C)

3.4. Intervening Conditions

Intervening conditions are the structural and extensive conditions affecting action and interaction, as well as the phenomenon. The research participants responded that inadequate support system and prejudice against adapted dance created barriers and frustrations against choreography. They also highlighted difficulties in the collaboration process as clash of opinions and complaints, which were occasionally raised between choreographers with and without disabilities in the choreography process. Moreover, when contacting with partners and selecting a partner in group dance moves they experienced difficulties due to physical and mental resistance; the safety of dancers also had to be considered. Therefore, elements of intervening conditions could be categorized into personal situations such as 'barrier and prejudice in choreography', 'conflicts in collaboration', and 'risk of injury and resistance'.

While working, disability was never a reference point for me. A person with a disability is the same human being as us, and I found it ironic labelling people with disabilities based on the perception that people without disabilities are the norm and the rest are not. It's merely a little difference, but we all are the same in talking to each other, sharing our minds, and expressing ourselves using our bodies as the medium. (Research participant B)

3.5. Action/Interaction Strategies

Action/interaction strategies are a method to handle a problematic phenomenon, and they refer to intentional and deliberate behaviors that must be taken to solve a problem in practice. As for the new approach to the body, the research participants reset their perspectives and premises regarding how impairments in body functions and structures are perceived by society and other people, and whether they could head in a positive direction. They also had to communicate endlessly and show respect among dancers and made constant attempts to see how movements were interpreted from various perspectives. "Mutual understanding and respect" was a strategy for work by the participants within adapted art to proceed in a more meaningful and appropriate direction in the context of creative intercorporeality. Based on communication and respect, as well as empathy and trust to understand differences, the research participants pursued ways to head in a new direction to accept the differences, breaking away from the negative perspective on these in bodies and movements. Therefore, choreographers working their peers with and without disabilities were accepting it by using strategies such as the "exploration of a new process of approach" and "mutual understanding and respect".

I believe that artists and dancers with disabilities daily experience unique challenges that derive from their discomfort. This is why I see disability art as a form of art that acknowledges the differences in each person. There will be uniqueness from such discomfort and differences, and the empathy that deems such uniqueness as the novelty will arise. (Research participant C)

3.6. Consequences

Consequences indicate outcomes or results of action/interaction to cope with a certain phenomenon or to manage and maintain such the phenomenon. The experience of accepting creative intercorporeality for choreographers with and without disabilities participating in the collaborative work resulted in the consequences of "synchronizing and empathy", "creative reciprocity and interaction", "discovery/re-discovery of potential", and "future sustainability of disability art".

The strategy "creative reciprocity" explored coexistence through creative expression and discovered what creates the conditions for inclusive dance by acquiring trust and empathy from reciprocity. "Interactive synchronization and empathy" showed how the research participants discovered new interpretations of the body and various possibilities of movements through disability art, instead of considering a disability equals to incompetence. Moreover, "future sustainability of disability art" indicates that, for continuous disability art activities, it is necessary to activate actual projects in addition to policy support, and to establish an inclusive environment for the coexistence of dancers.

Even in adapted dance, I am not moved by seeing dancers with disabilities on the stage, but purely by the work itself and the competence of those dancers. I want to say that, to change the stereotypical perception, dancers with disabilities need to grow their competency in creating a balance and harmony with choreographers and performers without disabilities. (Research participant F)

4. Result (2) Core Category and Situation Model

4.1. Core Category

This study conducted selective coding for the acceptance process of the research participants in collaborative work of choreographers with and without disabilities in the context of creative intercorporeality, ultimately forming a paradigm model and the story outline. As a result, the core category was "creative intercorporeality in dancers with and without disabilities".

Through such a process, it was possible to determine how the integrated approach that embraces is due to the collaborative work of choreographers with and without disabilities, and how the collaboration is formed.

First, choreographers began to look for new works originating from fundamental concerns such as exploration of the body, audience development, and dance. While the focus had been on working with dance specialists before, now the targets changed to various non-specialists such as an old lady, a middle-aged man, or a teenager, thereby expanding the scope of activities and naturally participating in collaborative work of choreographers with and without disabilities. Some dancers participated with interest in adapted dance after watching a performance by overseas a dancer with a disability, and others were recommended by other dancers who had already participated in adapted dance or began disability art upon the request of an adapted dance organization. Participating in collaborative work of choreographers with and without disabilities could be regarded as a starting point for many choreographers and performers to start a new form of work through various types of approaches, while also having the opportunity to gain disability awareness.

Second, the choreographers considered that disability awareness is important for participating in disability art. However, since education on disability awareness has not existed for a long time, many individuals without a disability still cannot easily approach to a disability condition. Nevertheless, the research participants showed an immediate response to change through education on disability awareness. The research participants who have collaborative work experience of choreographers with and without disabilities were experiencing change in naturally accepting disabilities in education on disability awareness.

Third, the research participants were able to take part in national events and projects of public institutions as an opportunity to expose a disability using disability art as a medium. With national and public art events, it was possible to not only be exposed to many people but also approach them in a less awkward way. Currently, there is a great interest in cultural diversity worldwide, and South Korea is also making a move to extensively improve disability awareness through policies and projects of public institutions. In this process, dancers linked their work with artistic value to the public sector, thereby creating an opportunity to promote positive disability awareness through internal and external public events.

Fourth, for the research participants who have experience in collaborative work, the form of disability and ability was an opportunity to have a new understanding of what was becoming meaning through their work. According to the research participants, the fundamental idea of becoming one through movement away from the dichotomy of disability and ability created great synergy in cooperative work. All agreed that perception of disability could never be a barrier to bringing about creative choreography or harmonizing among dancers.

4.2. Situation Model

The situation model is the stage in which the consequences thus far are summarized and integrated to promote the understanding of the core category and provide a more convincing explanation [41]. This study built the situation model for "creative intercorporeality in collaborative work of choreographers with and without disabilities" at the individual, artistic, and social levels. Figure 1 shows how the integrated approach that embraces intercorporeality is formed through collaboration between choreographers with and without disabilities. The oval-shaped lines in Figure 1 are marked as individual, arts community, and society & nation, and the dotted lines among the lines represent how the factors of each level affect the integrated approach that embraces diversity.

This situation model includes causal conditions as well as contextual, intervening conditions, action/interaction strategies, and consequences. Cases such as "new approach to the body", "motivation for new idea", "acquiring mutually integrated choreography", "methodological agenda of support system", that are hovering between the individual and artistic levels, that are hovering between the artistic and social levels indicate that the category appears in each one. Also, the consequences and stages of the process in which dancers participating in collaborative work of choreographers with and without disabilities accept creative intercorporeality and the core category were presented in order at the bottom of the figure.

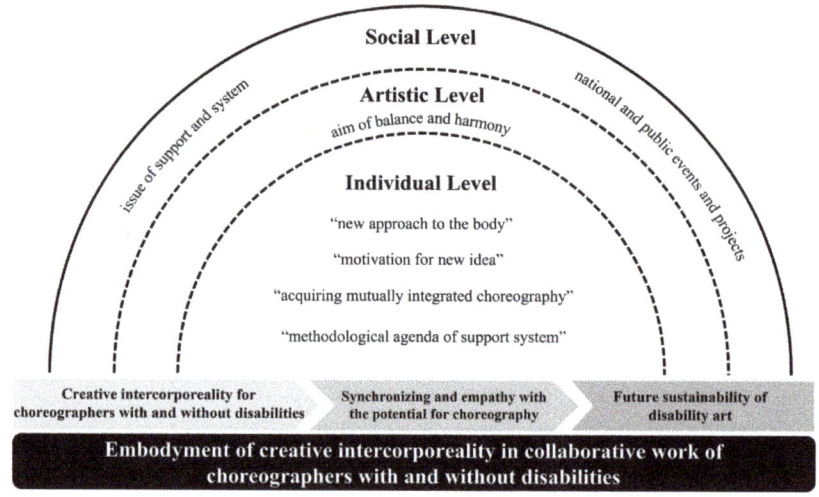

Figure 1. Situation model.

5. Discussion

Until now, choreographers and performers who participate in disability art tended to improve their understanding of disability or gain new insights when they had more experience [21,42]. On the other hand, when the activity did not last, the dancers simply confirmed that they knew about the disability and had no opportunity to gain a new understanding [43,44]. This was supported by Marsh [45] who argued that there was not enough research evidence on adapted dance yet and that there was a lack of knowledge of collaboration among choreographers with and without disabilities. Ames, Benjamin, and Whatley have studied the vivid experiences of artists with disabilities and the dance activities of performers with disabilities [20,21,46], but they have shown that the development of adapted dance is uncertain unless all performers cooperate and show continued interest and participation [47,48]. This indicates that artistic opportunities and continuous activities in which the collaborations should continue [3,7,49].

This study was intended to present an academic discourse on the process of experiencing creative intercorporeality in the collaborative choreography process for choreographers with and without disabilities. This study analyzed the raw data on the experiences of ten dancers who participated in cooperative choreography between dancers with and without disabilities and derived a total of 190 conceptual words. Based on this, the axial coding method of Strauss and Corbin [41] was classified into 14 upper categories and 30 lower categories, and "creative intercorporeality in collaborative work of choreographers with and without disabilities" was derived as a core phenomenon forming the paradigm.

As shown in Figure 2, as factors influencing this core phenomenon, personal situations such as new motivation in choreography, collaboration of choreographers with and without disabilities and a new approach to the choreography of methodological agenda were found in common contexts. This led to questions such as "How far is the artistic possibility that human can express with their bodies?" and "Have we not limited the artistic beauty expressed with their bodies too much in stereotypes?" It was about the choreographer's intellectual curiosity and value of beauty toward new and rare movements, as well as ventilation of socially prevalent prejudices. In particular, this study found that the beginning of cooperative work between choreographers with and without disabilities stems from creative attempts to escape stereotypes and challenges to themselves. It can be seen as an effort to expand the language of movement in various ways by not limiting the artistry of dance to the technical framework through "inclusive" dance of performers with and without disabilities [4,19].

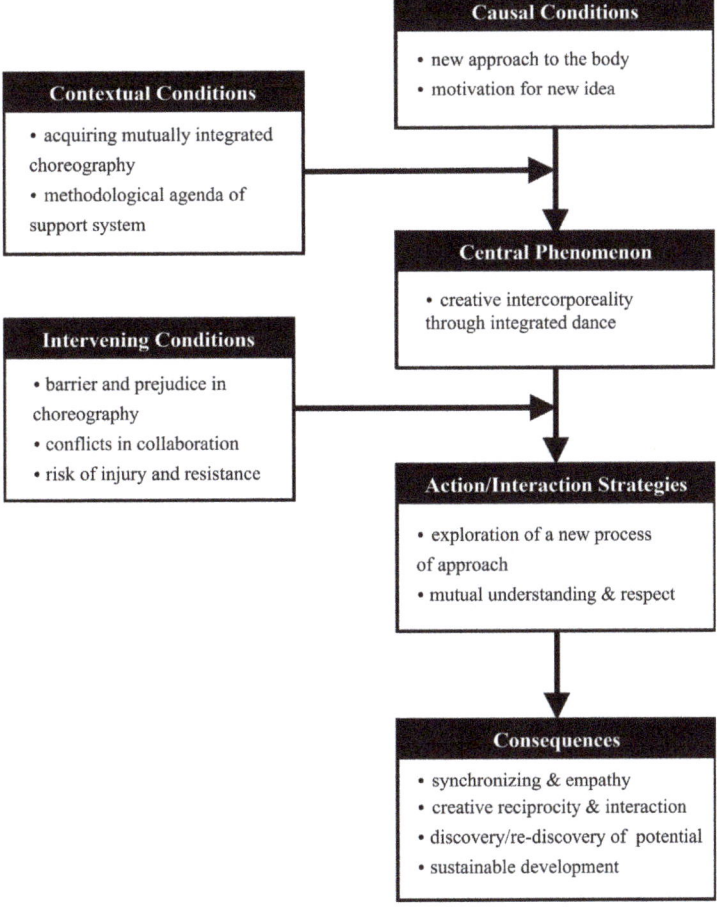

Figure 2. Paradigm model.

However, unlike the motivation to participate, the process was never easy. "How do two choreographers with different thoughts and physical environments communicate with each other and solve problems of movement?" It said that the more they aimed for professional performance, the more difficulties they faced. In other words, constraint factors that mediate the synergy of collaborative choreography were derived. Cooperative choreography among choreographers with and without disabilities should avoid excessive technical expression in consideration of the physical risk of injury and resistance, difficulty and conflict of cooperation and obstruction and prejudice against disability that may arise. This dilemma in terms of working choreographers with and without disabilities has already been appeared in previous studies [4,20,21], so it can occur as much as possible and should be fully considered [24]. However, finding empirical insights on how to deal with the dilemma and defects and solving problems in the collaborative choreography process of the research participants are a meaningful work suggested by this study.

This study focused on the action/interaction strategy that alleviated the interventional element. A "new approach" different from the general choreography process was found. Rather than entering the composition of the scenes and movements of the choreography related to the subject in earnest, each focused on exchanging existing activities in dance. They said they have studied the process of criticizing each other's strengths and weaknesses about choreography and finding common denominators that can be matched by trying each other with their preferred styles for quite a long time. The process necessarily involved an emotional consensus of "mutual understanding and respect". It can be seen that these mutual efforts presuppose not only the physical aspect but also emotional, cognitive, and social interactions in the cooperative choreography in the relationship between two choreographers.

The result of the current study can be presented as a situation model as "creative intercorporeality through collaborative work of choreographers with and without disabilities" at the individual, artistic, and social levels. In other words, through a series of processes called cooperative choreography, "creative intercorporeality" was concluded to have experienced meaningful achievements such as creative intercorporeality, discovery/rediscovery of potential, and sustainability of interaction.

This study attempted a qualitative approach focusing on the experience and interaction process of collaborative work among choreographers with and without disabilities in that the quality of the experience is important, emphasizing the essential role of oneself and other egos in social understanding. To explain this in detail, this study borrowed Shogo Tanaka's concept of "intercorporeality" of "connection and empathy of cognition and behavior occurring in interrelationships between independent egos" [39].

In this study, the cooperative choreography between ones with and without disabilities had an important meaning in the serious creative process itself. In the cognitive process of trying to empathize with each other, the relationship between integration, empathy and trust was the basis, and this was implemented as an active and specific interactive behavior of unity through the body and harmonious choreography. In the process of cooperative choreography of choreographers with and without disabilities, "creative intercorporeality" could be defined as forming creative empathy and achievement through physical, emotional, cognitive, and behavioral interactions such as bond and intimacy between the two dancers.

This study was able to explain how choreographers with different conditions and situations in the context of diversity accept differences for the creative work of "choreography", and how the behavioral synergy of the two individuals creates creative achievements. In particular, this study, based on the experiences of choreographers who participated in collaborative choreography toward the proposition of "possible dance", is meaningful in that it practically showed the potential of inclusive dance and the possibility of inclusive gaze through creative dance.

6. Conclusions

There has been prejudice in the field of dance for a while. The participation of individuals with disabilities in dance was viewed as the domain of "community dance", or explained as the mainstream's "inclusive" attitude toward certain special people. But, it presupposes a contradiction that is already unilaterally limited, and diversity is not respected. In the challenge of implementing the art of 'creative intercorporeality,' there is not certain standards of how to move and express in dance. Moreover, disability is never a barrier in dance, an artist who delivers a message through various bodily movements, choreography, and a creative work develops the language of dance.

This study focused on the process in which cooperative work between choreographers with and without disabilities constantly forms emotional empathy and trust relationships through interactions for creative work. In particular, from the perspective of social cognitive theory, this process can be explained as presupposing 'creative intercorporeality' for the attitude of embracing each other's perspectives in the interaction between the two dancers. Therefore, in the process of collaborative work of choreographers with and without disabilities, 'creative intercorporeality' can be defined as a creative attitude and perspective that expresses harmony, concurrency, consistency, and balance through physical, emotional, cognitive, and behavioral empathy between the choreographers.

The change in dancers' perception of dance access to disability and methodology was significant in reaffirming the original aesthetic reflection of dance art as a creative expression of 'choreography' along with the trend of adapted dance. In particular, the intrinsic dynamism of creative intercorporeality in cooperative choreography reflects various trends as well as the philosophical background of dance. It is still prevalent to challenge blind cooperation work on the grounds of the movement's own methodological approach or national support system without understanding or deliberation on 'disability'. Disability art initiated against this background should be avoided. Along with this reflection, confirming the artistic performance and developing potential dancers with disabilities should also not be overlooked.

This study findings may make unique contributions to dance literature for the interactions between choreographers with and without disabilities, in that it provides insight to increase the value of dance arts. Along with the methodological attempts of various basis theories, it seems necessary to further discuss the a fundamental theory for the participation of individuals with disabilities in dance. Through this, it is suggested that a comprehensive review and discourse on dance for persons with disabilities should be presented, so that they keep participating in the art of dance.

Author Contributions: Conceptualization, J.K.; methodology, J.J. and A.H.; data collection, A.H.; data curation, J.K. and J.J.; writing—original draft preparation, J.K.; writing—review and editing, J.K., J.J. and A.H.; project administration, J.K.; funding acquisition, J.K., J.J. and A.H. All authors have read and agreed to the published version of the manuscript.

Funding: This research was supported by the Ministry of Education of Republic of Korea, the National Research Foundation of Korea (NRF-2020S1A5B8104241).

Institutional Review Board Statement: The study was conducted according to the guidelines of the Declaration of Helsinki and was approved by the Institutional Review Board (or Ethics Committee) of Sangmyung University (SMUIRB C-2020-017).

Informed Consent Statement: Informed consent was obtained from all subjects involved in the study.

Data Availability Statement: The data are not publicly available due to privacy issues.

Acknowledgments: The authors would like to thank the reviewers for their comments and suggestions that have significantly improved the initial version of the paper. We further acknowledge the contribution of the Ministry of Education of Republic of Korea, the National Research Foundation of Korea, GACE, University of Seoul, and Sangmyung University.

Conflicts of Interest: The authors declare no conflict of interest. The funders had no role in the design of the study; in the collection, analyses, or interpretation of data; in the writing of the manuscript, or in the decision to publish the results.

References

1. Brinson, P. *Dance as Education: Towards a National Dance Culture*; Falmer: Brighton, UK, 1991.
2. Cooper-Albright, A. *Choreographing Difference, the Body and Identity in Contemporary Dance*; Wesleyan University Press: Middletown, CT, USA, 1997.
3. Kim, J.Y.; Hong, A.R. How can we lead creative choreography?: Narrative inquiry of dance educators' teaching experiences in dance class for students with intellectual disabilities. *Res. Danc. Phys. Educ.* **2020**, *4*, 61–74. [CrossRef]
4. Benjamin, A. *Making an Entrance: Theory and Practice for Disabled and Non-Disabled Dancers*; Routledge: London, UK, 2013.
5. Aujla, I.; Needham-Beck, S. Subjective well-being among young dancers with disabilities. *Int. J. Disabil. Dev. Educ.* **2020**, *67*, 563–570. [CrossRef]
6. Hu, M.; Wang, J. Artificial intelligence in dance education: Dance for students with special educational needs. *Technol. Soc.* **2021**, *67*, 101784. [CrossRef]
7. May, T.; Chan, E.S.; Lindor, E.; McGinley, J.; Skouteris, H.; Austin, D.; McGillivray, J.; Rinehart, N.J. Physical, cognitive, psychological and social effects of dance in children with disabilities: Systematic review and meta-analysis. *Disabil. Rehabil.* **2021**, *43*, 13–26. [CrossRef]
8. Zitomer, M.R. Children's perceptions of disability in the context of elementary school dance education. *Rev. phénEPS/PHEnex J.* **2016**, *8*, 1–16.
9. Bryan, R.R.; McCubbin, J.A.; Van Der Mars, H. The ambiguous role of the paraeducator in the general physical education environment. *Adapt. Phys. Act. Q.* **2013**, *30*, 164–183. [CrossRef]
10. Kapodistria, L.; Chatzopoulos, D.A. Greek traditional dance program for improving balance of young children. *Res. Danc. Educ.* **2021**, 1–13. Available online: https://www.tandfonline.com/doi/abs/10.1080/14647893.2021.1980525?journalCode=crid20 (accessed on 26 February 2022). [CrossRef]
11. Raghupathy, M.K.; Divya, M.; Karthikbabu, S. Effects of Traditional Indian Dance on Motor Skills and Balance in Children with Down syndrome. *J. Mot. Behav.* **2022**, *54*, 212–221. [CrossRef]
12. Reinders, N.J.; Bryden, P.J.; Fletcher, P.C. 'Dance is something that anyone can do': Creating dance programs for all abilities. *Res. Danc. Educ.* **2019**, *20*, 257–274. [CrossRef]
13. Urmston, E.; Aujla, I.J. Values, attributes, and practices of dance artists in inclusive dance talent development contexts. *J. Danc. Educ.* **2021**, *21*, 14–23. [CrossRef]
14. Zitomer, M.R.; Reid, G. To be or not to be–able to dance: Integrated dance and children's perceptions of dance ability and disability. *Res. Danc. Educ.* **2011**, *12*, 137–156. [CrossRef]
15. Goodwin, D.L. I can be beautiful and graceful-dancing from a wheelchair. *Palaestra* **2004**, *20*, 5–7.
16. Goodwin, D. The voices of students with disabilities: Are they informing inclusive physical education practice? In *Disability and Youth Sport*; Routledge: London, UK, 2009; pp. 65–87.
17. Goodwin, D.L.; Krohn, J.; Kuhnle, A. Beyond the wheelchair: The experience of dance. *Adapt. Phys. Act. Q.* **2004**, *21*, 229–247. [CrossRef]
18. Goodwin, D.L.; Thurmeier, R.; Gustafson, P. Reactions to the metaphors of disability: The mediating effects of physical activity. *Adapt. Phys. Act. Q.* **2004**, *21*, 379–398. [CrossRef]
19. Watlington, E. Cripping choreography. *Art Am.* **2021**, *109*, 28–33.
20. Benjamin, A. Cabbages and kings: Disability, dance and some timely considerations. In *The Routledge Dance Studies Reader*; Routledge: Oxford, UK, 2010; pp. 129–139.
21. Whatley, S. Dance and disability: The dancer, the viewer and the presumption of difference. *Res. Danc. Educ.* **2007**, *8*, 5–25. [CrossRef]
22. Irving, H.R.; Giles, A.R. A dance revolution? Responding to dominant discourses in contemporary integrated dance. *Leisure/Loisir* **2011**, *35*, 371–389. [CrossRef]
23. Snow, K. Mainstreaming, integration, inclusion: Is there a difference. In *Disability is Natural E-Newsletter*; NIDRR: Washington, DC, USA, 2008.
24. Weisberg, R.W. Expertise and structured imagination in creative thinking: Reconsideration of an old question. In *The Cambridge Handbook of Expertise and Expert Performance*; Ericsson, K.A., Hoffman, R.W., Kozbelt, A., Williams, A.M., Eds.; Cambridge University Press: Cambridge, UK, 2018; pp. 812–834.
25. Nordin, S.M.; Cumming, J. Where, when, and how: A quantitative account of dance imagery. *Res. Q. Exerc. Sport* **2007**, *78*, 390–395. [CrossRef]
26. Sandahl, C. Disability arts. In *Encyclopedia of Disability*; Albrecht, G., Ed.; Sage: Thousand Oaks, CA, USA, 2005; pp. 405–406.
27. Sandahl, C. Disability art and artistic expression. In *Encyclopedia of American Disability History*; Burch, S., Ed.; Facts on File: New York, NY, USA, 2009; pp. 246–268.
28. Sandahl, C.; Auslander, P. *Bodies in Commotion: Disability & Performance*; University of Michigan Press: Ann Arbor, MI, USA, 2005.
29. Smith, O. Shifting Apollo's frame: Challenging the body aesthetic in theater dance. In *Bodies in Commotion: Disability and Performance*; Sandahl, C., Auslander, P., Eds.; University of Michigan Press: Ann Arbor, MI, USA, 2005; pp. 73–85.
30. Goldstein, E.B. *Cognitive Psychology: Connecting Mind, Research and Everyday Experience*; Cengage Learning: Stamford, CT, USA, 2011.
31. Fuchs, T.; De Jaegher, H. Enactive intersubjectivity: Participatory sense-making and mutual incorporation. *Phenomenol. Cogn. Sci.* **2009**, *8*, 465–486. [CrossRef]

32. Gallagher, S. The practice of mind: Theory, simulation or primary interaction? *J. Conscious. Stud.* **2001**, *8*, 83–108.
33. Gallagher, S. Understanding interpersonal problems in autism: Interaction theory as an alternative to theory of mind. *Philos. Psychiatry Psychol.* **2004**, *11*, 199–217. [CrossRef]
34. Gallagher, S.; Zahavi, D. *The Phenomenological Mind*, 2nd ed.; Routledge: London, UK, 2012.
35. Downs, D.S.; Hausenblas, H.A. The theories of reasoned action and planned behavior applied to exercise: A meta-analytic update. *J. Phys. Act. Health* **2005**, *2*, 76–97. [CrossRef]
36. Pavski, V.; Chakrabarti, C.L.; Sturgeon, R.E. Spatial imaging of the furnace atomization plasma emission spectrometry source. *J. Anal. At. Spectrom.* **1994**, *9*, 1399–1409. [CrossRef]
37. Motl, R.W.; Snook, E.M.; Wynn, D. Physical activity behavior in individuals with secondary progressive multiple sclerosis. *Int. J. MS Care* **2007**, *9*, 139–142. [CrossRef]
38. Merleau-Ponty, M. *The Primacy of Perception: And Other Essays on Phenomenological Psychology, the Philosophy of Art, History, and Politics*; Northwestern University Press: Evanston, IL, USA, 1964.
39. Tanaka, S. Intercorporeality as a theory of social cognition. *Theory Psychol.* **2015**, *25*, 455–472. [CrossRef] [PubMed]
40. Glaser, B.G.; Strauss, A.L. *The Discovery of Grounded Theory: Strategies for Qualitative Research*; Aldine: Chicago, IL, USA, 1967.
41. Strauss, A.; Corbin, J. *Basics of Qualitative Research Techniques*; Sage Publications, Inc.: London, UK, 1998.
42. Cheesman, S. Dance and Disability: Embracing difference, tensions and complexities. *Danc. Res. Aotearoa* **2014**, *2*, 20–30. [CrossRef]
43. Albright, A.C. *Strategic Abilities: Negotiating the Disabled Body in Dance*; Michigan Publishing, University of Michigan Library: Ann Arbor, MI, USA, 1998.
44. Loots, L. "You don't look like a dancer!": Gender and disability politics in the arena of dance as performance and as a tool for learning in South Africa. *Agenda* **2015**, *29*, 122–132. [CrossRef]
45. Marsh, K. Taking Charge: Dance, Disability and Leadership: Exploring the Shifting Role of the Disabled Dance Artist. Ph.D. Thesis, Coventry University, Coventry, UK, 2016.
46. Ames, M. Performing between intention and unconscious daily gesture. How might disabled dancers offer us a new aesthetic sensibility? *Performance* **2012**, *11*, 143–158.
47. Downie, A. Equity-Informed Dancer Wellness. *J. Danc. Educ.* **2022**, *23*, 1–11. [CrossRef]
48. Kuppers, P. Accessible education: Aesthetics, bodies and disability. *Res. Danc. Educ.* **2000**, *1*, 119–131. [CrossRef]
49. Lee, Y.; Kim, J.; Hong, A. Multiple mediation effects of peer relationship and social withdrawal in relationship between self-esteem and multicultural acceptance in multicultural youth participating in physical activity. *Int. J. Sport Psychol.* **2022**, *53*, 83–97.

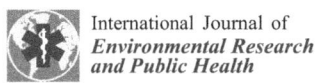

International Journal of
Environmental Research and Public Health

Review

A Systematic Review on the Biomechanics of Breakfall Technique (Ukemi) in Relation to Injury in Judo within the Adult Judoka Population

Ruqayya Lockhart [1], Wiesław Błach [2], Manuela Angioi [1], Tadeusz Ambroży [3], Łukasz Rydzik [3,*] and Nikos Malliaropoulos [1,4,5]

1. Centre for Sports and Exercise Medicine, William Harvey Research Institute, Queen Mary University of London, London E1 4DG, UK; r.lockhart@smd17.qmul.ac.uk (R.L.); m.angioi@qmul.ac.uk (M.A.); contact@sportsmed.gr (N.M.)
2. Faculty of Sport, University School of Physical Education in Wroclaw, 51-612 Wroclaw, Poland; wieslaw.judo@wp.pl
3. Institute of Sports Sciences, University of Physical Education, 31-571 Krakow, Poland; tadek@ambrozy.pl
4. Sports Clinic, Rheumatology Department, Barts Health NHS Trust, London E1 4DG, UK
5. Sports and Exercise Medicine Clinic, 4639 Thessaloniki, Greece
* Correspondence: lukasz.rydzik@awf.krakow.pl

Abstract: Objectives: To investigate the biomechanics of Ukemi in relation to head and neck injury in adult judokas with varying skill sets. Design: Narrative systematic review. Methods: An extensive literature search was performed using PubMed, Google Scholar, Science direct and EMBASE from inception to April 2021. Studies were included if they: (1) reported biomechanical analysis of judo throws and Ukemi; (2) were on adult judoka populations; (3) discussed injury related to judo technique. The included studies were assessed for risk of bias using a five-part modified STROBE checklist. A narrative synthesis was performed due to the heterogeneity of included studies. Results: 173 titles and abstracts were screened with 16 studies (158 judokas, 9 of which were female) included. All studies used 3D biomechanical analysis to assess Ukemi. Ukemi implementation produced reduced kinematic data in comparison to direct occipital contact, which was always below the injury threshold. Analysis of lower limb and trunk kinematics revealed variances in Ukemi between novice and experienced judoka. Whilst no significant differences were seen in neck flexion angles, hip, knee and trunk angle time plots revealed greater extension angles in experienced judokas. Conclusions: Ukemi is essential in preventing head and neck injuries; however, technique differs between experienced and novice judoka. Larger flexion angles of the hip, knee and trunk are seen in novice judoka, which correlate with increased kinematic data. The association of greater neck muscle strength with improved Ukemi is weak. However, a negative correlation was established between fatigue and breakfall skill by one study.

Keywords: sports injuries; judo; Ukemi

1. Introduction

Judo is an extremely popular martial art; it is an official Olympic and Paralympic sport, practised in over 200 countries worldwide [1,2]. It was first developed in 1882 by Professor Jugoro Kao, who created a more defensive style of martial art, going beyond sport, represented by three fundamental principles: (1) physical education; (2) contest proficiency and (3) mental training—all with the goal of being a better individual in society [2]. However, like with any sport, there are associated injury risks.

The aim of judo is to pin your opponent to the ground using grappling and throwing techniques [1,3]. Despite this more defensive style, an observational study from 2008 to 2016 recorded injury incidence rates in judo of 9.6 per 1000 min of exposure. Furthermore, in comparison to other combat sports such as boxing, taekwondo and wrestling, judo had the highest injury rate; this warrants investigation [4]. Common injuries include strains, sprains and contusions of the knee, shoulders and fingers [3,5]. Less frequent are injuries affecting the brain and spinal cord, such as acute subdural haematoma (ASDH); however, they are more prevalent in young and novice judokas [6,7]. In Japan, there has been a decline in judo participation in schools due to fear of severe injury. Over the past 30 years, approximately 300 students have been made disabled or comatose due to traumatic brain injuries (TBI) in Japan [8].

Judo consists of standing and ground fighting; however, the majority of injuries are mostly associated with standing, grappling and throwing moves [3,5]. Studies reporting the prevalence of injury suggest a greater association of injury to the uke (athlete being thrown) in comparison to the tori (throwing athlete) [9]. A 2016 study reported an injury rate of 43.8% in the uke population, as opposed to an injury rate of 25% seen in the tori population [10]. Osoto-gari (OS), Seoi-nage (SN) and Ouchi-gari (OU) are frequently used throwing techniques in high-level competitions. Amongst these techniques, SN is the most common throwing technique amongst judokas who sustained head and neck injury (42.9%) [11,12]. Head and neck injuries usually result from head impact onto the judo mat (tatami). It is believed that sudden rotational acceleration in the sagittal plane causes rupture of bridging veins resulting in TBI on impact [13–16].

Ukemi, or 'safe falling', is a breakfall motion technique that is emphasised in judo [17]. Before participating in combat practice (randori), judokas must perfect Ukemi [18,19]. Judokas learn variations of Ukemi to prepare them for randori; this includes sideways breakfall (Yoko Ukemi) [20], forward breakfall (Mae-Ukemi) [21], backwards breakfall (Ushiro Ukemi) and forward breakfall with a roll (Mae Maware Ukemi) [22]. However, this discipline has not prevented severe injuries from taking place [6,11,16], leading us to question the effectiveness of Ukemi. Hence, this study will assess the efficacy of Ukemi through an analysis of impact on the head and neck and evaluate whether improvements in technique can be made to reduce injury rates.

This systematic review aims to provide a clear understanding of the biomechanics of Ukemi, when implemented by experienced and novice judoka, and establish whether it is suitable protection from severe injury. A comprehensive review of the biomechanics of Ukemi has never been published. Several descriptive and observational studies of Ukemi have been undertaken in recent years. Many of these use advanced 3D kinematic analysis to understand breakfall motion associated with different throws in various populations [23–39]. Therefore, there is a need to review the current understanding of the biomechanics of Ukemi. From this, we will provide recommendations for further research topics and practical suggestions to prevent injury during practice.

2. Materials and Methods

2.1. Study Design

This systematic review was conducted and reported according to the Preferred Reporting Items for Systematic Reviews and Meta-Analyses (PRISMA) guidelines [40].

2.2. Inclusion and Exclusion Criteria

Articles were included if the following criteria were met: (1) reported biomechanical analysis of judo breakfall technique (Ukemi); (2) adult judoka population; (3) discussion of injury related to judo technique; (4) English papers.

Articles were excluded if the following criteria were met: (1) review and retrospective type articles; (2) computerised biomechanical models; (3) non-English papers; (4) judokas aged <18; (5) studies with no available abstract; (6) biomechanical analysis of the tori's actions; (7) biomechanical analysis of other combat sports (jujitsu, karate and MMA). The inclusion-exclusion criteria are shown in Table 1.

Table 1. Inclusion and exclusion criteria.

Inclusion	Exclusion
• Reported Biomechanical analysis of judo breakfall technique (Ukemi) • Adult judoka participants (>18 years old) • Discussion of injury related to judo practice • English papers	• Review and retrospective articles • Computerised biomechanical models • Non-English papers • Child participants (<18 years old) • Studies with no available abstract • Biomechanical analysis of the tori's actions • Biomechanical analysis of other combat sports

2.3. Literature Search Strategy

An extensive literature search was performed using PubMed, Google Scholar, Science Direct and EMBASE from inception to April 2021. Articles on the biomechanics of judo techniques relating to injury in judo in the adult judoka population were selected and reviewed. A broad search was used as the literature on this topic is sparse; a more specific search produced too few results. The following Boolean combination of terms was used [41]: ('Biomechanic*'OR 'Biomechanical analysis' OR 'Biomechanical injury' AND 'Kinetics' OR 'Kinematics' AND 'Injury' AND 'Judo*'). MeSH subject headings were not used to narrow or broaden the search [42]. Due to the large difference between results in google scholar and the other databases, we chose to only use the first 200 results as sorted by relevance of Google Scholar ranking [43]. Two reviewers (RL and MP) independently performed the search to ensure the results of the literature search were identical.

All publications were exported to Mendeley reference desktop Version1.19.4 (Elsevier, New York, NY, USA), where all duplicates were removed by the first author [44]. The papers were then imported to Rayyan, a web and mobile screening tool for systematic reviews (version 2016), where the reviewers collaboratively screened the articles [45]. A third reviewer was available if a consensus could not be reached.

2.4. Literature Screening

Articles were screened in a step-by-step process in the order of title, abstract and full text, in line with the predetermined study criteria. The two authors (RL, MP) screened all titles and abstracts independently and selected potential studies. When all potential studies were agreed on by both authors, full texts were reviewed for articles that met the inclusion criteria or for papers that could not explicitly be excluded. Further articles were excluded if the full text revealed they did not meet the inclusion or met exclusion criteria.

2.5. Data Extraction and Analysis

Data from eligible studies were extracted by one reviewer (RL) and independently verified by the second reviewer (MP). Data elements recorded included: author, year of publication, study design and basic participant characteristics (age, years; height, cm; and weight, kg), anthropomorphic test device (ATD) data, experience level (all judokas who had not reached their 1st Dan were considered novice) [46], throws being used and biomechanical assessment method. A narrative synthesis of the data was performed; a meta-analysis was not possible due to the heterogeneity between studies.

2.6. Quality Assessment of Literature

A five-item study checklist developed by another systematic review analysing observational studies was used to assess the risk of bias in the individual studies [47,48]. The five items included were modified from the 'strengthening the reporting of observational studies in epidemiology' (STROBE) statement [49]. The items were (1) study setting, location and study period; (2) eligibility criteria, sources and methods of participant selection; (3) exposure definition and measurement; (4) study outcome definition and measurement; and (5) main results and precision (e.g., 95% confidence interval). Each study was analysed as having a low or high risk of bias for each statement. If reporting of said item was lacking or unclear, it would warrant a high risk of bias; low bias items were scored 1, high bias items were scored 0. Reviewers agreed that a total score > 3 was considered low bias, a score of 3 was considered moderate bias, a score of 2 was high bias and a score of 1 warranted exclusion due to extremely high bias. The explanation and elaboration article was used to give examples and methodology for examining articles [50]. The two researchers assessed quality independently and then resolved disagreements to form the current assessment. One study was excluded based on the risk of bias assessment.

3. Results

3.1. Study Selection

The online database search identified 1493 titles from PubMed, Google Scholar, Science Direct and EMBASE, respectively, the following number of publications were found in each database (7,19,37,1430). After duplicates were removed, 1403 remained; following the screening process, a total of 37 studies were assessed for eligibility, 16 of these [23–38] were included in the systematic review. Included studies were agreed upon by the two reviewers; a third reviewer was not needed to reach a consensus. Figure 1 represents the 2020 PRISMA flow diagram [51].

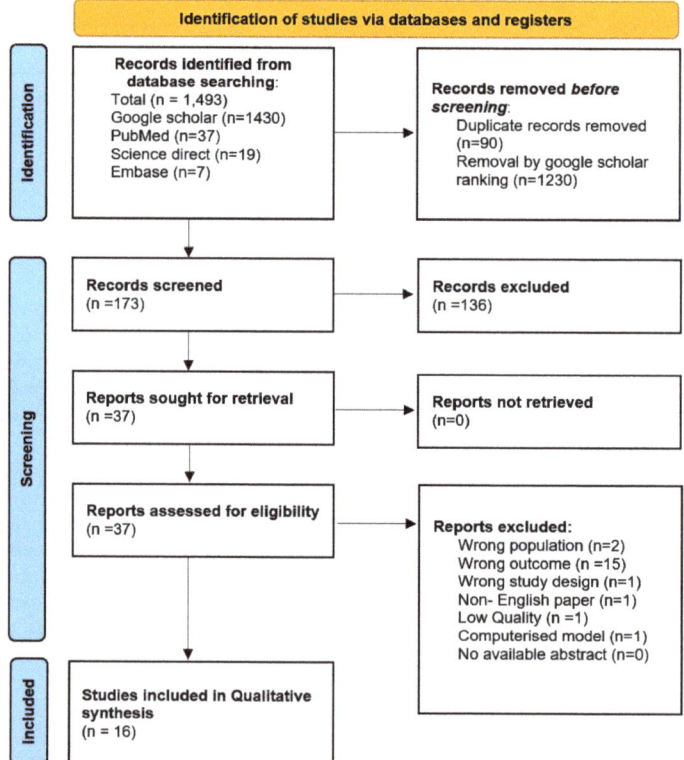

Figure 1. PRISMA flow diagram.

3.2. Study Characteristics and Data Extraction

A total of 158 judokas were included in this review, 9 were female and 149 were male, 54 were elite and 104 were novice judokas. All tori's were elite judoka who knew how to correctly perform the throw. The age (years), weight (kg) and height (cm) mean and range were the following: 24 (18–65) years, 166.2 (164.2–184.7) kg and 68.6 (64.9–101.7) cm. Four studies (25%) investigated Ukemi comparing experienced and novice judokas; five studies (31%) investigated throws without Ukemi, using ATD dummies; four studies (25%) evaluated the Breakfall technique with no associated throw. Twelve (75%) studies evaluated breakfall with an associated throw (OS, OU, SN and Tai-otoshi (TO)); all studies (100%) used 3D biomechanical analysis, two studies (12.5%) evaluated EMG activity; two studies (12.5%) evaluated neck strength and four studies (25%) evaluated multi-planer motion. See Appendix A for outcome groupings and Tables 2–5 for study characteristics and outcomes.

Table 2. Study characteristics and outcomes.

Study Reference	Hashimoto, et al., 2015	Hitosugi, et al., 2014	Ishikawa, et al., 2018	Ishikawa, et al., 2020
Study design	Observational	Observational	Observational	Observational
Participant characteristics: Number, gender, (Elite/Novice), (Tori/Uke), Age (years), Height (cm), Weight (kg)	N = 8, Male 3, Elite Uke:(27, 184.7, 101.7) 5, Elite Tori: 3, (25, 169, 66) and 2, (27, 177, 93)	1, Male Elite Tori: (26, 177, 90) ADT dummy Uke, (NA, 175, 75)	9 Male 8, Novice Uke: (17.5, 173, 72.4) 1, Elite Tori: (20, 165.0, 70.0)	15 Male 14 Elite Uke: (19.4, 168.1, 77.5) 1Elite Tori: (18, 173.0, 74.0)
Breakfall technique	Exemplary Ukemi following OS and OU	No breakfall, of OS and OU	Basic Ukemi of OS, OU, SN, TO	Exemplary Ukemi of OS
Biomechanical assessment method	Vertical Velocity of the Uke's head (kg m/s^2)	3D Linear (G) and angular acceleration (rad/s^2) of the uke's head	3D Rotational acceleration of the ukes head (rad/s^2)	3D angular acceleration of the ukes head (rad/s^2) Neck muscle strength during forward & backward flexion (N)
Measured Outcomes and key findings	Vertical velocity OS > OU (204.82 +/− 19.95 > 118.46 +/− 63.62) $p = 0.08$ Vertical Velocity reduced when body surface area increased. In OS the head reached its lowest point before the trunk and lower limbs, the opposite is true for OU	Occipital head contact = large force in the longitudinal direction for linear acceleration and sagittal plane angular acceleration. Linear acceleration values in the longitudinal direction: OU > OS (41.0 +/− 2.6 G and 86.5 +/− 4.3 G) Angular acceleration values in the sagittal plane: OS > OU (3315 +/− 168 and 1328 +/− 201)	Max rotational acceleration generated: TO: 368.3, SN: 276.2, OS: 693.2, OU: 401.6 Rotational Acceleration: OS > OU > TO > SN	The maximum angular acceleration of the head immediately increased after high-intensity exercise ($p < 0.01$) Neck forward flexion strength increased ($p < 0.05$)
Risk of bias	Low	Low	Low	Moderate

Table 3. Study characteristics and outcomes.

Study Reference	Koshida, et al., 2012	Koshida, et al., 2013	Koshida, et al., 2014	Koshida, et al., 2016
Study design	Observational	Observational	Observational	Observational
Participant characteristics: Number, gender, (Elite/Novice), (Tori/Uke), Age (years), Height (cm), Weight (kg)	10 Male 6, Elite Uke: (20.5, 171.9, 72.4) 4, Novice Uke: (20, 168.8, 68)	24 Male 11, Elite Uke:(19.9, 164.2, 70.1) 13, Novice Uke: (21.4,169.2, 68.6)	24 Male 11, Elite Uke: (19.9, 164.2, 70.1) 13, Novice Uke: (21.4,169.2, 68.6)	22 Male 12, Novice (21.3, 174, 71.3) 10 Elite, (19.9, 168, 70.1)

Table 3. Cont.

Study Reference	Koshida, et al., 2012	Koshida, et al., 2013	Koshida, et al., 2014	Koshida, et al., 2016
Breakfall technique	Basic Ukemi, no throw	Basic Ukemi, no throw	Basic Ukemi, no throw	Ukemi following OS
Biomechanical assessment method	Neck and Trunk flexion angle time curve (°) EMG amplitude (%) Of SCM, EO, RA	Head, neck-, trunk-, hip-, and knee-angle–time-curve profiles (°)	Peak Linear acceleration of the ukes head in the sagittal plane (g/s^2) Neck, head, trunk, hip and knee flexion angle time profiles (°) EMG amplitude (%) Of SCM, EO, RA	Peak angular momentum of neck extension ($kg\,m^2s^{-1}$) Neck, trunk, hip and knee flexion angles (°)
Measured Outcomes and key findings	Coefficient of multiple correlation (CMC) In neck and trunk values: (0.989 and 0.954), statistical significance (0.05) No significant difference between neck and Trunk flexion angle time curves and muscle activation between Novice and experienced judoka.	The results showed significant differences in knee ($p < 0.001$) and trunk ($p < 0.005$) flexion angle time curves, whereas no significant differences were found in head, neck, and hip kinematics between the novice and experienced judokas	No significant difference seen in mean peak linear acceleration in novice and elite judoka (1.69 +/− 0.48 g/s^2 and 2.11 +/− 0.57 g/s^2) $p = 0.06$ Neck, Hip and Trunk angles showed minimal differences between the groups A large significant difference was seen in knee extension movement. EMG activation patterns showed no significant difference between the two groups	Mean peak angular momentum of neck extension in the novice judokas (-1.29 ± 0.23) was significantly greater than that in the experienced judokas (-0.78 ± 0.28) No significant differences in the neck ($p = 0.6$) or right hip ($p = 0.4$) angles between the experienced and novice judokas pairwise comparison = significant differences in the trunk angle movement in OS ($p < 0.001$) significantly greater left hip flexion observed in the novice judokas in OS ($p < 0.01$) Greater knee flexion stability seen in experienced judokas ($p > 0.005$)
Risk of bias	Moderate	Low	Moderate	Moderate

Table 4. Study characteristics and outcomes.

Study Reference	Koshida, et al., 2/2017	Koshida, et al., 10/2017	Koshida, et al., 2018	Michnik, et al., 2014
Study design	Observational	Observational	Observational	Observational
Participant characteristics: Number, gender, (Elite/Novice), (Tori/Uke), Age (years), Height (cm), Weight (kg)	13 Male 12 Novice, Uke: (21.3, 174, 71.3) 1 Elite, Tori: (38, 170, 73)	22 Male 21 Novice, Uke, (20.1, 170, 68.6) 1Elite, Tori: (41, 170, 65)	23 Male, 9 Female 31 Novice Uke, (20.9, 167, 64.9) 1 Elite Tori,	2 Male 1 novice Uke, (24, 183, 77) 1 Elite Uke, (65, 181, 84)
Breakfall technique	Ukemi following OS and OU	Ukemi following OS	Ukemi following OS	Basic Ukemi, no throw but knocked out of balance by 3rd party
Biomechanical assessment method	Mean peak angular momentum of neck extension ($kg\,m^2s^{-1}$) neck, hip, Trunk, knee angle time plots (°)	Peak angular momentum of neck extension ($kg\,m^2s^{-1}$) Neck flexion angles (°) Forward flexion neck muscle strength (N)	Peak neck angular momentum ($kg\,m^2s^{-1}$) Trunk COM angular velocity (rad/s^2)	Velocity of centre of mass Torso Angle of centre of mass (°)

Table 4. Cont.

Study Reference	Koshida, et al., 2/2017	Koshida, et al., 10/2017	Koshida, et al., 2018	Michnik, et al., 2014
Measured Outcomes and key findings	Mean peak angular momentum of neck extension in OS > OU: (1.29 +/− 0.23 And 0.84 +/− 0.29) $p < 0.01$ A significant difference was seen between OS and OU in neck, hip, and knee angle time plots ($p < 0.01$). No variances seen in trunk angles between OS and OU	Neck flexion angle increased until peak flexion, followed by abrupt extension at end. Neck flexion in OS is multidirectional, Peak angular momentum of the sagittal plane was greatest, but the Horizontal and frontal plane accounted for 30% of neck extension. No linear relationship between neck strength and angular momentum.	A significant correlation was seen between the trunk COM velocity and the peak neck angular momentum in novice judoka.	No difference was seen in the speed of the centre of mass between novice + elite. Differences were seen between Torso angles of novice and experienced judoka.
Risk of bias	Moderate	Moderate	Low	Low

Table 5. Study characteristics and outcomes.

Study Reference	Murayama, et al., 2013	Murayama, et al., 2014	Murayama, et al., 2019	Murayama, et al., 2020
Study design	Observational	Observational	Observational	Observational
Participant characteristics: Number, gender, (Elite/Novice), (Tori/Uke), Age (years), Height (cm), Weight (kg)	1 Male 1 Elite, Tori, (26, 177, 90) ADT dummy Uke, (NA, 175, 75)	1 Male 1 Elite, Tori, (26, 177, 90) ADT dummy Uke, (NA, 175, 75)	1 Male 1 Elite, Tori, (33, 166, 82) ADT dummy Uke, (NA, 175, 75)	2 Male 1 Elite Tori, (29, 177, 90) 1 Elite Uke
Breakfall technique	No breakfall, of OS and OU With and without under-mat	No breakfall, of OS and OU With and without under-mat	No breakfall, of SN	Basic Ukemi, following OS
Biomechanical assessment method	Resultant Head acceleration (G) Head injury Criterion (HIC)	Peak translational (G) and rotational acceleration (rad/s^2)	Peak linear (G) and angular (rad/s^2) acceleration	Translational (G) and Rotational (rad/s^2) acceleration
Measured Outcomes and key findings	Head acceleration in the longitudinal direction: OU > OS HIC values without under mat: OU and OS (1174.7 +/− 246.7) and (330.0 +/− 78.3) HIC values with under mat: OU and OS (539.3 +/− 43.5) and (156.1 +/− 30.4)	Translational acceleration: OU > OS, (130.0 +/− 13.2 and 74.4 +/− 9.8) Rotational acceleration: OS > OU (5081.3 +/− 691.8 and 1906.0 +/− 280.1) Translational acceleration was significantly reduced by use of an under-mat ($p = 0.021$) Rotational acceleration was not significantly reduced by use of an under-mat ($p = 0.29$)	Peak values of linear and angular acceleration did not significantly differ between 3 directional axes. High angular acceleration was observed (1890.1 +/− 1151.9) Increase in linear acceleration in the longitudinal direction and angular acceleration in the sagittal plane was not seen	No significant difference was seen in the three axis directions for both accelerations. Peak resultant rotational and translational accelerations (679.4 +/− 173.6 and 10.3 +/− 1.6) were significantly lower than previous ADT Study. ($p = 0.0021$)
Risk of bias	Moderate	Moderate	Moderate	Moderate

3.3. Study Quality Assessment

Of the 16 studies included, six [23–25,28,33,34] were high-quality studies and ten were moderate [26,27,29–32,35–38]. One study [39] was removed from the review due to the extremely high bias identified by the modified strobe criteria. The mean modified strobe score was 3.4, study quality ranged from 3 to 4. None of the studies described the study setting, location or period; 5 out of 16 (5/16) did not adequately describe the eligibility criteria and sources and methods of participant selection. All studies described exposure definition and measurement; 4/16 did not describe the study outcome definition and measurement sufficiently and 1/16 studies did not describe the main results with precision, see Figure 2.

All included studies (N= 22)	(1) Study setting, location and study period	(2) Eligibility criteria, and sources and methods of participant selection.	(3) Exposure definition and measuremt	(4) Study ocutcome definition and measurement	(5) Main results and precision (e.g. 95% confidence interval)	Number of items with low risk of bias	Quality	Study reference Number
Hashimoto, et al., 2015	0	1	1	1	1	4	H	23
Hitosugi, et al., 2014	0	1	1	1	1	4	H	24
Ishikawa, et al., 2018	0	1	1	1	1	4	H	25
Ishikawa, et al., 2020	0	1	1	0	1	3	M	26
Koshida, et al., 2012	0	1	1	1	0	3	M	27
Koshida, et al., 2013	0	1	1	1	1	4	H	28
Koshida, et al., 2014	0	0	1	1	1	3	M	29
Koshida, et al., 2/ 2017	0	1	1	0	1	3	M	31
Koshida, et al., 2016	0	1	1	0	1	3	M	30
Koshida, et al., 10/2017	0	1	1	0	1	3	M	32
Koshida, et al., 2018	0	1	1	1	1	4	H	33
Michnik, et al., 2014	0	1	1	1	1	4	H	34
Murayama, et al., 2013	0	0	1	1	1	3	M	35
Murayama, et al., 2014	0	0	1	1	1	3	M	36
Murayama, et al., 2019	0	0	1	1	1	3	M	37
Murayama, et al., 2020	0	0	1	1	1	3	M	38
Sacripanti, et al., 2010	0	0	1	0	0	1	VL	39

Figure 2. Modified STROBE criteria quality assessment. H = High quality. M = Moderate Quality. L = Low Quality. VL = Very Low Quality = Excluded.

4. Discussion and Suggestions—Narrative Synthesis

This review is the first to summarise the relationship between Ukemi and the impact of falls on the head and neck. Analysis of Ukemi biomechanics evaluates the effectiveness of Ukemi in reducing the impact of falls in judo as well as ascertaining the injury risk to the uke during a throw. Direct occipital contact onto the tatami (judo mat) produced greater acceleration and momentum values in comparison to when Ukemi was implemented. Kinematic data assessing impact was always below the injury threshold when Ukemi was performed. Further kinematic data revealed differences in breakfall technique between novice and experienced judoka. Whilst no significant differences were seen in neck flexion angles (NFA), hip, knee and trunk angle time plots revealed greater flexion angles in novice judokas.

4.1. Head Kinematics of Breakfall Motion

Direct impact of the head on the tatami is a major cause of head and neck injury [52]; it accounts for approximately 60% of ASDH in judo [38]. Impact responses of the head have frequently been described in terms of acceleration in cadaver and mechanical studies [53,54]. The current gold standard to assess head injury is the head injury criterion (HIC), determined by translational rotation. The US National Football League reported a HIC value of 250 for concussions [55].

4.1.1. Translational (Linear) and Rotational (Angular) Acceleration

ATD studies revealed that occipital contact on the tatami during OS and OU induces high translational acceleration in the longitudinal direction [24,35,36]. However, Ukemi, following OS, dramatically reduced peak resultant translational acceleration (maximum value: 10.3 G), well below the HIC value for concussion [29,38]. This implies that Ukemi is a sufficient measure to prevent severe head injury.

However, the HIC does not consider rotational acceleration, which plays a role in head injury mechanisms [56,57]. Rotational acceleration is associated with traumatic brain injury, concussion, ASDH and axonal injury; therefore, it should be a variable in the head injury criterion [25,36,56–58]. ATD studies discovered that without Ukemi, the head experiences high rotational acceleration during OS (maximum value 5081.3 +/− 691.8 rad/s^2) that would result in injury; translational acceleration of the same throw did not meet the HIC [24,36,38]. All throws assessed in this study (OS, OU, Seoi-Nage (SN) and Tai-Otoshi (TO)) produced peak resultant rotational acceleration values below the concussion limit (4500 (rad/s^2) once Ukemi was applied [25,26,37]. A comparison of rotational acceleration in ATD and expert studies saw a five-fold reduction in acceleration [25,36,38]. In addition, the use of an under-mat significantly reduced translational acceleration in OS and OU [35,36] but had no effect on rotational acceleration [36]. This infers that an under-mat is a deficient shock absorber to reduce impact to the head [36]. Furthermore, the development of a new HIC that takes into account translational and rotational acceleration is needed.

Additionally, sagittal plane rotational acceleration has been linked to more severe outcomes than coronal and horizontal plane rotation [13,14,59], whilst ATD studies support this notion [24,36]; sagittal plane rotation may be reduced by Ukemi. Murayama found no difference between acceleration in the three planes during Ukemi implementation [38]. However, Ishikawa saw a greater acceleration in the sagittal plane following OS during Ukemi [26]. To assess whether Ukemi affects sagittal plane rotation, this relationship must be investigated further.

Our data on rotational acceleration highlights that the sudden backwards head rotation is a key component of severe head injury in addition to linear acceleration. Furthermore, correct Ukemi significantly reduces both acceleration values below limits relating to concussion; therefore, it is effective in protecting judoka from severe head and neck injury.

4.1.2. Neck Muscle Strength

Neck muscle strength is thought to play a role in the prevention of head and neck injury [26,60]. It is assumed that greater neck strength equates to better control of neck muscles and, therefore, a better ability to prevent neck extension momentum and angular acceleration of the head [61]. However, following high-intensity judo practice, the angular acceleration of the head increased, but neck muscle strength did not decrease [26]. Therefore, fatigue may have a greater influence on Ukemi than neck muscle strength. This study was performed on experienced adult judokas; therefore, it is unlikely that neck muscle strength would change significantly due to fatigue. In the case of novice judokas, neck muscle strength may be a greater contributor to head injury. A 2016 review highlighted an association between reduced neck muscle strength and greater injury risk [60]. Therefore, future research should focus on assessing this relationship in judo. Regardless, the importance of rest incorporated in training should not be underestimated [26].

4.2. Neck Kinematics during Breakfall Motion
4.2.1. Neck Flexion Angles (NFA)

From the studies included in this review, the most common measure of 'impact' to evaluate head and neck injury was the NFA time plots [27–32]. Neck flexion is taught as part of Ukemi to prevent head impact due to neck and head extension [61]. It is theorised that NFA will differ between elite and novice judoka as elite will have greater neck muscle strength and, therefore, a better ability to resist extension [26,27]. However, the majority of the literature suggests that towards the end of breakfall motion, there is no significant difference in NFA between novice and elite judoka [27,28,30]. One study found a minimal statistical difference between novice and experienced judoka. However, interpretation of these results warrants thought due to the small effect size [29]. No significant difference was seen in the head flexion angle between novice and elite judoka [28]. Whilst head and neck flexion may play a role in Ukemi, it may not be an adequate measure of Ukemi skill.

4.2.2. Peak Angular Momentum of Neck Extension (PAMNE)

PAMNE is another measure to assess the likelihood of head and neck injury. It is implied that the greater the magnitude of PAMNE, the more likely injury will result, as there is a greater application of force to the head and neck [30]. A significant difference in PAMNE was seen between novice and experienced judoka when thrown by OS [30], indicating experienced judokas have a more advanced breakfall technique. Analysis of peak angular momentum (PAM) of the neck in the sagittal, frontal and horizontal planes demonstrated a greater PAM in the sagittal plane. However, horizontal and frontal plane momentum accounted for 30% of peak flexion momentum, demonstrating the multi-planar movement of the neck during OS. Hence, improvement of neck strength in all three planes may improve breakfall motion [32]. Currently, no significant association has been seen between neck muscle strength and impact [26,32]; further analysis is needed to determine this relationship.

4.3. Correct Ukemi

It is proposed that skill of breakfall technique can be determined by observation of upper and lower limb kinematics [62,63] in addition to head and neck kinematics. Avoidance of head contact on the tatami through Ukemi is key to preventing head and neck injury. However, the positioning of the upper and lower limbs may determine the likelihood of head contact by predicting disordered falling [23]. It is proposed that advanced judoka have greater control of their limbs during breakfall in comparison to novice judoka; hence, why more severe outcomes are associated with the novice population [6,7]. Three-dimensional analysis of hip, knee and trunk angle time plots identified variances in breakfall technique between experienced and novice judoka.

4.3.1. Ushiro Ukemi

Ushiro Ukemi (backwards breakfall) is a motion where the uke strongly hits the tatami before the head reaches its lowest point [17,22]. This is deemed a protective mechanism for the cervical spine and head as it is believed to reduce the impact on the head and neck. Ushiro Ukemi, exhibited in OU, directly correlated with vertical velocity measures of the ukes head. At the beginning of the throw, vertical velocity increased until it reached its maximum value; the impact of the hand, forearm and trunk hitting the tatami induced a reduction in vertical velocity [23]. In contrast, in OS, the trunk and lower limbs hit the tatami after the head reached its lowest position—this is reflected in a greater vertical velocity [23] and rotational acceleration [38]. This signifies the importance of Ushiro Ukemi in preventing severe injury during backwards falls. Monitoring of Ukemi timing patterns would enable coaches to predict disordered falling and tailor training based on timing patterns.

4.3.2. Hip and Knee Angle Time Plots

Observation of basic backwards breakfall with no associated throw showed little [29] to no difference [28] in hip angle time curves between novice and experienced judoka. However, breakfall of OS showed greater left hip flexion in novice judoka [30,31]. A straighter hip positioning was seen in more experienced judoka [30], suggesting that greater hip flexion during Ukemi following OS is associated with a greater risk of injury. The analysis of Ukemi with no associated throw may not be useful in identifying differences in novice and advanced judokas as the momentum of the uke may significantly differ with and without the uke being thrown.

In addition, observation of knee flexion angle time curves, basic backwards breakfall and OS demonstrate a significant difference between novice and experienced judoka. During Ukemi, experienced judoka show faster knee extension [28], as well as greater knee extension values throughout the entire motion [29,30]. Faster and greater knee extension may contribute to better control during the backwards fall. Hence, coaches may need to pay more attention to hip and knee kinematics during training.

4.3.3. Trunk Angle Time Plots

It is proposed that trunk kinematics play an imperative role in breakfall technique as it demonstrates control during breakfall [64]. However, studies observing breakfall motion without an associated throw found no or minor differences in trunk flexion between novice and experienced judoka [27–29]. Both exhibited similar trunk flexion patterns, which remained stable towards the end of motion [27–29]. However, a slight increase in trunk flexion angle was observed in novice judokas over the same period [27,28]. The increase in flexion may indicate reduced trunk stability of the novice judoka; however, the effect size was small.

Further comparison of trunk flexion during OS demonstrated a greater flexed position in novice judoka; in comparison, experienced judoka maintained a straighter position throughout motion; however, trunk flexion was equivalent at the end phase of motion [30]. Evaluation of trunk kinematics during OS and OU, in elite judoka, revealed that the trunk and lower extremities hit the tatami after the head reached its lowest position in OS; the opposite was true for OU [23]. However, when these two throws were performed by novice judoka, no variances in trunk angle time plots were observed [31]. These findings infer that experienced judoka have greater trunk stability and, therefore, control over trunk flexion. The flexed position adopted by novice judokas is comparable to the 'squat protective mechanism', which enables the lower limb to absorb the potential energy and reduce the impact force. However, in OS, the lower extremities are unable to provide the breaking force using the squatting position as the body is mid-air whilst falling backwards [30]. Moreover, greater trunk flexion amplifies the risk of head and neck injury by increasing angular velocity [33]. Trunk extension acts as a protective mechanism; therefore, judokas should enhance core strength to be able to maintain trunk extension during Ukemi. In addition, it is suggested that strengthening the peripheral scapular and cervical muscles will support a stable relationship between the head and trunk, allowing judoka to have greater control during a fall [65]. However, the literature only implies a potential association between neck and trunk muscle function, which needs further investigation.

A comparative report analysing variances of body control of an older experienced and younger novice judoka found that after collision, the novice judoka was motionless, reflected by a torso angle of 0°. Whereas the experienced judoka rolled the trunk on collision, allowing for dispersal of energy, reflected by a torso angle of −25°. Whilst there were no differences in the speed of the centre of mass, the experienced judokas technique resulted in a reduction in 'impact'. Further research is needed to assess the trunk roll technique in Ukemi and its association with reduced injury risk [34].

4.4. Clinical Implication

We can draw several clinical implications from this review; however, these should be interpreted with caution. All included studies were of high to moderate quality; however, heterogeneity of the methodology of the included studies made formulating concise conclusions challenging. The thresholds stated in this review are subject to change based on calculations of risk curves, which would change the interpretation of results [66]. Nevertheless, this review suggests that when Ukemi is performed correctly, a considerable reduction in impact on the head and neck is seen. This emphasises the importance of the practice in a sport that is changing. It is believed that adaption of the traditional Ukemi, known as 'unorthodox Ukemi', can elicit dangerous behaviours, such as head rolls, which call for the uke to purposefully land on their head as opposed to avoiding head contact [19]. One study in this review recognised an association between fatigue and greater impact on the head and neck. This study elicits that fatigue can reduce the control the uke has during the fall. Hence, the simple solution of coaches ensuring that judokas are not overly fatigued during practice can limit severe injury risk to the uke. An awareness of the coach's responsibility towards the judoka as well as certification of coaches by the international judo federation is necessary to prevent injury [8]. This should especially be the case when coaching younger judoka, who are less experienced and require safeguarding. The association of a greater flexed position seen in novice judoka can be used by coaches to assess their skillset and predict dangerous falling patterns. Judoka who show these patterns, should not be encouraged to practice throws that are associated with severe injuries (OS). Furthermore, the practice of Ukemi should be introduced as early as possible in young judokas, as this is a preventative measure for injury. Further analysis of neck muscle strength is needed to examine the relationship with impact on the head and neck.

4.5. Limitations

There are some limitations of this review to consider. Firstly, biomechanical measurements of impact on the head and neck vary between studies (i.e., velocity, acceleration, momentum); whilst we grouped studies based on these measurements' comparison of different variables of severe injury was not possible. Only nine participants were female; therefore, this data can be said to represent the male population but is not representative of female judoka, especially since differences between male and female judoka have been highlighted [67]. Lastly, the impact of a fall and, therefore, Ukemi response is likely to differ when the fall is associated with and without a throw; this review did not fully explore this topic.

4.6. Future Work

Future research should focus on Ukemi biomechanics during competitions and move away from comparative studies which involve breakfall motion analysis without an associated throw. The relationship between neck strength and the performance of Ukemi should also be explored. Only one study in this review directly measured neck strength as a variable. More research may suggest that greater neck strength could play a significant role in preventing head and neck injury. Similarly, only one study touched on the link between fatigue and its effect on the performance of Ukemi; this should be explored further as it is an easily applicable protective measure. Furthermore, the studies to date are not representative of the biomechanics of Ukemi in the female population; therefore, future research should include data from this cohort. In addition, setting up prospective studies analysing how Ukemi can prevent the number of injuries amongst judoka could further research.

Lastly, Ukemi practice can not only impact judo injury prevention but can also be implemented in the general population. Research can be directed at implementing Ukemi techniques to reduce the consequences of falls in the elderly population.

5. Conclusions

This review clarifies that Ukemi is essential in preventing severe injuries by reducing the 'impact' on the head and neck of the uke. The use of an under-mat did not prove to be adequate in reducing head impact. Good breakfall technique is associated with control of the whole body, including upper and lower limbs in addition to the head and neck. Small differences were seen in hip, knee and trunk angle time curves between novice and advanced judokas. Greater extension of the hip, knee and trunk in advanced judokas indicate that greater extension of the trunk and lower limb may act as a protective mechanism. Variance in lower body dynamic strength profiles between elite and novice judoka suggests greater strength provides better control. Timing patterns should therefore be analysed by coaches to predict disordered falling and highlight improvements that can be made. No study in this review found a correlation between greater neck strength and improved Ukemi. Improving neck strength is clearly not the simple solution to reducing 'impact' on the head and neck. However, more research is needed to assess this relationship. Fatigue has been shown to negatively impact Ukemi; therefore, the provision of appropriate breaks in training sessions and competitions may significantly reduce injury risk.

Author Contributions: Conceptualisation, R.L., W.B., M.A. and N.M.; methodology, R.L., W.B., M.A. and N.M.; software, R.L. and N.M.; validation, R.L. and N.M., formal analysis, R.L., W.B. and N.M.; investigation, R.L., M.A. and N.M.; resources, R.L. and N.M.; data curation, R.L. and N.M.; writing—original draft preparation, R.L., W.B., M.A. and N.M.; writing—review and editing, R.L., W.B., T.A., Ł.R. and N.M.; visualisation, R.L. and N.M.; supervision, R.L., W.B. and N.M.; project administration, R.L., W.B., T.A., Ł.R. and N.M.; funding acquisition, R.L., W.B., T.A., Ł.R. and N.M. All authors have read and agreed to the published version of the manuscript.

Funding: This research received no external funding.

Institutional Review Board Statement: The study was conducted according to the guidelines of the Declaration of Helsinki and approved by the Ethics Committee of the Regional Medical Board in Krakow (approval No. 287/KBL/OIL/2020).

Informed Consent Statement: Informed consent was obtained from all subjects involved in the study.

Data Availability Statement: The data presented in this study are available on request from the corresponding author.

Conflicts of Interest: The authors declare no conflict of interest.

Abbreviations

Key for Tables 2–4
COM: Centre of mass
HIC: Head injury criterion
G: Unit of measure for resultant head acceleration
N: Newtons
ATD: Anthropomorphic test device
EMG: Electromyography
SCM: Sternocleido-mastoid
EO: External oblique
RA: Rectus abdominis

Appendix A

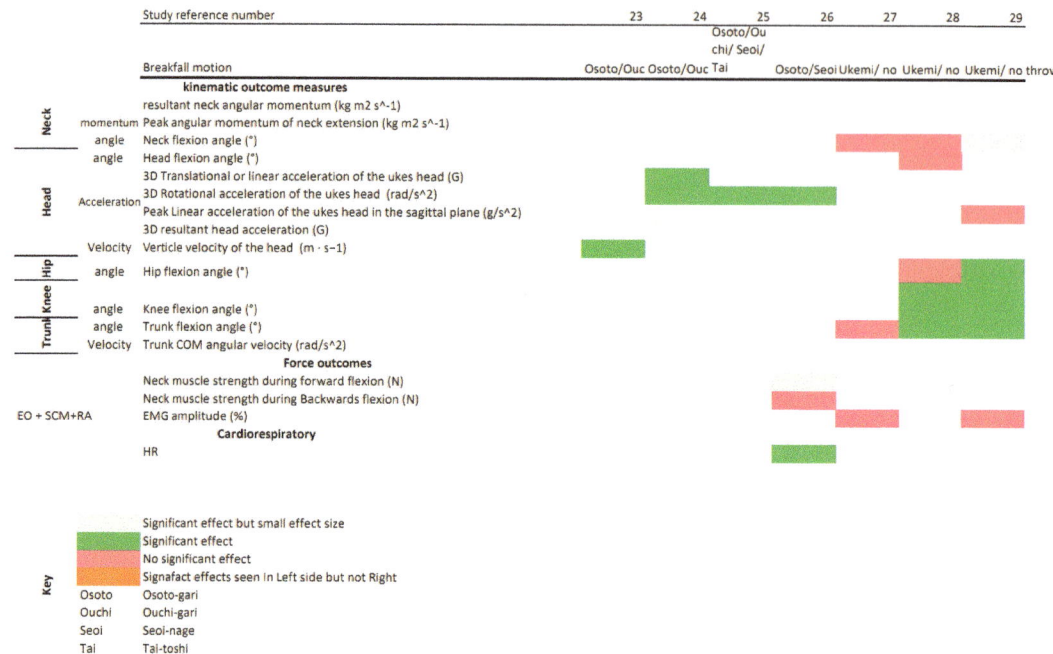

Figure A1. Outcome groupings.

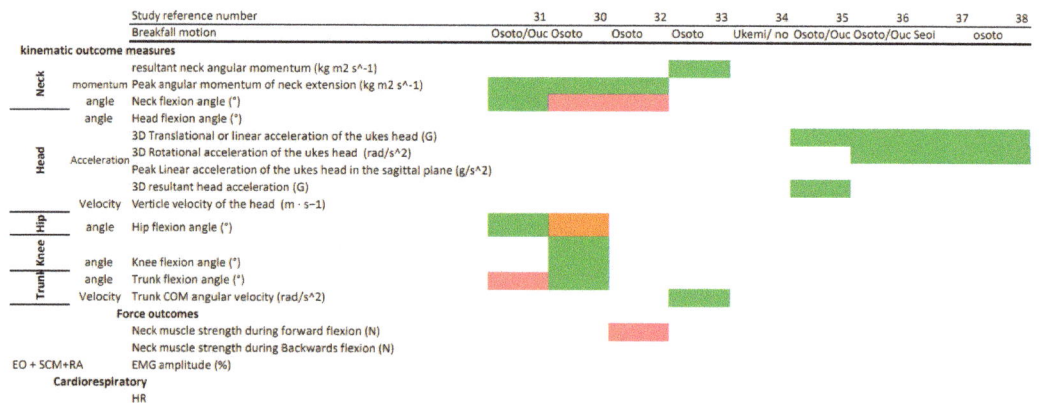

Figure A2. Outcome groupings.

References

1. Sato, S. The sportification of judo: Global convergence and evolution. *J. Glob. Hist.* **2013**, *8*, 299. [CrossRef]
2. History/IJF.org [Internet]. Ijf.org. 2021. Available online: https://www.ijf.org/history (accessed on 15 May 2021).
3. Pocecco, E.; Ruedl, G.; Stankovic, N.; Sterkowicz, S.; Del Vecchio, F.B.; García, C.G.; Rousseau, R.; Wolf, M.; Kopp, M.; Miarka, B.; et al. Injuries in judo: A systematic literature review including suggestions for prevention. *Br. J. Sports Med.* **2013**, *47*, 1139–1143. [CrossRef]

4. Lystad, R.P.; Alevras, A.; Rudy, I.; Soligard, T.; Engebretsen, L. Injury incidence, severity and profile in Olympic combat sports: A comparative analysis of 7712 athlete exposures from three consecutive Olympic Games. *Br. J. Sports Med.* **2021**, *55*, 1077–1083. [CrossRef]
5. Błach, W.; Smolders, P.; Rydzik, Ł.; Bikos, G.; Maffulli, N.; Malliaropoulos, N.; Jagiełło, W.; Maćkała, K.; Ambroży, T. Judo Injuries Frequency in Europe's Top-Level Competitions in the Period 2005–2020. *J. Clin. Med.* **2021**, *10*, 852. [CrossRef] [PubMed]
6. Kamitani, T.; Nimura, Y.; Nagahiro, S.; Miyazaki, S.; Tomatsu, T. Catastrophic head and neck injuries in judo players in Japan from 2003 to 2010. *Am. J. Sports Med.* **2013**, *41*, 1915–1921. [CrossRef]
7. Koiwai, E.K. Fatalities associated with judo. *Physician Sportsmed.* **1981**, *9*, 61–66. [CrossRef] [PubMed]
8. Krieger, D.; Norica, N.; Kitano, P. Japan Confronts Hazards of Judo (Published 2013) [Internet]. Nytimes.com. 2021. Available online: https://www.nytimes.com/2013/04/18/sports/japan-confronts-hazards-of-judo.html (accessed on 16 May 2021).
9. Frey, A.; Lambert, C.; Vesselle, B.; Rousseau, R.; Dor, F.; Marquet, L.A.; Toussaint, J.F.; Crema, M.D. Epidemiology of judo-related injuries in 21 seasons of competitions in France: A prospective study of relevant traumatic injuries. *Orthop. J. Sports Med.* **2019**, *7*, 2325967119847470. [CrossRef] [PubMed]
10. Minghelli, B.; Isidoro, R. Prevalence of injuries in Jiu-Jitsu and Judo athletes of Portugal South: Associated injury mechanisms. *J. Community Med. Health Educ.* **2016**, *6*, 10–4172.
11. Nakanishi, T.; Hitosugi, M.; Murayama, H.; Takeda, A.; Motozawa, Y.; Ogino, M.; Koyama, K. Biomechanical analysis of serious neck injuries resulting from judo. *Healthcare* **2021**, *9*, 214. [CrossRef] [PubMed]
12. Santos, L.; Fernandez-Rio, J.; Ruiz, M.L.; Del Valle, M.; Callan, M.; Challis, D.; Sterkowicz, S. Three-dimensional assessment of the judo throwing techniques frequently used in competition. *Arch. Budo* **2014**, *10*, 107–115.
13. Gennarelli, T.A.; Thibault, L.E. Biomechanics of acute subdural hematoma. *J. Trauma* **1982**, *22*, 680–686. [CrossRef]
14. Ommaya, A.K.; Gennarelli, T.A. Cerebral concussion and traumatic unconsciousness: Correlation of experimental and clinical observations on blunt head injuries. *Brain* **1974**, *97*, 633–654. [CrossRef]
15. Unterharnscheidt, F.; Higgins, L.S. Traumatic lesions of brain and spinal cord due to nondeforming angular acceleration of the head. *Tex. Rep. Biol. Med.* **1969**, *27*, 127–166.
16. Nagahiro, S.; Mizobuchi, Y.; Hondo, H.; Kasuya, H.; Kamitani, T.; Shinbara, Y.; Nimura, Y.; Tomatsu, T. Severe head injuries during Judo practice. *No shinkei geka. Neurol. Surg.* **2011**, *39*, 1139–1147.
17. Kanō, J. *Kodokan Judo*; Kodansha International: Tokyo, Japan, 1994.
18. Franchini, E.; Brito, C.J.; Fukuda, D.H.; Artioli, G.G. The physiology of judo-specific training modalities. *J. Strength Cond. Res.* **2014**, *28*, 1474–1481. [CrossRef]
19. Lee, B. Understanding Ukemi (Falling Techniques) By Brandon Lee | Judo Info [Internet]. Judoinfo.com. 2021. Available online: https://judoinfo.com/lee/ (accessed on 16 May 2021).
20. Kim, E.H.; Kim, S.S. A Kinematic Comparative Analysis of Yoko Ukemi (side breakfall) by Each Stage in Judo. *Korean J. Sport Biomech.* **2004**, *14*, 203–218.
21. Kim, E.H.; Kim, J.T. A Kinematical Analysis of Mae-ukemi (forward breakfall) in Judo. *Korean J. Sport Biomech.* **2002**, *12*, 131–142. [CrossRef]
22. Minamitani, N.; Yamamoto, H. A case study of cai applied to ukemi practice in judo. In Proceedings of the ISBS-Conference Proceedings Archive, 16 international Symposium on Biomechanics in Sports, Konstanz, Germany, 21–25 July 1998.
23. Hashimoto, T.; Ishii, T.; Okada, N.; Itoh, M. Impulsive force on the head during performance of typical ukemi techniques following different judo throws. *J. Sports Sci.* **2015**, *33*, 1356–1365. [CrossRef]
24. Hitosugi, M.; Murayama, H.; Motozawa, Y.; Ishii, K.; Ogino, M.; Koyama, K. Biomechanical analysis of acute subdural hematoma resulting from judo. *Biomed. Res.* **2014**, *35*, 339–344. [CrossRef]
25. Ishikawa, Y.; Anata, K.; Hayashi, H.; Yokoyama, T.; Ono, T.; Okada, S. Effects of different throwing techniques in judo on rotational acceleration of uke's head. *Int. J. Sport Health Sci.* **2018**, *16*, 173–179. [CrossRef]
26. Ishikawa, Y.; Anata, K.; Hayashi, H.; Uchimura, N.; Okada, S. Influence of fatigue on head angular acceleration in judo high-intensity exercise. *Arch. Budo* **2020**, *16*, 99–106.
27. Koshida, S.; Matsuda, T. Neck and Trunk Kinematics and Electromyographic Activity during Judo Backward Breakfalls. In Proceedings of the ISBS-Conference Proceedings Archive, 30th Annual Conference of Biomechanics in Sport, Melbourne, Australia, 2–6 July 2012.
28. Koshida, S.; Matsuda, T.; Ishii, T.; Hashimoto, T. Kinematics of judo backward breakfall: Comparison between novice and experienced judokas. In Proceedings of the ISBS-Conference Proceedings Archive, 31 International Conference on Biomechanics in Sport: Taipei, Taiwan, 7–11 July 2013.
29. Koshida, S.; Ishii, T.; Matsuda, T.; Hashimoto, T. Biomechanics of the judo backward breakfall: Comparison between experienced and novice judokas. *Arch. Budo* **2014**, *10*, 187–194.
30. Koshida, S.; Ishii, T.; Matsuda, T.; Hashimoto, T. Kinematics of judo breakfall for osoto-gari: Considerations for head injury prevention. *J. Sports Sci.* **2016**, *35*, 1059–1065. [CrossRef] [PubMed]
31. Koshida, S.; Ishii, T.; Matsuda, T.; Hashimoto, T. Biomechanics of judo backward breakfall for different throwing techniques in novice judokas. *Eur. J. Sport Sci.* **2016**, *17*, 417–424. [CrossRef] [PubMed]

32. Koshida, S.; Ishii, T.; Matsuda, T.; Hashimoto, T. Three-dimentional neck kinematics during breakfall for osoto-gari and its association with neck flexion strength in novice judokas. *ISBS Proc. Arch.* **2017**, *35*, 14.
33. Koshida, S.; Ishii, T.; Matsuda, T.; Hashimoto, T. Trunk biomechanics during breakfall for osoto-gari and its association with judo-related head injury risk in novice judokas. *ISBS Proc. Arch.* **2018**, *36*, 146.
34. Michnik, R.; Jurkojc, J.; Wodarski, P.; Mosler, D.; Kalina, R.M. Similarities and differences of body control during professional, externally forced fall to the side performed by men aged 24 and 65 years. *Arch. Budo* **2014**, *10*, 233–243.
35. Murayama, H.; Hitosugi, M.; Motozawa, Y.; Ogino, M.; Koyama, K. Simple strategy to prevent severe head trauma in Judo. *Neurol. Med.-Chir.* **2013**, *53*, 580–584. [CrossRef] [PubMed]
36. Murayama, H.; Hitosugi, M.; Motozawa, Y.; Ogino, M.; Koyama, K. Rotational acceleration during head impact resulting from different judo throwing techniques. *Neurol. Med.-Chir.* **2014**, *54*, 374–378. [CrossRef]
37. Murayama, H.; Hitosugi, M.; Motozawa, Y.; Ogino, M.; Koyama, K. Biomechanical analysis of the head movements of a person thrown by the judo technique 'Seoi-nage'. *Neurol. Med.-Chir.* **2019**, *60*, 101–106. [CrossRef]
38. Murayama, H.; Hitosugi, M.; Motozawa, Y.; Ogino, M.; Koyama, K. Ukemi Technique Prevents the Elevation of Head Acceleration of a Person Thrown by the Judo Technique 'Osoto-gari'. *Neurol. Med.-Chir.* **2020**, *60*, 307–312. [CrossRef] [PubMed]
39. Sacripanti, A. Biomechanics of kuzushi-tsukuri and interaction in competition (A new global didactic Judo vision). In Proceedings of the SPASS International Conference, Lignano Sabbiadoro, Italy, 5–9 September 2010; pp. 1–125.
40. Liberati, A.; Altman, D.G.; Tetzlaff, J.; Mulrow, C.; Gøtzsche, P.C.; Ioannidis, J.P.; Clarke, M.; Devereaux, P.J.; Kleijnen, J.; Moher, D. The PRISMA statement for reporting systematic reviews and meta-analyses of studies that evaluate healthcare interventions: Explanation and elaboration. *BMJ* **2009**, *339*, b2700. [CrossRef] [PubMed]
41. Bramer, W.M.; de Jonge, G.B.; Rethlefsen, M.L.; Mast, F.; Kleijnen, J. A systematic approach to searching: An efficient and complete method to develop literature searches. *J. Med. Libr. Assoc. JMLA* **2018**, *106*, 531. [CrossRef]
42. Salvador-Oliván, J.A.; Marco-Cuenca, G.; Arquero-Avilés, R. Errors in search strategies used in systematic reviews and their effects on information retrieval. *J. Med. Libr. Assoc. JMLA* **2019**, *107*, 210. [CrossRef] [PubMed]
43. Bramer, W.M.; Rethlefsen, M.L.; Kleijnen, J.; Franco, O.H. Optimal database combinations for literature searches in systematic reviews: A prospective exploratory study. *Syst. Rev.* **2017**, *6*, 245. [CrossRef]
44. Reiswig, J. Mendeley. *J. Med. Libr. Assoc. JMLA* **2010**, *98*, 193. [CrossRef]
45. Ouzzani, M.; Hammady, H.; Fedorowicz, Z.; Elmagarmid, A. Rayyan—A web and mobile app for systematic reviews. *Syst. Rev.* **2016**, *5*, 210. [CrossRef] [PubMed]
46. Dan British Judo [Internet]. Available online: https://www.britishjudo.org.uk/my-judo/grading/grades/dan/?msclkid=7fff8f25ac2911eca2cff2e6ca481dce (accessed on 25 March 2022).
47. Waldén, M.; Hägglund, M.; Ekstrand, J. The epidemiology of groin injury in senior football: A systematic review of prospective studies. *Br. J. Sports Med.* **2015**, *49*, 792–797. [CrossRef] [PubMed]
48. Malta, M.; Cardoso, L.O.; Bastos, F.I.; Magnanini, M.M.; Silva, C.M. STROBE initiative: Guidelines on reporting observational studies. *Rev.3 Saude Publica* **2010**, *44*, 559–565. [CrossRef]
49. Von Elm, E.; Altman, D.G.; Egger, M.; Pocock, S.J.; Gotzsche, P.C.; Vandenbroucke, J.P. Strobe Initiative. The Strengthening the Reporting of Observational Studies in Epidemiology (STROBE) Statement: Guidelines for reporting observational studies. *Int. J. Surg.* **2014**, *12*, 1495–1499. [CrossRef]
50. Vandenbroucke, J.P.; Von Elm, E.; Altman, D.G.; Gotzsche, P.C.; Mulrow, C.D.; Pocock, S.J.; Poole, C.; Schlesselman, J.J.; Egger, M. Strobe Initiative. Strengthening the Reporting of Observational Studies in Epidemiology (STROBE): Explanation and elaboration. *PLoS Med.* **2007**, *4*, e297. [CrossRef] [PubMed]
51. Page, M.J.; E McKenzie, J.; Bossuyt, P.M.; Boutron, I.; Hoffmann, T.C.; Mulrow, C.D.; Shamseer, L.; Tetzlaff, J.M.; Moher, D. Updating guidance for reporting systematic reviews: Development of the PRISMA 2020 statement. *J. Clin. Epidemiol.* **2021**, *134*, 103–112. [CrossRef] [PubMed]
52. Viano, D.C.; Parenteau, C.S. Analysis of head impacts causing neck compression injury. *Traffic Inj. Prev.* **2008**, *9*, 144–152. [CrossRef]
53. Schmitt, K.U.; Niederer, P.F.; Cronin, D.S.; Morrison, B., III; Muser, M.H.; Walz, F. *Trauma Biomechanics: An Introduction to Injury Biomechanics*; Springer: Berlin/Heidelberg, Germany, 2019.
54. Siswanto, W.A.; Hua, C.S. Strength analysis of human skull on high speed impact. *Int. Rev. Mech. Eng.* **2012**, *6*, 1508–1514.
55. Marjoux, D.; Baumgartner, D.; Deck, C.; Willinger, R. Head injury prediction capability of the HIC, HIP, SIMon and ULP criteria. *Accid. Anal. Prev.* **2008**, *40*, 1135–1148. [CrossRef] [PubMed]
56. Shafiee, A.; Ahmadian, M.T.; Hoursan, H.; Hoviat Talab, M. Effect of linear and rotational acceleration on human brain. *Modares Mech. Eng.* **2015**, *15*, 248–260.
57. King, A.I.; Yang, K.H.; Zhang, L.; Hardy, W.; Viano, D.C. Is head injury caused by linear or angular acceleration. In Proceedings of the IRCOBI Conference, Lisbon, Portugal, 25 September 2003; Volume 12.
58. Hansen, K.; Dau, N.; Feist, F.; Deck, C.; Willinger, R.; Madey, S.M.; Bottlang, M. Angular Impact Mitigation system for bicycle helmets to reduce head acceleration and risk of traumatic brain injury. *Accid. Anal. Prev.* **2013**, *59*, 109–117. [CrossRef] [PubMed]
59. Franchini, E.; Del Vecchio, F.B.; Matsushigue, K.A.; Artioli, G.G. Physiological profiles of elite judo athletes. *Sports Med.* **2011**, *41*, 147–166. [CrossRef] [PubMed]

60. Hrysomallis, C. Neck muscular strength, training, performance and sport injury risk: A review. *Sports Med.* **2016**, *46*, 1111–1124. [CrossRef] [PubMed]
61. Ivancic, P.C. Neck injury response to direct head impact. *Accid. Anal. Prev.* **2013**, *50*, 323–329. [CrossRef] [PubMed]
62. Shin, J.W.; Kim, K.D. The effect of enhanced trunk control on balance and falls through bilateral upper extremity exercises among chronic stroke patients in a standing position. *J. Phys. Ther. Sci.* **2016**, *28*, 194–197. [CrossRef] [PubMed]
63. Kim, S.; Joo, K.S.; Liu, J.; Sohn, J.H. Lower extremity kinematics during forward heel-slip. *Technol. Heal. Care* **2019**, *27*, 345–356. [CrossRef] [PubMed]
64. Nevisipour, M.; Grabiner, M.D.; Honeycutt, C.F. A single session of trip-specific training modifies trunk control following treadmill induced balance perturbations in stroke survivors. *Gait Posture* **2019**, *70*, 222–228. [CrossRef] [PubMed]
65. Kavanagh, J.J.; Morrison, S.; Barrett, R.S. Coordination of head and trunk accelerations during walking. *Eur. J. Appl. Physiol.* **2005**, *94*, 468–475. [CrossRef]
66. Funk, J.R.; Duma, S.M.; Manoogian, S.J.; Rowson, S. Biomechanical risk estimates for mild traumatic brain injury. In Proceedings of the Annual Proceedings/Association for the Advancement of Automotive Medicine, Melbourne, Australia, 15–17 October 2007; Volume 51, p. 343.
67. Sterkowicz, S. Differences in the schooling tendencies of men and women practicing judo (based on the analysis of the judo bouts during the 1996 Olympic Games). *J. Hum. Kinet.* **1998**, *1*, 99–113.

Article

Differences between Treadmill and Cycle Ergometer Cardiopulmonary Exercise Testing Results in Triathletes and Their Association with Body Composition and Body Mass Index

Szymon Price [1], Szczepan Wiecha [2,*], Igor Cieśliński [2], Daniel Śliż [1,3,*], Przemysław Seweryn Kasiak [4], Jacek Lach [1], Grzegorz Gruba [4], Tomasz Kowalski [5] and Artur Mamcarz [1]

1. 3rd Department of Internal Medicine and Cardiology, Medical University of Warsaw, 02-091 Warsaw, Poland; szymonprice@gmail.com (S.P.); jacek.lach@wum.edu.pl (J.L.); artur.mamcarz@wum.edu.pl (A.M.)
2. Department of Physical Education and Health in Biala Podlaska, Faculty in Biala Podlaska, Jozef Pilsudski University of Physical Education in Warsaw, 21-500 Biala Podlaska, Poland; igor.cieslinski@awf.edu.pl
3. Public Health School Centrum Medyczne Kształcenia Podyplomowego (CMKP), 01-813 Warsaw, Poland
4. Students' Scientific Group of Lifestyle Medicine, 3rd Department of Internal Medicine and Cardiology, Medical University of Warsaw, 02-091 Warsaw, Poland; przemyslaw.kasiak1@gmail.com (P.S.K.); gregorygpl@gmail.com (G.G.)
5. Institute of Sport-National Research Institute, 01-982 Warsaw, Poland; tomekbielany@gmail.com
* Correspondence: authors: szczepan.wiecha@awf.edu.pl (S.W.); daniel.sliz@wum.edu.pl (D.Ś.)

Abstract: Cardiopulmonary exercise testing (CPET) is the method of choice to assess aerobic fitness. Previous research was ambiguous as to whether treadmill (TE) and cycle ergometry (CE) results are transferrable or different between testing modalities in triathletes. The aim of this paper was to investigate the differences in HR and VO_2 at maximum exertion between TE and CE, at anaerobic threshold (AT) and respiratory compensation point (RCP) and evaluate their association with body fat (BF), fat-free mass (FFM) and body mass index (BMI). In total, 143 adult (n = 18 female), Caucasian triathletes had both Tr and CE CPET performed. The male group was divided into <40 years (n = 80) and >40 years (n = 45). Females were aged between 18 and 46 years. Body composition was measured with bioelectrical impedance before tests. Differences were evaluated using paired t-tests, and associations were evaluated in males using multiple linear regression (MLR). Significant differences were found in VO_2 and HR at maximum exertion, at AT and at RCP between CE and TE testing, in both males and females. VO_{2AT} was 38.8 (±4.6) mL/kg/min in TE vs. 32.8 (±5.4) in CE in males and 36.0 (±3.6) vs. 32.1 (±3.8) in females (p < 0.001). HR_{AT} was 149 (±10) bpm in TE vs. 136 (±11) in CE in males and 156 (±7) vs. 146 (±11) in females (p < 0.001). VO_2max was 52 (±6) mL/kg/min vs. 49 (±7) in CE in males and 45.3 (±4.9) in Tr vs. 43.9 (±5.2) in females (p < 0.001). HRmax was 183 (±10) bpm in TE vs. 177 (±10) in CE in males and 183 (±9) vs. 179 (±10) in females (p < 0.001). MLR showed that BMI, BF and FFM are significantly associated with differences in HR and VO_2 at maximum, AT and RCP in males aged >40. Both tests should be used independently to achieve optimal fitness assessments and further training planning.

Keywords: triathlon training; heart rate; ventilation

1. Introduction

Cardiopulmonary exercise testing (CPET) is a dynamic, non-invasive method to assess the cardiopulmonary system at rest and during exercise [1]. It may be applied in medicine to evaluate the degree of cardiovascular function impairment and plan rehabilitation and in sports science to assess participants' fitness [2]. Key variables measured in CPET include heart rate (HR), oxygen consumption (VO_2), respiratory rate (RR), pulmonary ventilation (VE), oxygen pulse, respiratory exchange ratio (RER), ventilatory equivalents for oxygen (VE/VO_2) and carbon dioxide (VE/VCO_2) [3]. The most frequently compared variable is the maximum oxygen uptake (VO$_2$max), which may be defined as the highest value reached, despite progressive increase of the load applied, with the development of a plateau in the VO$_2$ [3]. Another important value is the VO$_2$ at the anaerobic threshold (AT), corresponding to the threshold between moderate and high-intensity exercise, which is the point when the lack of sufficient oxygen supply to the exercising muscles necessitates glycolytic ATP production and the accumulation of lactic acid [4]. Thus, in exercise at an intensity below AT, lactate remains at resting levels, while in high-intensity exercise above AT, lactate rises until an elevated steady state is attained [4]. The respiratory compensation point (RCP) is identified as the second breakpoint in the ventilation response and is a measurable variable most closely related to the concept of critical power (CP), which in turn represents the point separating power outputs that can be sustained for a prolonged time from power outputs, which lead to a certain maximum after which exercise intolerance occurs [4,5]. CP is especially relevant in high-intensity training or intermittent highintensity training [5].

The most commonly used testing modalities are the cycle ergometer (CE) and treadmill (TE), with various protocols or self-paced [6,7]. These training modalities both have unique strengths and weaknesses. The TE activates more muscle groups, and VO$_2$max is generally higher than in the cycle ergometer by 7–18%, varying between studies, although there exist many conflicting papers, and results are inconsistent [8]. The cycle ergometer allows better electrocardiographic (ECG) analysis due to fewer artefacts from upper body motion [6]. The relationship between testing modality and VO$_2$ max is ambiguous. Triathletes with previous experience in cycling may obtain results on the cycle ergometer that are equal to or even higher than those obtained on the treadmill, while trained runners display higher results in treadmill testing [9–11]. Usually, for triathletes the testing modality is selected specifically to fit the discipline trained by the examinee, i.e., a treadmill for runners or a cycle ergometer for cyclists [12]. A unique challenge is posed by triathletes, who have no single mode of training, but rather devote a portion of their training to swimming, cycling and running [8]. The monitoring of training would therefore ideally be carried out with all of the specific tests for the most accurate results, but this would be highly impractical given that testing is time consuming, costly and must be repeated regularly [12]. It is therefore important to know whether there is a significant difference between treadmill and cycle ergometry results in triathletes. Few studies have been conducted to assess this, and existing studies often included small studied groups of fewer than twenty participants [8]. The results of previous studies are inconclusive, showing that VO$_2$ max in triathletes may be equal [13–17], higher [18,19] or even lower [20] in treadmill testing compared with cycle ergometry. The anaerobic threshold (AT) and lactate threshold (LT) were also either reported as higher, in the treadmill test [21], or similar, in both tests [22]. Millet et al. point out that study methods were often unclear and the study group sizes were limited in many of the existing studies [8].

Maximal heart rate (HRmax) is either reported as similar [15,18,21,23], or slightly higher in treadmill testing compared with cycle ergometry [20,21,24]. It is also unclear whether this relationship is true for males and females alike, or only for males [8]. Another important parameter to consider is the HR corresponding to the AT, which is often used to prescribe submaximal exercise training loads [8]. This value has previously been generally reported as higher in treadmill tests compared with cycle ergometry [15,24–26]. However, some studies yielded no significant difference [13,27].The sex differences between triathletes in running and cycling are also unclear. Most studies did not evaluate these differences at all, and the ones that did yield no difference between cycling and running for both males and females [16,28].

It is also unclear how age affects the differences between testing modalities. Aerobic capacity decreases rapidly after the age of 40 years in males and is related to muscle mass [29–31]. Older age is also associated with a decreased exercise efficiency and an increase in the oxygen cost of exercise, which contribute to a decreased exercise capacity. These age-related changes may be reversed with exercise training, which improves efficiency to a greater degree in the elderly than in the young [32]. It has been proposed that the difference in VO$_2$max between treadmill and cycle ergometry between runners and triathletes may be due to the higher muscle mass of triathletes, especially in the upper body, and not to running economy [8]. Body composition has been shown to impact triathlon performance. Fat mass and fat percentage are positively associated with race time (i.e., the race time is greater in participants with higher fat mass), while fat-free mass is negatively related to race time [33]. Another paper demonstrated that body fat is associated with race time in male Ironman triathletes but not in females [34].

To the best of our knowledge, no studies evaluated whether an association exists between body composition (BC) and differences in VO$_2$max in different testing modalities in triathletes. Despite previous research on the topic, it remains unclear whether treadmill and cycle ergometry may be used interchangeably for the monitoring of training in triathletes, largely due to insufficient data on the differences in results obtained from both testing modalities [8,23,35].

The main aim of this study was to assess the difference in VO$_2$ and HR at maximum exertion and at AT and RCP in cycle ergometry and treadmill testing in triathletes of various levels. A further aim was to evaluate whether an association exists between these parameters and BC or body mass index (BMI). Based on previous literature, we hypothesized that results are different in different testing modalities in triathletes and that they are influenced by body composition.

2. Materials and Methods

2.1. Participants Preliminary Inclusion Criteria

The study involving human participants was reviewed and approved by the Bioethical Committee of the Medical University of Warsaw. The patients/participants provided their written informed consent to participate in this study. All procedures were carried out in accordance with the Declaration of Helsinki. The data of participants was gathered from records of commercial CPET performed in the years 2013–2020. They were recruited via the internet and social media advertisements or via recommendations from trainers or other clients. The tests were carried out on the personal request of the participants as part of training optimization and diagnostics. The participants were triathletes who had participated in competitive events. Inclusion criteria for the study were: age over 18 years, triathlon training for at least three months, having a treadmill test and a cycle ergometer test performed within a maximum two months' timeframe and meeting the maximum exertion criteria described below. Exclusion criteria were any chronic or acute medical conditions (including musculoskeletal system disorders such as new fractures and sprains, as well as addiction to nicotine, alcohol or other substances) or the ongoing intake of any medication. Identical study methods and procedures were used during the entire period from which data were gathered. Participants were informed via e-mail on how to prepare for the test. They were advised to avoid any exercise 2 h prior to the test, eat a light carbohydrate meal 2–3 h before the test and stay hydrated by drinking isotonic beverages. They were also instructed to avoid medicines, caffeine and cigarettes before the test.

2.2. Selected Subjects

From the database, we obtained 238 individual cases of people who carried out the study twice (cycling and running separately). After verifying the inclusion criteria, we obtained 143 cases included in further analysis. The average time interval between both tests was 2.44 ± 3.10 days in female and 5.29 ± 6.81 in male triathletes. The order of testing was random. For 86 cases, running protocol was the first test performed. Populational data were calculated as means with standard deviation (SD) and are presented in Table 1. Documented competition experience from the earliest competition to the day of the first test was an average of 94.1 ± 38.8 months; 95% CI from 74.2 to 113.9 in females and an average of 103.3 ± 42.8 months and 95% CI from 95.6 to 110.9 in male triathletes (Table 2).

The population was also divided according to age into two groups, <40 years and >40 years (age was not included as an independent variable in these models).

Table 1. Population characteristics for males and females, including characteristics of the age groups ≤40 and >40 years of age in males and the mean differences between them.

		Female Triathletes				
Characteristic		All n = 18 [1]				
Age		33 (7)				
Height		169 (4)				
Weight		61.9 (4.4)				
BMI		21.70 (1.37)				
BF		23.3 (3.5)				
FM		14.55 (2.93)				
FFM		47.38 (2.61)				
		Male triathletes				
Characteristic	All n = 125	≤40, n = 80 [1]	>40, n = 45 [1]	Difference [2]	95% CI [2,3]	p-Value [2]
Age	38 (10)	32 (5)	46 (8)	15.39	12.10–15.67	<0.001
Height	181 (7)	181.0 (7.0)	180.0 (6.0)	1.40	−1.00, 3.80	0.3
Weight	79 (9)	78.0 (10.0)	79.0 (8.0)	−0.67	−4.00, 2.70	0.7
BMI	24.04 (2.19)	23.8 (2.4)	24.4 (1.7)	−0.56	−1.30, 0.18	0.13
BF	15.4 (4.2)	15.2 (4.2)	15.8 (4.3)	−0.60	−2.20, 1.00	0.5
FM	12.3 (4.6)	12.2 (4.8)	12.6 (4.1)	−0.47	−2.10, 1.10	0.6
FFM	66 (6)	66.0 (6.0)	66.0 (6.0)	−0.21	−2.40, 2.00	0.9

[1] Mean (SD); [2] Welch Two Sample t-test; [3] CI = Confidence Interval. Abbreviations: height (cm); weight (kg); BMI, body masa index; BF, body fat (%); FM, fat mass (kg); FFM, fat-free mass (kg).

Table 2. Participant's training experience and competition results.

	Males, n = 125		Females, n = 18	
Distance between CPET	5.29 (6.81)		2.44 (3.10)	
Training experience	103.32 (42.63)		94.11 (38.80)	
	Competition results			
Type of competition	n of records	Result	n of records	Result
1/8 Iron Man	21	01:18:37 (00:20:38)	1	01:35:27 (00:00:00)
1/4 Iron Man	41	02:29:17 (00:14:31)	6	02:34:18 (00:14:57)
1/2 Iron Man	33	04:57:01 (00:37:04)	4	05:33:17 (00:25:59)
Sprinter's distance	10	01:09:01 (00:07:13)	2	01:18:28 (00:10:40)
Olympic distance	20	02:33:59 (00:19:57)	5	02:48:43 (00:05:21)

Data are presented as mean (SD). Distance between CPET is presented in days. Training experience is presented in months. All types of competition refer to triathlon distances. The sports result was investigated in a period not longer than three months from the CPET. Competition results are presented as hours:minutes:seconds. Abbreviations: CPET, cardiopulmonary exercise testing.

2.3. Measures

Body mass (BM) and fat mass (FM) were measured with the use of a BC analyzer (Tanita, MC 718, Tokyo, Japan) before every test with the multifrequency 5 kHz/50 kHz/250 kHz electrical bioimpedance method. The BC tests were conducted directly prior to each CPET if the interval between tests was >48 h, and mean values from both tests were further analyzed. In cases where two CPET tests were carried out on the following days, only one BC analysis was performed prior to the first CPET. All measurements (BC and CPET) took place under similar conditions in the medical clinic Sportslab (www.sportslab.pl; accessed on 2 February 2022, Warsaw, Poland). The conditions were 40 m² of indoor, air-conditioned space, altitude 100 m MSL, temperature 20–22 degrees Centigrade and 40–60% humidity.

2.4. CPET Equipment

Exercise tests were performed on a cycle ergometer Cyclus−2 (RBM elektronik-automation GmbH, Leipzig, Germany) and on a mechanical treadmill (h/p/Cosmos quasar, Germany), within one day–two months of one another. During all tests, cardiopulmonary indices were recorded using a Cosmed Quark CPET device (Rome, Italy), calibrated before each test according to the manufacturer's instructions. HR was measured using the ANT+ chest strap, which is part of the Cosmed Quark CPET device (declared accuracy similar to ECG, ±1 bpm.). The Cosmed Quark CPET software has been updated regularly over the years (from PFT Suite to Omnia 10.0 E.). During the entire data collection period, three Cosmed Quark CPET gas analyzers were used (each replaced after three to four years of use). All the mechanical equipment used in CPET testing procedures was serviced and checked by the producer every year to keep their technical passports valid in accordance with local regulations for medical facilities. Each test was preceded by a 5 min adaptation (walking or pedaling with no resistance). To account for the different exercise capacity of the triathletes, the initial power (Watt) or speed (km/h) were determined based on an interview carried out before each individual test. The lowest power at which the participant subjectively felt resistance was selected as the initial power for cycle ergometer tests (60–150 W). The power was then increased by 20–30 W every 2 min. For treadmill tests, the start speed was an individually selected slow running pace, between 7 and 12 km/h based on the interviews, and 1% incline was applied. The speed was then increased by 1 km/h every 2 min. To assess the maximum level of aerobic fitness, participants were instructed to maintain the effort for as long as possible, encouraged verbally to the greatest possible effort. They could terminate the test at any moment if they felt they could no longer maintain the exertion level.

Participants were under cardiopulmonary monitoring during the entire test. Before each CPET, after each change of load and 3 min after the test, 20 µL of blood were collected from the fingertip for determination of lactate concentration (LA) using the Super GL2 analyzer (Müller Gerätebau GmbH, Freital, Germany) calibrated before each series of samples. There were no interruptions in the CPET during the collection of blood samples. During the running test, the triathletes, while running, put their hands on the rail attached to the treadmill and a technician took a blood sample. Before the sample was drawn into the capillary, the first drops of blood were carefully squeezed into a swab. Similarly, during the cycling test, the subject was asked to relax their hands for about 20–30 s before the collection, and then the first drops of blood were discarded before taking the sample into a capillary.

2.5. CPET Protocol

The test was terminated by the operator if either VO_2 or HR showed no further increase with increasing speed/power. The results of the BC analysis and CPET were saved as an Excel (Microsoft Corporation, Washington, United States) spreadsheet for further analysis. The raw data were anonymized and processed with the use of a custom program created in Python software to identify data at AT, RCP and maximum exertion. In accordance with current standards, CPET data were recorded breath by breath and then averaged across 15 s intervals; the highest HR in the interval was recoded, and HR values were not averaged [36]. For statistical evaluation, we included only cases where three of four following criteria were met: RER during test reaching > 1.10, VO_2 plateau (an increase in VO_2 with increasing speed/power lower than 100 mL/min), respiratory frequency over 45/min and perceived exertion over 18 in Borg scale [37]. AT and RCP were located from visual inspection. It was assumed that AT was reached after the following criteria were met: (1) VE/VO_2 curve begins to rise with constant VE/VCO_2 curve and (2) end-tidal partial pressure of oxygen begins to rise with constant end-tidal partial pressure of carbon dioxide [38]. It was assumed that RCP was reached after the following criteria were met: (1) a decrease in partial pressure of end-tidal CO_2 ($PetCO_2$) after reaching a maximal level; (2) a rapid nonlinear increase in VE (second deflection); (3) the VE/VCO_2 ratio reached a minimum and began to increase and (4) a nonlinear increase in VCO_2 versus VO_2 (departure from linearity) [38].

2.6. Retrospective Performance Data

Competition experience was assessed using the enduhub.com (accessed on 15 December 2021) database (Enduhub Corporation, Newark, DE, USA). It is a commonly available website where official scores of participants' competitions on standardized distances (1/8, 1/4, 1/2 Ironman, Sprinter and Olympic distances of triathlons were included) are uploaded by event organizers. Each score in this database was thoroughly validated by professional companies specialized in time measuring during sports events (Datasport, Szczawno Zdrój, Poland and STS-Timing, Łubianka, Poland). Results are verified before publication by enduhub.com editors. We used the earliest officially available score from a distance-standardized triathlon and used it as a starting point to assess competition experience, which was presented in months (month of competition and CPET were both included). These times were applied to calculate how long each sportsman is engaged in regular training and actively take part in public competitions.

2.7. Data Analysis

Statistical analysis has been conducted in R environment/programming language for statistical computing (R Core Team, Vienna, Austria; version 3.6.4;) and lmtest and gtsummary libraries [39,40]. Missing data were identified in lactate values in seven cases and imputation was performed with random forests [41]. Normality was tested with the Anderson-Darling test. Data were calculated as means with SD and 95% confidence intervals (CI). Differences between results of both testing modalities were calculated using paired t-tests. A significance level of $p < 0.05$ was adopted for all results.

MLR models were created to evaluate the relationship between the differences in results from treadmill and cycle ergometry (dependent variables), body fat (BF), fat-free mass (FFM) and BMI. Several regression models were initially tested and MLR was selected as the best fit based on the Akaike information criterion. The models were only created for the male population due to group sizes. The Harvey-Collier test was used to test linearity. R-squared (R^2) was used to assess the quality of the models.

3. Results

The differences between CPET results in cycle ergometry and treadmill testing are presented in Table 3 for females and Tables 4–6 for males. Results of MLR are presented in Table 7. Only regression results in the two age subgroups are presented, as no significant relationships were found in the whole male population. All statistically significant results are marked bold. Selected (based on highest R^2) relationships are presented as linear regression graphs (Figure 1); it illustrates the linear relationship between BMI and body fat with CPET parameters in the older population. Moreover, we assessed the effect of theta (θ) interval as well as training advancement and previous experience, and no significant differences were observed for the differences between VO_2max, VEmax and HRmax. Thus it suggests the homogeneity of our study group.

Table 3. Differences between cycle ergometry (CE) and treadmill (Tr) CPET results in female participants; significant results are bold.

Characteristic	CE, n = 18 [1]	Tr, n = 18 [1]	Difference [2]	95% CI [2,3]	p-Value [2]
VO_{2AT}	32.1 (3.8)	36.0 (3.6)	−3.9	−5.4, −2.5	**<0.001**
VO_{2ATa}	1976 (257)	2216 (221)	−240	−328, −152	**<0.001**
RER_{AT}	0.87 (0.05)	0.88 (0.03)	−0.01	−0.04, 0.02	0.5
HR_{AT}	**146 (11)**	**156 (7)**	**−10**	**−14, −6.1**	**<0.001**
O_2pulse_{AT}	13.64 (2.07)	14.28 (1.84)	−0.65	−1.2, −0.07	**0.031**
VE_{AT}	53 (7)	62 (8)	−8.5	−12, −4.4	**<0.001**
RR_{AT}	29 (5)	36 (8)	−6.7	−9.5, −3.9	**<0.001**
Lac_{AT}	1.77 (0.54)	1.87 (0.46)	−0.11	−0.32, 0.10	0.3
VO_{2RCP}	40.2 (4.5)	42.9 (4.7)	−2.8	−4.1, −1.4	**<0.001**
VO_{2RCPa}	2471 (279)	2642 (283)	−170	−255, −85	**<0.001**
VCO_{2RCP}	2468 (282)	2643 (283)	−174	−262, −87	**<0.001**
HR_{RCP}	169 (9)	175 (8)	−6.7	−8.3, −5.1	**<0.001**
VE_{RCP}	80 (10)	86 (9)	−5.3	−11, 0.32	0.063
RR_{RCP}	38 (6)	44 (7)	−5.7	−7.7, −3.6	**<0.001**
O_2pulse_{RCP}	14.69 (1.80)	15.13 (1.98)	−0.44	−0.82, −0.05	**0.029**
Lac_{RCP}	4.30 (0.69)	4.50 (0.82)	−0.20	−0.72, 0.31	0.4
VO_2max	43.9 (5.2)	45.3 (4.9)	−1.4	−2.8, −0.02	**0.047**
VO_2max_a	2704 (319)	2791 (305)	−87	−169, −4.2	**0.040**
RERmax	1.13 (0.03)	1.11 (0.03)	0.01	−0.01, 0.04	0.3
O_2pulse_{max}	15.12 (1.96)	15.33 (2.03)	−0.20	−0.59, 0.18	0.3
HRmax	179 (10)	183 (9)	−3.5	−5.2, −1.8	**<0.001**
VEmax	110 (18)	104 (13)	6.0	−1.8, 14	0.12
RRmax	55 (11)	55 (9)	−0.11	−2.4, 2.2	>0.9
Lacmax	10.76 (1.94)	9.40 (1.28)	1.4	0.47, 2.2	**0.005**

[1] Mean (SD); [2] Paired t-test; [3] CI = Confidence Interval. Abbreviations: VO_2, oxygen uptake; AT, anaerobic threshold; VO_{2AT}, relative VO_2 at AT (mL/kg/min); VO_{2ATa}, absolute VO_2 at AT (mL/min); RER_{AT}, respiratory exchange ratio at AT; HR_{AT}, heart rate at AT (bpm); O_2pulse_{AT}, oxygen pulse at AT (mL/beat); VE_{AT}, pulmonary ventilation at AT (L/min); RR_{AT}, respiratory rate at AT (breaths per minute); Lac_{AT}, lactate concentration at AT (mmol/L); RCP, respiratory compensation point; VO_{2RCP}, relative VO_2 at RCP (mL/kg/min); VO_{2RCPa}, absolute VO_2 at RCP (mL/min); VCO_{2RCP}, carbon dioxide production at RCP(mL/min); HR_{RCP}, heart rate at RCP (bpm); VE_{RCP}, pulmonary ventilation at RCP(L/min); RR_{RCP}, respiratory rate at RCP (breaths per minute); O_2pulse_{RCP}, oxygen pulse at RCP (mL/beat); Lac_{RCP}, lactate concentration at RCP(mmol/L); VO_2max, relative maximum VO_2 (mL/kg/min); VO_2max_a, absolute maximum VO_2 (mL/min); RERmax, maximal respiratory exchange ratio; O_2pulse_{max}, maximal oxygen pulse (mL/beat); HRmax, maximal heart rate (bpm); VEmax, maximal pulmonary ventilation (L/min); RRmax, maximal respiratory rate (breaths per minute); Lacmax, maximal lactate concentration (mmol/L).

Table 4. Differences between cycle ergometry (CE) and treadmill (TE) CPET results in male participants; significant results are bold.

Characteristic	CE, n = 125 [1]	TE, n = 125 [1]	Difference [2]	95% CI [2,3]	p-Value [2]
VO_{2AT}	32.8 (5.4)	38.8 (4.6)	−6.0	−6.7, −5.3	**<0.001**
VO_{2ATa}	2530 (366)	3012 (345)	−482	−541, −424	**<0.001**
RER_{AT}	0.86 (0.06)	0.89 (0.04)	−0.02	−0.04, −0.01	**<0.001**
HR_{AT}	136 (11)	149 (10)	−13	−15, −11	**<0.001**
O_2pulse_{AT}	18.73 (2.88)	20.32 (2.36)	−1.6	−1.9, −1.2	**<0.001**
VE_{AT}	66 (10)	83 (11)	−17	−18, −15	**<0.001**
RR_{AT}	28 (5)	37 (8)	−8.2	−9.3, −7.1	**<0.001**
Lac_{AT}	1.70 (0.37)	1.77 (0.40)	−0.07	−0.14, 0.00	**0.043**
VO_{2RCP}	44 (8)	48 (6)	−4.1	−5.1, −3.1	**<0.001**
VO_{2RCPa}	3372 (533)	3707 (420)	−335	−411, −259	**<0.001**
VCO_{2RCP}	3378 (539)	3708 (420)	−329	−406, −252	**<0.001**
HR_{RCP}	163 (10)	172 (9)	−9.4	−11, −8.2	**<0.001**
VE_{RCP}	110 (17)	119 (15)	−9.4	−12, −6.9	**<0.001**
RR_{RCP}	39 (7)	46 (10)	−6.7	−8.1, −5.2	**<0.001**
O_2pulse_{RCP}	20.78 (3.44)	21.59 (2.65)	−0.81	−1.2, −0.39	**<0.001**

Table 4. Cont.

Characteristic	CE, $n = 125$ [1]	TE, $n = 125$ [1]	Difference [2]	95% CI [2,3]	p-Value [2]
Lac$_{RCP}$	4.21 (0.60)	4.29 (0.74)	−0.08	−0.23, 0.06	0.3
VO$_2$max	49 (7)	52 (6)	−2.9	−3.6, −2.1	<0.001
VO$_2$max$_a$	3808 (476)	4045 (435)	−238	−300, −175	<0.001
RERmax	1.13 (0.04)	1.11 (0.03)	0.02	0.02, 0.03	<0.001
O$_2$pulse$_{max}$	21.54 (2.91)	22.16 (2.66)	−0.62	−0.94, −0.29	<0.001
HRmax	177 (10)	183 (10)	−5.9	−6.8, −5.0	<0.001
VEmax	158 (24)	152 (18)	6.6	3.4, 9.8	<0.001
RRmax	57 (10)	58 (10)	−1.8	−3.6, −0.05	0.044
Lacmax	10.93 (1.82)	9.68 (1.65)	1.2	0.91, 1.6	<0.001

[1] Mean (SD); [2] Welch Two Sample t-test; [3] CI = Confidence Interval. Abbreviations: VO$_2$, oxygen uptake; AT, anaerobic threshold; VO$_{2AT}$, relative VO$_2$ at AT (ml/kg/min); VO$_{2ATa}$, absolute VO$_2$ at AT (ml/min); RER$_{AT}$, respiratory exchange ratio at AT; HR$_{AT}$, heart rate at AT (bpm); O$_2$pulse$_{AT}$, oxygen pulse at AT (ml/beat); VE$_{AT}$, pulmonary ventilation at AT (L/min); RR$_{AT}$, respiratory rate at AT (breaths per minute); Lac$_{AT}$, lactate concentration at AT (mmol/L); RCP, respiratory compensation point; VO$_{2RCP}$, relative VO$_2$ at RCP (ml/kg/min); VO$_{2RCPa}$, absolute VO$_2$ at RCP (ml/min); VCO$_{2RCP}$, carbon dioxide production at RCP(ml/min); HR$_{RCP}$, heart rate at RCP (bpm); VE$_{RCP}$, pulmonary ventilation at RCP(L/min); RR$_{RCP}$, respiratory rate at RCP (breaths per minute); O$_2$pulse$_{RCP}$, oxygen pulse at RCP (ml/beat); Lac$_{RCP}$, lactate concentration at RCP(mmol/L); VO$_2$max, relative maximum VO$_2$ (ml/kg/min); VO$_2$max$_a$, absolute maximum VO$_2$ (ml/min); RERmax, maximal respiratory exchange ratio; O$_2$pulsemax, maximal oygen pulse (ml/beat); HRmax, maximal heart rate (bpm); VEmax, maximal pulmonary ventilation (L/min); RRmax, maximal respiratory rate (breaths per minute); Lacmax, maximal lactate concentration (mmol/L).

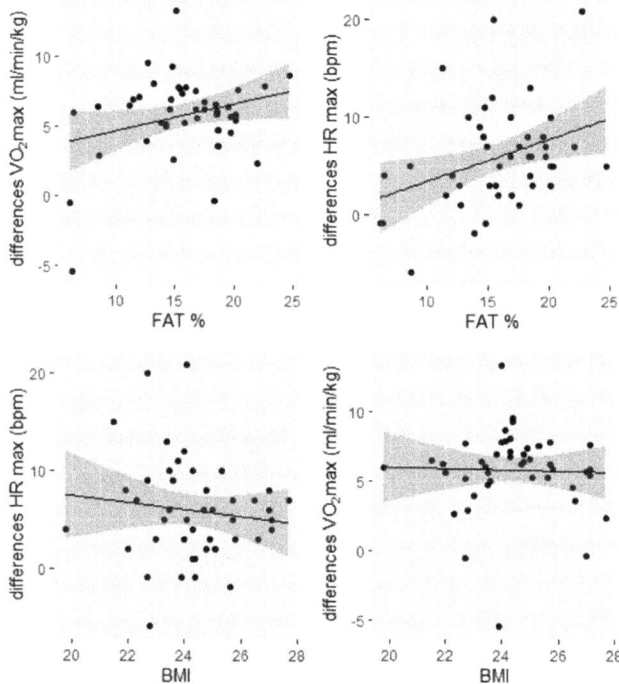

Figure 1. Regression analysis for males in subgroup >40 years. Legend: Multiple linear regression was performed to evaluate the association between differences in treadmill and cycle ergometer test results, and BMI, body fat and fat-free mass in amateur male triathletes. The figure presents the most important (highest R^2) relationships in the group of males >40 years of age ($n = 40$) as linear regression graphs. Abbreviations: BMI, body mass index (kg/m^2); HR max, maximal heart rate (bpm); VO$_2$ max, maximum oxygen uptake (mL/min/kg).

Table 5. Differences between cycle ergometry (CE) and treadmill (TE) CPET results in male participants ≤ 40 years; significant results are bold.

Characteristic	CE, n = 80 [1]	TE, n = 80 [1]	Difference [2]	95% CI [2,3]	p-Value [2]
VO_{2AT}	**34 (6)**	**40 (5)**	**−6.2**	**−7.2, −5.1**	**<0.001**
VO_{2ATa}	**2584 (363)**	**3078 (350)**	**−494**	**−577, −412**	**<0.001**
RER_{AT}	**0.87 (0.06)**	**0.88 (0.04)**	**−0.02**	**−0.03, 0.00**	**0.047**
HR_{AT}	**140 (11)**	**151 (10)**	**−12**	**−14, −9.5**	**<0.001**
O_2pulse_{AT}	**18.60 (2.86)**	**20.40 (2.41)**	**−1.8**	**−2.3, −1.3**	**<0.001**
VE_{AT}	**66 (10)**	**82 (11)**	**−17**	**−19, −14**	**<0.001**
RR_{AT}	**28 (6)**	**36 (7)**	**−8.2**	**−9.5, −6.9**	**<0.001**
Lac_{AT}	1.67 (0.37)	1.76 (0.40)	−0.08	−0.17, 0.00	0.057
VO_{2RCP}	**45 (7)**	**49 (6)**	**−4.0**	**−5.0, −2.9**	**<0.001**
VO_{2RCPa}	**3461 (447)**	**3790 (417)**	**−328**	**−415, −242**	**<0.001**
VCO_{2RCP}	**3463 (458)**	**3791 (417)**	**−328**	**−417, −239**	**<0.001**
HR_{RCP}	**166 (10)**	**175 (9)**	**−8.9**	**−10, −7.4**	**<0.001**
VE_{RCP}	**109 (16)**	**119 (15)**	**−10**	**−13, −7.0**	**<0.001**
RR_{RCP}	**38 (7)**	**45 (9)**	**−6.4**	**−8.0, −4.9**	**<0.001**
O_2pulse_{RCP}	**20.90 (2.94)**	**21.71 (2.69)**	**−0.81**	**−1.3, −0.36**	**<0.001**
Lac_{RCP}	4.15 (0.63)	4.24 (0.72)	−0.08	−0.26, 0.10	0.4
VO_2max	**51 (7)**	**53 (7)**	**−2.8**	**−3.8, −1.7**	**<0.001**
VO_2max_a	**3885 (471)**	**4118 (418)**	**−233**	**−316, −149**	**<0.001**
$RERmax$	**1.13 (0.04)**	**1.11 (0.03)**	**0.02**	**0.01, 0.03**	**<0.001**
O_2pulse_{max}	**21.65 (2.94)**	**22.22 (2.62)**	**−0.57**	**−1.0, −0.14**	**0.010**
$HRmax$	**180 (9)**	**186 (9)**	**−5.9**	**−7.0, −4.8**	**<0.001**
$VEmax$	**159 (24)**	**152 (16)**	**7.3**	**2.9, 12**	**0.001**
$RRmax$	56 (11)	58 (8)	−1.3	−3.3, 0.69	0.2
$Lacmax$	**10.94 (1.91)**	**9.81 (1.53)**	**1.1**	**0.59, 1.7**	**<0.001**

[1] Mean (SD); [2] Welch Two Sample t-test; [3] CI = Confidence Interval. Abbreviations: VO_2, oxygen uptake; AT, anaerobic threshold; VO_{2AT}, relative VO_2 at AT (ml/kg/min); VO_{2ATa}, absolute VO_2 at AT (ml/min); RER_{AT}, respiratory exchange ratio at AT; HR_{AT}, heart rate at AT (bpm); O_2pulse_{AT}, oxygen pulse at AT (ml/beat); VE_{AT}, pulmonary ventilation at AT (L/min); RR_{AT}, respiratory rate at AT (breaths per minute); Lac_{AT}, lactate concentration at AT (mmol/L); RCP, respiratory compensation point; VO_{2RCP}, relative VO_2 at RCP (ml/kg/min); VO_{2RCPa}, absolute VO_2 at RCP (ml/min); VCO_{2RCP}, carbon dioxide production at RCP(ml/min); HR_{RCP}, heart rate at RCP (bpm); VE_{RCP}, pulmonary ventilation at RCP(L/min); RR_{RCP}, respiratory rate at RCP (breaths per minute); O_2pulse_{RCP}, oxygen pulse at RCP (ml/beat); Lac_{RCP}, lactate concentration at RCP(mmol/L); VO_2max, relative maximum VO_2 (ml/kg/min); VO_2max_a, absolute maximum VO_2 (ml/min); $RERmax$, maximal respiratory exchange ratio; $O_2pulsemax$, maximal oyegn pulse (ml/beat); $HRmax$, maximal heart rate (bpm); $VEmax$, maximal pulmonary ventilation (L/min); $RRmax$, maximal respiratory rate (breaths per minute); $Lacmax$, maximal lactate concentration (mmol/L).

Table 6. Differences between cycle ergometry (CE) and treadmill (TE) CPET results in male participants >40 years; significant results are bold.

Characteristic	CE, n = 45 [1]	TE, n = 45 [1]	Difference [2]	95% CI [2,3]	p-Value [2]
VO_{2AT}	**31.1 (4.6)**	**36.9 (3.1)**	**−5.8**	**−6.6, −4.9**	**<0.001**
VO_{2ATa}	**2434 (354)**	**2895 (305)**	**−461**	**−532, −390**	**<0.001**
RER_{AT}	**0.86 (0.05)**	**0.89 (0.04)**	**−0.03**	**−0.05, −0.02**	**<0.001**
HR_{AT}	**129 (10)**	**144 (9)**	**−15**	**−17, −12**	**<0.001**
O_2pulse_{AT}	**18.96 (2.93)**	**20.18 (2.29)**	**−1.2**	**−1.7, −0.75**	**<0.001**
VE_{AT}	**67 (11)**	**83 (10)**	**−16**	**−19, −14**	**<0.001**
RR_{AT}	**29.1 (4.7)**	**37.3 (8.4)**	**−8.2**	**−10, −6.2**	**<0.001**
Lac_{AT}	1.75 (0.36)	1.80 (0.39)	−0.05	−0.16, 0.07	0.4
VO_{2RCP}	**41.1 (8.4)**	**45.4 (4.3)**	**−4.3**	**−6.2, −2.4**	**<0.001**
VO_{2RCPa}	**3213 (634)**	**3559 (387)**	**−346**	**−494, −198**	**<0.001**
VCO_{2RCP}	**3228 (637)**	**3560 (387)**	**−332**	**−481, −182**	**<0.001**
HR_{RCP}	**157 (9)**	**167 (8)**	**−10**	**−12, −8.3**	**<0.001**
VE_{RCP}	**112 (19)**	**119 (16)**	**−7.8**	**−12, −3.7**	**<0.001**
RR_{RCP}	**40 (7)**	**47 (11)**	**−7.1**	**−10, −4.1**	**<0.001**

Table 6. Cont.

Characteristic	CE, $n = 45$ [1]	TE, $n = 45$ [1]	Difference [2]	95% CI [2,3]	p-Value [2]
O_2pulse_{RCP}	20.55 (4.21)	21.36 (2.59)	−0.82	−1.7, 0.08	0.073
Lac_{RCP}	4.31 (0.53)	4.40 (0.78)	−0.09	−0.36, 0.19	0.5
VO_2max	**46.9 (6.0)**	49.9 (4.8)	−3.0	−4.2, −1.8	<0.001
VO_2max_a	**3670 (459)**	3916 (439)	−246	−343, −149	<0.001
RERmax	**1.13 (0.03)**	1.11 (0.03)	0.03	0.01, 0.04	<0.001
O_2pulse_{max}	21.35 (2.88)	22.05 (2.76)	−0.71	−1.2, −0.20	0.008
HRmax	**172 (8)**	178 (9)	−5.9	−7.5, −4.3	<0.001
VEmax	157 (25)	151 (22)	5.5	1.0, 9.9	0.018
RRmax	57 (10)	59 (12)	−2.7	−6.6, −4.9	<0.001
Lacmax	**10.90 (1.65)**	9.45 (1.82)	1.5	0.72, 2.2	<0.001

[1] Mean (SD); [2] Welch Two Sample t-test; [3] CI = Confidence Interval. Abbreviations: VO_2, oxygen uptake; AT, anaerobic threshold; VO_{2AT}, relative VO_2 at AT (ml/kg/min); VO_{2ATa}, absolute VO_2 at AT (ml/min); RER_{AT}, respiratory exchange ratio at AT; HR_{AT}, heart rate at AT (bpm); O_2pulse_{AT}, oxygen pulse at AT (ml/beat); VE_{AT}, pulmonary ventilation at AT (L/min); RR_{AT}, respiratory rate at AT (breaths per minute); Lac_{AT}, lactate concentration at AT (mmol/L); RCP, respiratory compensation point; VO_{2RCP}, relative VO_2 at RCP (ml/kg/min); VO_{2RCPa}, absolute VO_2 at RCP (ml/min); VCO_{2RCP}, carbon dioxide production at RCP(ml/min); HR_{RCP}, heart rate at RCP (bpm); VE_{RCP}, pulmonary ventilation at RCP(L/min); RR_{RCP}, respiratory rate at RCP (breaths per minute); O_2pulse_{RCP}, oxygen pulse at RCP (ml/beat); Lac_{RCP}, lactate concentration at RCP(mmol/L); VO_2max, relative maximum VO_2 (ml/kg/min); VO_2max_a, absolute maximum VO_2 (ml/min); RERmax, maximal respiratory exchange ratio; $O_2pulsemax$, maximal oygen pulse (ml/beat); HRmax, maximal heart rate (bpm); VEmax, maximal pulmonary ventilation (L/min); RRmax, maximal respiratory rate (breaths per minute); Lacmax, maximal lactate concentration (mmol/L).

Table 7. Regression analysis for males in two subgroups (≤40 years and >40 years).

Age Group	≤40 Years			>40 Years		
Predictors	BMI	BF	FFM	BMI	BF	FFM
VO_2AT						
b	0.02	0.15	0.01	−0.92	0.39	0.16
95% CI	−0.94, 1.0	−0.33, 0.63	−0.19, 0.22	−1.7, −0.15	0.13, 0.64	−0.03, 0.34
p-value	>0.9	0.5	>0.9	0.020	0.004	0.089
R^2		0.023			0.197	
HRAT						
b	0.23	−0.10	−0.06	−1.3	1.0	0.17
95% CI	−1.8, 2.3	−1.1, 0.93	−0.49, 0.38	−3.5, 0.93	0.29, 1.8	−0.36, 0.71
p-value	0.8	0.9	0.8	0.2	0.008	0.5
R^2		0.001			0.172	
VO_2RCP						
b	−0.16	0.30	0.05	−1.4	0.80	0.15
95% CI	−1.1, 0.82	−0.19, 0.80	−0.16, 0.26	−3.1, 0.26	0.24, 1.4	−0.25, 0.56
p-value	0.8	0.2	0.6	0.095	0.006	0.4
R^2		0.055			0.169	
HRRCP						
b	0.47	−0.16	−0.01	−1.3	0.79	0.13
95% CI	−1.0, 1.9	−0.89, 0.57	−0.32, 0.30	−3.0, 0.34	0.24, 1.4	−0.27, 0.54
p-value	0.5	0.7	>0.9	0.11	0.006	0.5
R^2		0.008			0.035	

Table 7. Cont.

Age Group	≤40 Years			>40 Years		
Predictors	BMI	BF	FFM	BMI	BF	FFM
VO_2max						
b	0.35	0.11	0.09	1.3	0.47	0.24
95% CI	−0.60, 1.3	−0.37, 0.59	−0.29, 0.12	−2.4, −0.19	0.11, 0.83	−0.03, 0.50
p-value	0.5	0.6	0.4	0.022	0.012	0.078
R^2		0.054			0.163	
HRmax						
b	−0.13	0.10	0.12	−1.5	0.78	−0.01
95% CI	−1.1, 0.87	−0.40, 0.61	−0.09, 0.31	−2.8, −0.16	0.35, 1.2	−0.32, 0.30
p-value	0.8	0.7	0.3	0.028	<0.001	0.9
R^2		0.028			0.28	

Abbreviations: BMI, body masa index; BF, body fat (%); FFM, fat-free mass (kg); VO_2AT, oxygen consumption at anaerobic threshold (ml/kg/min); HRAT, heart rate at anaerobic threshold (bpm); VO2RCP, oxygen consumption at respiratory compensation point(ml/kg/min); HRRCP, heart rate at respiratory compensation point(bpm); VO_2max, maximum oxygen uptake (ml/kg/min); HRmax, maximal heart rate (bpm).

4. Discussion

The hypothesis for the study was mostly confirmed; we demonstrated significant differences in cardiorespiratory parameters at AT, RCP and maximum exertion between cycle ergometry and treadmill testing. Regression models demonstrated significant relationships between BC, BMI and training experience, as well as differences in VO_2max in cycle ergometry and treadmill testing, especially in the older population of triathletes. However, the coefficient of determination (R^2) in the regression models ranged from 0.035 to 0.28, which indicates a low regression fit to the observed data. To the best of our knowledge, this is the first study to evaluate the differences between treadmill and cycle ergometer CPET in a large group of triathletes and the first to analyze factors associated with these differences. The results of our study show that both male and female triathletes have a significantly higher VO_2/AT in the treadmill than in the cycle ergometer tests. The AT is a crucial parameter in determining performance and in training monitoring in endurance sports, as it indicates the level of exertion a triathlete can sustain for a prolonged period of time during competition without rapid lactate build-up [8,42]. Training at the anaerobic threshold (AnT) intensity improves the peak oxygen uptake and the AT level [43]. Recent studies also demonstrate that a large volume of low-intensity training (i.e., below the AT) is important for endurance triathletes [44,45].

Previous research was ambiguous as to whether VO_{2AT} differs between testing modalities in triathletes [8]. The present paper shows significant differences in VO_{2AT}. This contradicts the results of several previous studies that found no differences in VO_2 at AT but were conducted on very small groups (14 participants at most) [8,14,22,25,46]. Some results were similar to our study [21]. The large mean difference in relative VO_{2AT} of 6 mL/kg/min in males shown in our study indicates that the values obtained from both testing modalities likely cannot be used interchangeably. The large difference in HR at AT of 13 bpm in males and 10 bpm in females is a further factor limiting the interchangeability of results from different testing modalities. The large discrepancies would hinder the accurate prescription of low-intensity (below AT) training based on HR zones. This is contrary to results from the studies of Hue and Bolognesi, who found differences of ~7 bpm, but without statistical significance, perhaps due to limited numbers of participants [13,27].

We found that the VO_2/RCP was significantly higher in treadmills than in cycle ergometry both in males and females, although the differences were smaller than in the

AT. We also found a large and significant difference in HR at RCP of 7–10 bpm, again limiting the transferability of results between modalities. To the best of our knowledge, no previous study evaluated RCP in triathletes in treadmill and cycle ergometry testing. The maximum exertion is the most commonly used parameter to assess the aerobic capacity of triathletes [8]. As with the other parameters (VO_2AT, VO_2RCP), we found VO_2max to be significantly higher in treadmill testing than in cycle ergometry. Millet et al. concluded from previous studies that VO_2max is generally similar in treadmill and cycle ergometry testing in triathletes, and that triathletes' training adaptation is therefore similar to that of cyclists [8]. This is contrary to the results of our study. Small sample sizes in previous studies are likely the cause for statistically significant differences not having been observed. In the present study, the differences in AT were larger than at maximum exertion. This may explain why significant differences were observed more often at AT than at maximum. The VO_2max in our studied population is lower than that reported in most previous studies, probably due to the higher mean age of the participants, which is a known factor limiting VO_2max [8,37]. HRmax was also significantly higher in treadmill testing than in cycle ergometry in both males and females. The results of previous studies on males were conflicting, some indicating HRmax to be lower in cycle ergometry by 6–10 bpm [13,20,21,24] and some finding no significant difference [14,15,18,23,47]. Few studies included females and the evidence was also conflicting; HRmax was observed to be either similar or higher in cycling [25,48].

We found that the VE was higher in cycle ergometry than on the treadmill, despite a slightly lower ventilation frequency, indicating a higher tidal volume. This is contrary to the lower VE and Vf in cyclists at both AT and RCP. The differences may correspond to higher lactate accumulation and an acidosis-induced respiratory response in cycle ergometry at maximum, but not at AT and RCP, where lactate levels were similar. This is partly similar to the findings of Koyal et al., who described a higher respiratory response due to higher acidosis in cycle ergometry during the low, moderate and high intensity of exercise in untrained subjects [49]. The differences at low and moderate intensity are most likely due to our subjects' experience in triathlon training and therefore lower lactate build-up when cycling at submaximal levels, as it has previously been demonstrated that trained cyclists accumulate less lactate in cycle ergometry [10]. The lower VE and Vf in cycle ergometry at AT and RCP are likely due to the lower VO_2. Some of the differences between CE and TE may also be due to different breathing patterns in TE and CE. VE increases more steeply in CE, and maximal VE is reached at a lower VT [50]. It has also been shown that cycling leads to a larger decrease in respiratory muscle endurance than using a treadmill, and it has been proposed that the differences in breathing mechanics may be due to a different entrainment of breath in CE and TE [4,30]. Studies showed that triathletes display a higher entrainment of breathing in CE than TE, and that entrainment decreases with increasing load in CE [31]. Altered breath patterns may result in different energy use for breathing and subsequently to differences in lactate levels. Optimizing the breathing patterns could lead to an improved economy in both cycling and running [51]. Overall, the large differences across all measured CPET parameters justify performing two separate tests on CE and TE. The differences may prevent accurate prescription of exercise loads and accurate training progress monitoring in the preparation for competitive events. Further research is needed for swimming.

The variance in differences in VO_2max obtained from treadmill and cycle ergometer testing was significantly explained by BMI, FATP, FFM and training experience in the group >40 years of age with an R^2 of 0.25. It has previously been shown that BM and BC are related to aerobic capacity and that the physiological ability to consume oxygen is negatively associated with FM [52–54]. However, to the best of our knowledge, this is the first study to demonstrate an association between BC, BMI and the differences in treadmill and cycle ergometry CPET results. We hypothesize that this relationship may be caused by the physiological differences between cycling and running. Cycling is a non-weight-bearing activity, with far less eccentric activity than during running [55]. Therefore, BM and BC may be more important in treadmill testing than in cycle ergometry. It is unclear why the observed differences are better explained by anthropometric variables in the older group compared to the younger group. We may suspect that the difference in the younger population would be better explained by other factors, perhaps by training volume in cycling or running, which were not evaluated in this study. It is also possible that the differences in BC, especially FFM, reflect differences in cardiovascular function, which might play a more important role in older triathletes and could have a different importance in cycle ergometry and treadmill testing [56,57]. Differences in HRmax were significantly explained by BMI and FATP in the older population. It has previously been shown that HRmax is related to BC and BMI, but it remains unclear what the cause for this relationship is or why BC is related to the differences in HRmax between treadmill and cycle ergometry [57].

5. Study Limitations

The time intervals between tests varied significantly. Tests were carried out at various times of the season. Training data, except months of experience in triathlon, were unavailable. The female group was too small for meaningful regression analysis, but it was larger than in many previous studies and large enough to observe many significant differences. It was not meaningful to divide females into younger and older age groups, as only 2 females were over 40 years of age. BC was measured with bioelectrical impedance, which may be less accurate than some other methods such as CT/MRI BC analysis, but it is commonly used in sports and therefore may be more practically applicable than more advanced methods. Varied results of CPET may be achieved, and those scores depend on the participant's endurance level. Preliminary preferred discipline (running or cycling) may also alter our findings. This relates mostly to novice subjects or beginners at lower levels of experience. Future research could address this issue. This study did not evaluate swimming further studies would be needed to determine differences in CPET between TE, CE and swimming.

6. Conclusions

VO_2 and HR are higher in treadmill testing than cycle ergometry at AT, RCP and maximum exertion in both male and female triathletes. The differences are partly explained by BMI, BF and FFM in the population above 40 years of age. These factors were not important in the younger group. The practical implication of this study is that, given the large differences between TE and CE testing, both tests should be carried out in triathletes.

Author Contributions: S.P., S.W. and D.Ś.: conceptualization and resources. J.L., S.W., D.Ś. and A.M.: investigation. I.C., G.G. and P.S.K.: statistical analysis. S.P., S.W., G.G. and P.S.K.: writing—original draft preparation. S.P., S.W., D.Ś., P.S.K., G.G., J.L. and T.K.: writing—review and editing. A.M.: supervision. All authors have read and agreed to the published version of the manuscript.

Funding: This research received no external funding.

Institutional Review Board Statement: The study was conducted according to the guidelines of the Declaration of Helsinki and approved by the Institutional Review Board: Komisja Bioetyczna przy Warszawskim Uniwersytecie Medycznym, AKBE/32/2021; date of approval: 15 March 2021.

Informed Consent Statement: Informed consent was obtained from all subjects involved in the study.

Data Availability Statement: The datasets generated during and/or analyzed during the current study are available from the corresponding author on reasonable request.

Conflicts of Interest: SW is the owner of the Sportslab clinic. Other authors have no conflict to declare.

References

1. Chambers, D.J.; Wisely, N.A. Cardiopulmonary exercise testing-a beginner's guide to the nine-panel plot. *BJA Educ.* **2019**, *19*, 158–164. [CrossRef]

2. Guazzi, M.; Adams, V.; Conraads, V.; Halle, M.; Mezzani, A.; Vanhees, L.; Arena, R.; Fletcher, G.F.; Forman, D.E.; Kitzman, D.W.; et al. EACPR/AHA Scientific Statement. Clinical recommendations for cardiopulmonary exercise testing data assessment in specific patient populations. *Circulation* **2012**, *126*, 2261–2274. [CrossRef] [PubMed]
3. Herdy, A.H.; Ritt, L.E.F.; Stein, R.; de Araújo, C.G.S.; Milani, M.; Meneghelo, R.S.; Ferraz, A.S.; Hossri, C.; de Almeida, A.E.M.; Fernandes-Silva, M.M.; et al. Cardiopulmonary Exercise Test: Background, Applicability and Interpretation. *Arq. Bras. Cardiol.* **2016**, *107*, 467–481. [PubMed]
4. Galán-Rioja, M.Á.; González-Mohíno, F.; Poole, D.C.; González-Ravé, J.M. Relative Proximity of Critical Power and Metabolic/Ventilatory Thresholds: Systematic Review and Meta-Analysis. *Sports Med.* **2020**, *50*, 1771–1783. [CrossRef] [PubMed]
5. Jones, A.M.; Vanhatalo, A. The 'Critical Power' Concept: Applications to Sports Performance with a Focus on Intermittent High-Intensity Exercise. *Sports Med.* **2017**, *47*, 65–78. [CrossRef] [PubMed]
6. Löllgen, H.; Leyk, D. Exercise Testing in Sports Medicine. *Dtsch. Arztebl. Int.* **2018**, *115*, 409–416. [CrossRef]
7. Hanson, N.; Scheadler, C.M.; Lee, T.L.; Neuenfeldt, N.C.; Michael, T.J.; Miller, M.G. Modality determines VO2max achieved in self-paced exercise tests: Validation with the Bruce protocol. *Eur. J. Appl. Physiol.* **2016**, *116*, 1313–1319. [CrossRef] [PubMed]
8. Millet, G.; Vleck, V.; Bentley, D. Physiological Differences Between Cycling and Running. *Sports Med.* **2009**, *39*, 179–206. [CrossRef]
9. Costa, M.M.; Russo, A.K.; Pićarro, I.C.; Neto, T.L.B.; Silva, A.C.; Tarasantchi, J. Oxygen consumption and ventilation during constant-load exercise in runners and cyclists. *J. Sports Med. Phys. Fit.* **1989**, *29*, 36–44.
10. Bouckaert, J.; Vrijens, J.; Pannier, J.L. Effect of specific test procedures on plasma lactate concentration and peak oxygen uptake in endurance athletes. *J. Sports Med. Phys. Fit.* **1990**, *30*, 13–18.
11. Marko, D.; Bahenský, P.; Snarr, R.L.; Malátová, R. VO2peak Comparison of a Treadmill Vs. Cycling Protocol in Elite Teenage Competitive Runners, Cyclists, and Swimmers. *J. Strength Cond. Res.* **2021**. [CrossRef]
12. Basset, F.; Boulay, M. Specificity of treadmill and cycle ergometer tests in triathletes, runners and cyclists. *Eur. J. Appl. Physiol.* **2000**, *81*, 214–221. [CrossRef] [PubMed]
13. Hue, O.; Le Gallais, D.; Chollet, D.; Préfaut, C. Ventilatory threshold and maximal oxygen uptake in present triathletes. *Can. J. Appl. Physiol.* **2000**, *25*, 102–113. [CrossRef] [PubMed]
14. Medelli, J.; Maingourd, Y.; Bouferrache, B.; Bach, V.; Freville, M.; Libert, J.P. Maximal oxygen uptake and aerobic-anaerobic transition on treadmill and bicycle in triathletes. *Jpn. J. Physiol.* **1993**, *43*, 347–360. [CrossRef]
15. Zhou, S.; Robson, S.J.; King, M.J.; Davie, A.J. Correlations between short-course triathlon performance and physiological variables determined in laboratory cycle and treadmill tests. *J. Sports Med. Phys. Fit.* **1997**, *37*, 122–130.
16. Sleivert, G.G.; Wenger, H.A. Physiological predictors of short-course triathlon performance. *Med. Sci. Sports Exerc.* **1993**, *25*, 871–876. [CrossRef]
17. Miura, H.; Kitagawa, K.; Ishiko, T. Economy during a simulated laboratory test triathlon is highly related to Olympic distance triathlon. *Int. J. Sports Med.* **1997**, *18*, 276–280. [CrossRef] [PubMed]
18. Kohrt, W.M.; Morgan, D.W.; Bates, B.; Skinner, J.S. Physiological responses of triathletes to maximal swimming, cycling, and running. *Med. Sci. Sports Exerc.* **1987**, *19*, 51–55. [CrossRef] [PubMed]
19. Schabort, E.J.; Killian, S.C.; St Clair Gibson, A.; Hawley, J.A.; Noakes, T.D. Prediction of triathlon race time from laboratory testing in national triathletes. *Med. Sci. Sports Exerc.* **2000**, *32*, 844–849. [CrossRef] [PubMed]
20. Hue, O.; Le Gallais, D.; Chollet, D.; Boussana, A.; Préfaut, C. The influence of prior cycling on biomechanical and cardiorespiratory response profiles during running in triathletes. *Eur. J. Appl. Physiol. Occup. Physiol.* **1998**, *77*, 98–105. [CrossRef] [PubMed]
21. Kohrt, W.M.; O'Connor, J.S.; Skinner, J.S. Longitudinal assessment of responses by triathletes to swimming, cycling, and running. *Med. Sci. Sports Exerc.* **1989**, *21*, 569–575. [CrossRef]
22. Albrecht, T.J.; Foster, V.L.; Dickinson, A.L.; DeBever, J.M. Triathletes, exercise parameters measured during bicycle, swim bench, and treadmill testing. *Med. Sci. Sports Exerc.* **1986**, *18*, S86. [CrossRef]
23. Basset, F.; Boulay, M. Treadmill and Cycle Ergometer Tests are Interchangeable to Monitor Triathletes Annual Training. *J. Sports Sci. Med.* **2003**, *2*, 110–116. [PubMed]
24. Roecker, K.; Striegel, H.; Dickhuth, H.-H. Heart-Rate Recommendations: Transfer Between Running and Cycling Exercise? *Int. J. Sports Med.* **2003**, *24*, 173–178. [CrossRef] [PubMed]
25. Schneider, D.A.; Lacroix, K.A.; Atkinson, G.R.; Troped, P.J.; Pollack, J. Ventilatory threshold and maximal oxygen uptake during cycling and running in triathletes. *Med. Sci. Sports Exerc.* **1990**, *22*, 257–264. [CrossRef] [PubMed]
26. Galy, O.; Le Gallais, D.; Hue, O.; Boussana, A.; Préfaut, C. Is exercise-induced arterial hypoxemia in triathletes dependent on exercise modality? *Int. J. Sports Med.* **2005**, *26*, 719–726. [CrossRef] [PubMed]
27. Bolognesi, M. Ventilatory Threshold and Maximal Oxygen Uptake During Cycling and Running in Duathletes. *Med. Sport* **1997**, *50*, 209–216.
28. O'Toole, M.L.; Hiller, D.B.; Crosby, L.O.; Douglas, P.S. The ultraendurance triathlete: A physiological profile. *Med. Sci. Sports Exerc.* **1987**, *19*, 45–50. [PubMed]
29. Fleg, J.L.; Lakatta, E.G. Role of muscle loss in the age-associated reduction in VO2 max. *J. Appl. Physiol.* **1988**, *65*, 1147–1151. [CrossRef] [PubMed]
30. Ades, P.A.; Toth, M.J. Accelerated decline of aerobic fitness with healthy aging: What is the good news? *Circulation* **2005**, *112*, 624–626. [CrossRef] [PubMed]

31. Koch, B.; Schäper, C.; Ittermann, T.; Spielhagen, T.; Dörr, M.; Völzke, H.; Opitz, C.F.; Ewert, R.; Gläser, S. Reference values for cardiopulmonary exercise testing in healthy volunteers: The SHIP study. *Eur. Respir. J.* **2009**, *33*, 389–397. [CrossRef]
32. Woo, J.S.; Derleth, C.; Stratton, J.R.; Levy, W.C. The Influence of Age, Gender, and Training on Exercise Efficiency. *J. Am. Coll. Cardiol.* **2006**, *47*, 1049–1057. [CrossRef] [PubMed]
33. Bilgin, Ü. Effects of Body Composition on Race Time in Triathletes. *Anthropology* **2016**, *23*, 406–413. [CrossRef]
34. Knechtle, B.; Wirth, A.; Baumann, B.; Knechtle, P.; Rosemann, T. Personal Best Time, Percent Body Fat, and Training Are Differently Associated With Race Time for Male and Female Ironman Triathletes. *Res. Q. Exerc. Sport* **2010**, *81*, 62–68. [CrossRef]
35. Carey, D.G.; Tofte, C.; Pliego, G.J.; Raymond, R.L. Transferability of running and cycling training zones in triathletes: Implications for steady-state exercise. *J. Strength Cond. Res.* **2009**, *23*, 251–258. [CrossRef] [PubMed]
36. Martin-Rincon, M.; Calbet, J.A.L. Progress Update and Challenges on V. O(2max) Testing and Interpretation. *Front. Physiol.* **2020**, *11*, 1070. [CrossRef] [PubMed]
37. Kaminsky, L.A.; Arena, R.; Myers, J. Reference Standards for Cardiorespiratory Fitness Measured With Cardiopulmonary Exercise Testing: Data From the Fitness Registry and the Importance of Exercise National Database. *Mayo Clin. Proc.* **2015**, *90*, 1515–1523. [CrossRef]
38. Beaver, W.L.; Wasserman, K.; Whipp, B.J. A new method for detecting anaerobic threshold by gas exchange. *J. Appl. Physiol.* **1989**, *60*, 2020–2027. [CrossRef]
39. R Core Team. *R: A Language and Environment for Statistical Computing*; R Foundation for Statistical Computing: Vienna, Austria, 2018.
40. Sjoberg, D.D.; Curry, M.; Hannum, M.; Larmarange, J.; Whiting, K.; Zabor, E.C. gtsummary: Presentation-Ready Data Summary and Analytic Result Tables. R Package Version 1.4.2. 2021. Available online: https://www.danieldsjoberg.com/gtsummary/ (accessed on 15 December 2021).
41. Stekhoven, D.J. missForest: Nonparametric Missing Value Imputation using Random Forest. R Package Version 1.4. 2013. Available online: https://cran.r-project.org/web/packages/missForest/missForest.pdf (accessed on 15 December 2021).
42. Ghosh, A.K. Anaerobic threshold: Its concept and role in endurance sport. *Malays. J. Med. Sci.* **2004**, *11*, 24–36. [PubMed]
43. Bourgois, J.G.; Bourgois, G.; Boone, J. Perspectives and determinants for training-intensity distribution in elite endurance athletes. *Int. J. Sports Physiol. Perform.* **2019**, *14*, 1151–1156. [CrossRef] [PubMed]
44. Casado, A.; Hanley, B.; Santos-Concejero, J.; Ruis-Pérez, L.M. World-class long-distance running performances are best predicted by volume of easy runs and deliberate practice of short interval and tempo runs. *J. Strength Cond. Res.* **2021**, *35*, 2525–2531. [CrossRef]
45. Kreider, R.B.; Boone, T.; Thompson, W.R.; Burkes, S.; Cortes, C.W. Cardiovascular and thermal responses of triathlon performance. *Med. Sci. Sports Exerc.* **1988**, *20*, 385–390. [CrossRef] [PubMed]
46. Bassett, D.R.; Howley, E.T. Limiting factors for maximum oxygen uptake and determinants of endurance performance. *Med. Sci. Sports Exerc.* **2000**, *32*, 70–84. [CrossRef] [PubMed]
47. Millet, G.; Vleck, V.; Bentley, D. Physiological requirements in triathlon. *J. Hum. Sport Exerc.* **2011**, *6*, 184–204. [CrossRef]
48. Koyal, S.N.; Whipp, B.J.; Huntsman, D.; Bray, G.A.; Wasserman, K. Ventilatory responses to the metabolic acidosis of treadmill and cycle ergometry. *J. Appl. Physiol.* **1976**, *40*, 864–867. [CrossRef]
49. Kalsås, K.; Thorsen, E. Breathing patterns during progressive incremental cycle and treadmill exercise are different. *Clin. Physiol. Funct. Imaging* **2009**, *29*, 335–338. [CrossRef]
50. Bahenský, P.; Bunc, V.; Malátová, R.; Marko, D.; Grosicki, G.J.; Schuster, J. Impact of a Breathing Intervention on Engagement of Abdominal, Thoracic, and Subclavian Musculature during Exercise, a Randomized Trial. *J. Clin. Med.* **2021**, *10*, 3514. [CrossRef]
51. Baker, J.S.; Bailey, D.M.; Davies, B. The relationship between total-body mass, fat-free mass and cycle ergometry power components during 20 s of maximal exercise. *J. Sci. Med. Sport* **2001**, *4*, 1–9. [CrossRef]
52. Minasian, V.; Marandi, S.M.; Kelishadi, R.; Abolhassani, H. Correlation between aerobic fitness and body composition in middle school students. *Int. J. Prev. Med.* **2014**, *5*, S102. [CrossRef] [PubMed]
53. Vargas, V.; Lira, C.; Vancini, R.; Rayes, A.; Andrade, M. Fat mass is negatively associated with the physiological ability of tissue to consume oxygen. *Mot. Rev. Educ. Física* **2018**, *24*, 4. [CrossRef]
54. Nicol, C.; Komi, P.; Marconnet, P. Fatigue effects of marathon running on neuromuscular performance: II. Changes in force, integrated electromyographic activity and endurance capacity. *Scand. J. Med. Sci. Sport* **2007**, *1*, 18–24. [CrossRef]
55. Zeng, Q.; Sun, X.-N.; Fan, L.; Ye, P. Correlation of body composition with cardiac function and arterial compliance. *Clin. Exp. Pharmacol. Physiol.* **2008**, *35*, 78–82. [CrossRef] [PubMed]
56. Carrick-Ranson, G.; Hastings, J.L.; Bhella, P.S.; Shibata, S.; Fujimoto, N.; Palmer, D.; Boyd, K.; Levine, B.D. The Effect of Age-related Differences in Body Size and Composition on Cardiovascular Determinants of VO2max. *J. Gerontol. Ser. A* **2013**, *68*, 608–616. [CrossRef] [PubMed]
57. Lach, J.; Wiecha, S.; Śliż, D.; Price, S.; Zaborski, M.; Cieśliński, I.; Postuła, M.; Knechtle, B.; Mamcarz, A. HR Max Prediction Based on Age, Body Composition, Fitness Level, Testing Modality and Sex in Physically Active Population. *Front. Physiol.* **2021**, *12*, 695950. [CrossRef]

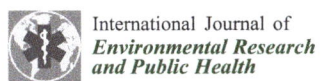

Review

Principles of Judo Training as an Organised Form of Physical Activity for Children

Monika Kowalczyk [1,*], Małgorzata Zgorzalewicz-Stachowiak [1], Wiesław Błach [2] and Maciej Kostrzewa [3,*]

[1] Department of Health Prophylaxis, University of Medical Sciences, 61-701 Poznan, Poland; neuro@ump.edu.pl
[2] Faculty of Physical Education & Sport, University School of Physical Education, 51-612 Wroclaw, Poland; wieslaw.judo@wp.pl
[3] Institute of Sport Science, The Jerzy Kukuczka Academy of Physical Education in Katowice, 40-065 Katowice, Poland
* Correspondence: monikakowalczyk@ump.edu.pl (M.K.); m.kostrzewa@awf.katowice.pl (M.K.)

Abstract: When organising judo training for children, it is essential to ensure maximum safety, and use an appropriate training methodology adapted to the age of the youngest judo athletes. This paper aims to review the current literature containing judo training principles and safety-related considerations for preschool (4–6 years) and school-age (7–12 years) children as an organised physical activity. Data were collected until October 2021 from eight international scientific databases (PubMed, Scopus, UpToDate, Web of Science, Cochrane, EBSCOhost, ScienceDirect, Google Scholar). In the overviews, we found various times and frequencies of judo training for children. In preschool, the training time was 30–60 min with a frequency of 2–3 times per week, whereas in the school-age group, the training time was extended from 45 to 90 min 3–4 times per week. The most common injuries included upper arm injuries, followed by those of the lower limbs. In the future, it would be an advantage to systematise the methodology of judo training as an organised form of physical activity that can complement the daily dose of exercises recommended by the World Health Organization for maintaining children's general health.

Keywords: judo; physical education and training; sports injuries; child

Citation: Kowalczyk, M.; Zgorzalewicz-Stachowiak, M.; Błach, W.; Kostrzewa, M. Principles of Judo Training as an Organised Form of Physical Activity for Children. *Int. J. Environ. Res. Public Health* **2022**, *19*, 1929. https://doi.org/10.3390/ijerph19041929

Academic Editor: Britton W. Brewer

Received: 30 December 2021
Accepted: 7 February 2022
Published: 9 February 2022

Publisher's Note: MDPI stays neutral with regard to jurisdictional claims in published maps and institutional affiliations.

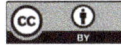

Copyright: © 2022 by the authors. Licensee MDPI, Basel, Switzerland. This article is an open access article distributed under the terms and conditions of the Creative Commons Attribution (CC BY) license (https://creativecommons.org/licenses/by/4.0/).

1. Introduction

The sedentary lifestyle of children is a serious problem in the 21st century. Fewer and fewer children participate in spontaneous outdoor games, and children are spending more time in front of multimedia screens. To maintain the psychophysical health of children aged 5–17 years, the World Health Organization (WHO) recommends physical activity (PA) for an average of 60 min per day at moderate to intense levels [1]. In the Polish curriculum, the weekly time allocated to physical education in the early school period (ages 7–10) is three classes per week for 45 min; in the school period (ages ten and above), it is four times per week for 45 min [2]. As a result, the PA time in school settings is insufficient to meet children's movement needs. Therefore, in addition to educational establishments, it is mainly the parents who should take care of their children's physical development.

Martial arts are now becoming increasingly popular around the world. These include judo, which is currently practised by millions of people. From the point of view of parents who enrol their children in training, judo is a PA that affects all aspects (physical, psychological and social) of practitioners' health [3]. Judo training can occur as an additional organised form of PA outside school, sports clubs, or physical education lessons. The International Judo Federation (IJF), taking into account the health and educational advantages of judo, created the "Judo in Schools" programme, which is available worldwide [4]. Its main goal is to present this martial art to as many children as possible, especially those aged 4–12, and to encourage them to train regularly. In addition, the programme's creators would like judo to become part of the core curriculum of physical education in schools globally.

History of Judo

Judo is a martial art created in Japan by Professor Jigoro Kano in the late 19th century. The word judo in Japanese translates as "the gentle way". Kano developed his techniques from various Japanese jujitsu schools [5]. Moreover, he described judo's educational and upbringing values based on the fundamental principles of Seiryoku-Zenyo and Jita-Kyoei [6–9]. According to these principles, the purpose of practising this martial art is to learn how to attack and defend with effective use of the body and mind energy (Seiryoku-Zenyo). Kano described it as the art of executing an effective technique during a fight appropriate to the action, where fighting is a learning process rather than the end in itself.

Furthermore, he emphasised the importance of self-improvement during training, resulting in mutual social benefits for all fellow practitioners on and off the mat (Jita-Kyoei). According to judo's philosophy, doing good, respect, harmony, discipline, and cooperation are essential in the training room and everyday life [10]. As a teenager, Jigoro Kano himself experienced violence from older classmates at jujitsu school [7]. To eliminate aggression and the use of force towards the weaker, he introduced white judo suits (judogi, equal for all), a division into belts (from white as a student's kyu to black as a master's dan). Kano also pointed out that fellow practitioners should be of similar weight and age to provide some protection for novices. In judo's etiquette, based on Japan's cultural traditions, he also included mutual bows to reflect respect for the other people training on the mat.

Following Jigoro Kano's philosophy "to the general good", judo training connects educational, social and health benefits [11]. De Crée [12] suggests that in training children, the initial intention of the founder of judo was to foster a progressive and complete form of physical and mental education. Kano's assumption through judo was the possibility of using the power of mind and body most effectively. Its training cultivates the body and spirit through the practice of attack and defence, and the essence of this principled moral code is learning through self-awareness. Judo has now evolved into a sport that focuses more on competition and winning. Therefore, it is essential to emphasise the fundamental principles of judo (Seiryoku-Zenyo and Jita-Kyoei), aiming at perfecting oneself and benefiting from life [13]. The educational benefit of judo is a value that should be cultivated among judo practitioners, especially the youngest.

Judo competitions are divided into age and weight categories [14]. In seniors (over the age of 20), there are seven weight categories for men and women. In the younger age categories, due to the biological development of children and adolescence, there are more designated weight categories according to the sports regulations of a given country, based on IJF rules. In Poland, children from 11 years of age (calendar age) can compete in regional competitions [14,15]. Children from the age of 14 (calendar year) can participate in national competitions. They must have a licence from the Polish Judo Association and up-to-date medical examinations.

Practitioners' clothing consists of judogi—trousers, jacket and belt. During official sports competitions, one competitor currently wears a white judogi and their opponent wears a blue one. The differently coloured judogi make it easier for the judges to distinguish and score the contestants during a fight.

This study aimed to review the current literature on the practical organisation and conduct of judo training for healthy children of preschool and school-age. The review analysed the purpose, forms and methods of training for children. The authors also took note of safety aspects and the risk of injury during such classes.

2. Materials and Methods

Until October 2021, publications were collected from eight international scientific databases (PubMed, Scopus, UpToDate, Web of Science, Cochrane, EBSCOhost, ScienceDirect, Google Scholar). Papers in English or Polish, dating from the 1st of January 2009 onwards, were considered. During the search of the relevant literature, "judo" in combination with the following terms: martial arts, children, young, youth, girls, boys, training, techniques, injuries, physical activity, was used. The analysis involved publications that presented forms and methods of judo-specific training for healthy preschool children (4–6 years old) and school-age children (7–12 years old) and the risk of injury. The references sections of these studies were also screened. There was no information found about injuries in judo in the 4–12 years old age group. Therefore, the available reports about injuries in children and adolescents up to 18 years of age were taken into account. Original research and reviews related to the presented topic were qualified.

3. Results

3.1. When Can Children Start Training Judo?

From the available literature, it can be seen that children start training from preschool age. Based on the available publications, it can be concluded that the youngest participants of judo lessons in Poland are between four and six years old [3,16,17]. Similarly, in her work, Demiral [18] proposes a primary judo curriculum for children aged 4–6. In the publication by Garcia et al. [19], describing a training programme of judo techniques for children, the authors indicate that of all children starting judo, 73% are aged 4–8, the majority of whom began training at the age of five or six (17.7% and 22.9%, respectively).

3.2. What Is the Recommended Duration and Frequency of Training?

Sterkowicz-Przybycień et al. [3] suggest that the duration of judo lessons for practitioners aged 4–6 should be 30–35 min twice per week. In studies by Walaszek et al. [16,17], children aged 5–6 exercised for 35–45 min 2–3 times per week. Neofit [20] describes recommendations based on feedback and coaching experience and suggests that judo training for a group of 4–6-year-olds should take place 2–3 times per week for 45 min. In Krustolovic et al.'s [21] study, children of an average age of six practised judo three times per week for 45 min, and in Djordjevic et al.'s [22] research, boys of an average age of six practised judo three times per week for 60 min. School practitioners in the study by Triki et al. [23], at the age of ten, trained in judo four times per week for 90 min. In Ludyga et al. [24], judokas with an average age of ten practised twice per week for 60 min. The judokas in Jankowicz-Szymanska et al.'s [25] and Maślinski et al.'s [26] studies were aged 11–12 and received judo lessons three times per week for 90 min. In the recent review of studies on the effectiveness of judo exercise in children, Gutierrez-Garcia et al. [10] point to different class methodologies for children aged 5–12. Their class duration was 35–90 min, and the frequency was between two and three times per week.

Throughout the judo training methodology, it is emphasised that activities should be adapted to children's abilities and psychomotor needs, and relate to their age. The Canadian Long Term Athlete Development (LTAD) judo training programme is based on children's so-called motor development windows [27]. The programme is designed to select athletes for practicing judo competitively and to achieve results at major sporting events. The first window of the programme covers the development of speed capabilities and occurs at 6–8 years for girls and 7–9 years for boys. The next window focuses on agility skills occurring in girls aged 8–11 and boys 9–12. For judoka under 11 years, it is recommended that the duration of training is 60–90 min 2–3 times per week; for those under the age of 13, it is suggested that training takes place 3–4 times per week for 60–90 min.

3.3. Purpose of the Training

In the early years, training should focus primarily on developing general physical fitness (coordination, speed, agility, efficiency and balance), learning how to safely break falls, and basic judo techniques [18,19,28,29].

The teaching of judo elements begins with learning how to fall (Ukemi), techniques on the ground (Ne-waza), through to learning grappling techniques (Katame-waza) and those when standing (Tachi-waza). The grappling group includes bracing, joint locking and choking techniques. Bracing techniques are taught first, and for safety reasons, joint locking and choking techniques are only allowed in sports competitions much later (in Poland from the age of 14 calendar years). Next, throwing techniques (Nage-waza) in the standing position are introduced (Tachi-waza). When practitioners have reached a sufficient level of fitness and skills, combat (Randori) elements are performed.

Moreover, training should not only focus on the development of physical attributes. Jigoro Kano, the founder of the first Kodokan School, also emphasised the formation of positive character traits such as discipline, responsibility and the ability to control emotions through training. According to the principles of Seiryoku-Zenyo and Jita-Kyoei, through judo, one should develop respect and modesty towards fellow practitioners, teachers, and also towards general social contacts [7,8].

3.4. Forms of Training

We found no standardised description in the literature of the forms of judo training in children as an organised form of activity. It would be beneficial if it involved a long-term evaluation of its effectiveness and influence on health. Currently, teachers choose these forms mainly based on their own knowledge and experience, adjusting the programme to the age and abilities of the persons exercising. Van Kooten [27] points out that in teaching judo children under 12 coaches should avoid "specialisation in judo, negative competitive experiences, and comparison with other children, while all activities should take the form of games".

Sterkowicz-Przybycień et al. [3], describing the curriculum for 4–6-year-olds, indicate that the main aim is to develop the movement skills through gymnastic and general development exercises. Moreover, the youngest children, when starting their training, learn proper judo bows, natural and defensive postures (Shisei), movement on the mat and, above all, falling on the mat (Ukemi). In the following stages, they learn basic holds (Honkesa-gatame, Yoko-shiho-gatame and Kami-shiho-gatame), body rotations (Tai-sabaki) and basic throws (O-goshi and O-soto-gari).

In their paper, Krustolovic et al. [21] present a judo programme for children with an average age of seven. In their nine-month programme, each 45-min workout is divided into three stages: warm-up (14–19 min), main part (25 min) and cool-down (5–8 min). The warm-up is based on general development, gymnastics and stretching exercises. In the main part, for 15 min, the following judo elements are practised: postures (Shisei), grasping the judogi (Kumi-kata), moving on the mat (Shintai), falls (Ukemi), throws (Nage-waza) and techniques on the ground (Ne-waza), and fighting (Randori). The next ten minutes are devoted to selecting games connected with learning judo techniques. The end of the session is a phase of calming down, relaxation and stretching.

A similar training scheme for children of an average age of ten for 45 to 60 min is presented by Missawi et al. [30]. The warm-up lasts 15–20 min with low-intensity games and stretching exercises, followed by the central part of the training session lasting 20–25 min. At this stage of training, pads (Ukemi), throws and combinations of these techniques (Uchi-komi, Renraku-waza) are perfected, followed by training fights (five minutes). The last 5–10 min are devoted to active regeneration. Ludyga et al. [24] also present a programme for school children beginning judo at an average age of ten. Each judo session consists of playful physical fitness exercises and judo techniques, including falling techniques and Randori (fighting).

Garcia et al. [19] propose a judo-teaching programme for children based on a survey conducted among 911 judo teachers from 19 countries. The trainers' responses were based on their knowledge and experience. The authors' most important point is adapting technical elements to the children's age and developmental abilities. The implementation of particular judo techniques should be based on two criteria: the safety of the fellow practitioner (Uke) and the ease of executing the throw. The teacher should observe if the person performing the throw (Tori) controls their and the Uke's movements while falling.

The authors suggest that the examination for the first white belt at the age of about six should include the ability to perform pads and move on the mat. Then, at about seven, trainers can start teaching children for their yellow belt using the most comfortable throws such as O-soto-gari, O-goshi, De-Ashi-barai, and Ko-soto-gari. The colours of the kyu training belts in Europe range from white through yellow, orange, green, blue and brown. After mastering the most difficult brown belt techniques, the student can take the master dan black belt exam. The authors emphasise the obtaining of a black belt and adequate physical fitness and technical skills. There are also minimum age criteria to maintain the child's safety. In Poland and Spain, the minimum age is 16 years old.

Games implemented in play are considered an exciting way to teach judo to children. This free activity has certain rules, and is performed in a specific place and time. The ending of games is not determined and allows learning to be adapted to solving problem situations during the game. The game may be used to introduce judo techniques separately or judo in its entirety with the ability to fight [31]. Children very much enjoy these games as they are motivating and receive praise when they correctly perform technique. Lukanova [32] and Masenko [33] describe judo training based on games and activities. According to these authors, training based on selected games should last between 24 and 45 min in total. However, short task games based on performing a single exercise should not be longer than 30–60 s, with a maximum of 3–5 repetitions. Simultaneously, the duration of longer games with a more complex exercise structure is 3–10 min with a similar number of repetitions [32,33]. In a recent report, Pereira et al. [31] present the systematisation of games through a network of complex connections. According to the authors, the proposed game system covers spheres from A to F, consisting of various functional units. The number of connections between the spheres and units of a given game affect its complexity and difficulty level. The presented network can be used for different learning levels, from judo beginners to professional participants. The authors indicate that such a teaching system may positively affect the teaching of judo techniques and their use in combat. Appropriately selected game elements can enrich movements and develop general physical fitness, judo tactics and technique elements. They also provide an introduction to the development of sports competition skills, which can be useful at a later stage of training.

3.5. Children Safety during Training

Trainers and the parents of children taking part in judo training must know about the associated injury risks. In the limited literature, the incidence of injuries was only observed together in the wider group aged under 18 [34,35]. According to Pocceco et al. [34] and Demorest et al. [35], reviews concern injuries for the whole group of those aged 5–17. The available data do not show any correlation between the ages of the children training and the incidence of injuries. The authors report that injuries are often associated with incorrect throwing and falling techniques and when there is too much of a difference in the body weights of those training. Moreover, they mention that the most common injuries are contusions, fractures, and sprains. These mainly affect the shoulder, elbow and wrist in the upper limb, and the foot and ankle in the lower limb. Demorest et al. [35] suggest that the more frequent upper limb injuries in judo, compared to other martial arts such as karate and taekwondo, where kicks are mainly performed, may occur due to judo-specificity. Judogi grabbing when throwing and falling on the mat are associated with more significant work of the upper limbs when performing judo techniques. Unfortunately, there are no data on related risk factors and judo injuries in younger children aged 4–12 years. The literature does not describe any injuries for the age group discussed that correlate with the length, intensity or difficulty of the techniques performed, or with the progress of the children.

In preventing injuries, the essential principle in judo training should be to ensure the maximum safety of the practitioners. According to Pocceco et al.'s [34] review, the trainer's qualifications, knowledge and experience in teaching this sport to children are of primary importance in injury prevention. The crucial element is to teach how to perform proper falling techniques, how to fall during throws and how to correctly execute throws. It is also essential to provide adequate, comprehensive physical development and prevent adepts from competing too early, that is, participating in sports competitions. Further, the mat intended for exercise should be of the appropriate quality and firmness to ensure proper cushioning for falls.

4. General Recommendations

Within this review, we found various methodologies for teaching judo to children. Some authors [3,16,19] suggest that judo classes could be started at the preschool age of between four and six years. Furthermore, analysing the available data [3,16,17,20,21] on the length and frequency of the training itself, the training time for preschool children (4–6 years) is between 30 min and up to even 60 min with a frequency of 2–3 times per week. At school age, authors [23–26] recommend extending the time from 45 to 90 min with a frequency of 3–4 times per week.

Numerous studies [5,19,21,27–29] conclude with similar aims when teaching judo as a way of developing physical fitness, learning judo elements and forming pro-social attitudes based on the original assumptions of the creator of judo, Jigoro Kano. However, the forms and methods of judo training are varied, depending on the teacher's plan [19]. Sterkowicz-Przybycień et al. [3] focus on developing physical fitness and learning basic judo elements such as falls, bracing techniques and basic throws (O-goshi and O-soto-gari). By comparison, Garcia et al. [19] propose a programme in which training children up to the age of six can develop general fitness, learn break-falls and how to move on the mat. They suggest starting by learning the most straightforward throws (O-soto-gari, O-goshi, De-Ashi-barai and Ko-soto-gari) from the age of seven. The description of the forms of training for the school groups in Krustolovic et al. [21] and Missawi et al. [30], despite the similar division of classes into three parts, differ in their duration. The warm-up time as an introduction to the class varies between 14 and 20 min. The main part of the training, dedicated to learning judo and training fight elements, last 20–25 min. Relaxation, calming down and stretching are performed in the class's last 5–10 min.

Smaruj et al. [36] and Kostrzewa et al. [37] mention strength, correct posture, effective movements and balance as critical elements in judo. Due to the activity's complexity, judo training can also be considered as a tool for increasing the strength of postural muscles, which should be taken into account when planning training for children.

Additionally, movement games and physical activities with judo elements are recommended as an exciting form of training for children [31–33]. The advantage of games and activities are that they simultaneously develop physical fitness while teaching the elements of judo, encourage the solving of problem situations during a game, and provide pleasure and satisfaction.

An important aspect during training, emphasised in the literature, is to provide an adequate safety level, for which the judo teacher is responsible [34]. Their professional qualifications and experience, and the equipment in the training halls, are important. Although, worldwide, children are more willingly practice, the risk of injuries should be taken into account when starting training. According to the reviews by Pocceco et al. [34] and Demorest et al. [35], the most common injuries are contusions, fractures or sprains of the upper limb, but these occur less often in the lower limb. In preventing injuries, it is essential to conduct regular medical check-ups that confirm no contraindications for practising judo and allow children to compete in sport according to the sports medicine regulations in force in a given country.

5. Conclusions

The advantage of judo is that it is a sport for participants of all ages and the cost of preparing a practice hall is low, with only mats being essential. However, although judo has existed for over 100 years, there are insufficient training guidelines for the youngest children, combined with assessments of its effectiveness and health benefits. The available publications show some methodological variation in this respect. Choosing a teaching programme is up to the teachers, based on their education, preparation and experience of working with children. It would be advantageous to create a relevant literature database of judo methodology for children with long-term observations of its effectiveness and influence on general health, which could be used primarily by young and less experienced teachers. In Poland, coaching can be provided by people who have adequate knowledge of judo, a minimum qualification of 1st Kyu (brown belt), have completed an appropriate training course or graduated in this field, and have registered with the Polish Judo Association and obtained a licence [15]. These people usually have a rich past as competitive athletes but are just beginning to gather coaching experience, generally by training the youngest children. It would be beneficial to systematise the forms and methods of judo training teachers. Additionally, as a supplement to the existing knowledge, an exciting research direction would also be assessing injuries in children aged 4–12 years, where activities are more recreational and there is less pressure on achieving sports results.

Judo, as a structured PA with the appropriate frequency, intensity and duration of exercise for preschool and school-age children, can supplement the WHO's recommendation for the amount of daily exercise to be undertaken. This is important for combating the sedentary lifestyles of this age group and the related rising tide of obesity.

Author Contributions: Conceptualisation, M.K. (Monika Kowalczyk); methodology, M.K. (Monika Kowalczyk); software, M.K. (Maciej Kostrzewa); validation, M.Z.-S. and W.B.; formal analysis, M.Z.-S. and W.B.; investigation, M.K. (Monika Kowalczyk); resources, M.K. (Monika Kowalczyk) and M.K. (Maciej Kostrzewa); data curation, M.K. (Monika Kowalczyk); writing—original draft preparation, M.K. (Monika Kowalczyk) and M.Z.-S.; writing—review and editing, M.Z.-S. and M.K. (Maciej Kostrzewa); visualisation, M.K. (Maciej Kostrzewa); supervision, M.Z.-S. and W.B.; project administration, M.Z.-S. All authors have read and agreed to the published version of the manuscript.

Funding: This research received no external funding.

Institutional Review Board Statement: Not applicable.

Informed Consent Statement: Not applicable.

Acknowledgments: The authors are most thankful to Czesław Koperski (7th DAN in Judo) for theoretical support and review of the paper in the area of Judo.

Conflicts of Interest: The authors declare no conflict of interest.

References

1. Bull, F.C.; Al-Ansari, S.S.; Biddle, S.; Borodulin, K.; Buman, M.P.; Cardon, G.; Carty, C.; Chaput, J.P.; Chastin, S.; Chou, R.; et al. World Health Organization 2020 guidelines on physical activity and sedentary behaviour. *Brit. J. Sports Med.* **2020**, *54*, 1451–1462. [CrossRef]
2. Minister of National Education. Ordinance of the Minister of National Education of 03.04.2019 on Framework Curricula for Public Schools. Available online: http://isap.sejm.gov.pl/isap.nsf/download.xsp/WDU20190000639/O/D20190639.pdf (accessed on 7 November 2021). (In Polish)
3. Sterkowicz-Przybycień, K.; Kłys, A.; Almansba, R. Educational judo benefits on the preschool children's behaviour. *J. Combat Sports Martial Arts* **2014**, *5*, 23–26. [CrossRef]
4. International Judo Federation. Judo in Schools. Available online: https://schools.ijf.org/ (accessed on 20 November 2021).
5. Fukuda, D.H.; Stout, J.R.; Burris, P.M.; Fukuda, R.S. Judo for children and adolescents: Benefits of combat sports. *Strength Cond. J.* **2011**, *33*, 60–63. [CrossRef]
6. Kozdraś, G. Sztuka walki judo jako forma edukacji dla dzieci żyjących w społeczeństwach otwartych. *Ido Mov. Culture. J. Martial Arts Anthrop.* **2014**, *14*, 29–38. (In Polish)

7. Matsunami, M. Traditional Sport in Japan. In *The Palgrave Handbook of Leisure Theory*; Spracklen, K., Lashua, B., Sharpe, E., Swain, S., Eds.; Palgrave Macmillan: London, UK, 2017. [CrossRef]
8. Sikorski, W.; Błach, W. Judo for health. *J. Combat Sports Martial Arts* **2010**, *1*, 123–124.
9. Geertz, W.; Dechow, A.S.; Pohl, E.; Zyriax, B.C.; Ganschow, R.; Schulz, K.H. Physical and psychological well-being in overweight children participating in a long-term intervention based on judo practice. *Adv. Phys. Educ.* **2017**, *7*, 85–100. [CrossRef]
10. Gutierrez-Garcia, C.; Astrain, I.; Izquierdo, E.; Gomez-Alonso, M.T.; Yague, J.M. Effects of judo participation in children: A systematic review. *Ido Mov. Culture J. Martial Arts Anthrop.* **2018**, *18*, 63–73. [CrossRef]
11. Kano, J. *Kodokan Judo*; Kodansha International, Inc.: Tokyo, Japan, 2013.
12. De Crée, C. ShōnenJūdō-no-kata ["Forms of Jūdōfor Juveniles"]—An experimental Japanese teaching approach to Jūdō skill acquisition in children considered from a historic-pedagogical perspective—Part 1. *J. Combat Sports Martial Arts* **2012**, *4*, 95–111. [CrossRef]
13. Takahashi, M. *Mastering Judo*; Human Kinetics: Champaign, IL, USA, 2005; pp. 2–10.
14. Kostka, T.; Furgal, W.; Gawroński, W.; Bugajski, A.; Czamara, A.; Klukowski, K.; Krysztofiak, H.; Lewicki, R.; Szyguła, Z.; Tomaszewski, W.; et al. Recommendations of the Polish Society of Sports Medicine on age criteria while qualifying children and youth for participation in various sports. *Brit. J. Sport. Med.* **2011**, *46*, 159–162. [CrossRef] [PubMed]
15. Polish Judo Association. Sports Regulations. Available online: http://web.pzjudo.pl/sites/default/files/zalaczniki/2020/regulamin_sportowy_pzj_200303_0.pdf (accessed on 19 November 2021). (In Polish)
16. Walaszek, R.; Sterkowicz, S.; Chwala, W.; Sterkowicz-Przybycień, K.; Burdacka, M.; Burdacki, M.; Kurowski, P. Photogrammetric evaluation of body posture of 6-year-old boys training judo, in three repeated assessments. *ActaBioeng. Biomech.* **2019**, *21*, 149–157. [CrossRef]
17. Walaszek, R.; Sterkowicz, S.; Chwala, W.; Sterkowicz-Przybycień, K.; Walaszek, K.; Burdacki, M.; Kłys, A. Assessment of the impact of regular judo practice on body posture, balance, and lower limbs mechanical output in six-year-old boys. *J. Sports Med. Phys. Fit.* **2017**, *57*, 1579–1589. [CrossRef] [PubMed]
18. Demiral, S. LTAD model active beginning stage adaptation in judo basic education program (Ukemi, Tachiwaza&Newaza basic drills) for 4–6 aged kids. *J. Educ. Train. Stud.* **2018**, *6*, 1–6. [CrossRef]
19. Garcia, J.G.; Deval, V.C.; Sterkowicz, S.; Molina, R. A study of the difficulties involved in introducing young children to judo techniques: A proposed teaching programme. *Arch. Budo* **2009**, *5*, 121–126.
20. Neofit, A. Survey on training in judo for children of preschool age (4–6/7 years). *Ann. Dunarea JosUniv. Galati Fascicle* **2010**, *15*, 23–27.
21. Krstulović, S.; Maleš, B.; Žuvela, F.; Erceg, M.; Miletić, D. Judo, soccer and track-and-field differential effects on some anthropological characteristics in seven-year-old boys. *Kinesiology* **2010**, *42*, 56–64.
22. Djordjević, I.; Valková, H.; Nurkić, F.; Djordjević, S.; Dolga, M. Motor proficiency of preschool boys related to organized physical activity July. *J. Phys. Educ. Sport* **2021**, *21*, 2258–2265. [CrossRef]
23. Triki, M.; Rebai, H.; Aouichaoui, C.; Shamssain, M.; Masmoudi, K.; Fellmann, N.; Zouari, H.; Zouari, N.; Tabka, Z. Comparative study of bronchial hyperresponsiveness between football and judo groups in prepubertal boys. *Asian J. Sports Med.* **2015**, *6*, e24043. [CrossRef]
24. Ludyga, S.; Tränkner, S.; Gerber, M.; Pühse, U. Effects of judo on neurocognitive indices of response inhibition in preadolescent children. *Med. Sci. Sports Exerc.* **2021**, *53*, 1648–1655. [CrossRef] [PubMed]
25. Jankowska-Szymańska, A.; Mikołajczyk, E.; Wardzała, R. Arch of the foot and postural balance in young judokas and peers. *J. Pediatr. Orthop. B* **2015**, *24*, 456–460. [CrossRef]
26. Maslinski, J.; Witkowski, K.; Jatowtt, A.; Cieslinski, W.; Piepiora, P. Physical fitness 11–12 years boys who train judo and those who do not practise sport. *Arch. Budo Sci. Martial Art Extrem. Sport* **2015**, *11*, 41–46.
27. Van Kooten, G.C. Re-considering Long-Term Athlete Development on coach education: An illustration from judo. *Int. Sport Coach. J.* **2016**, *3*, 83–89. [CrossRef]
28. Protic-Gava, B.; Drid, P.; Krkeljas, Z. Effects of judo participation on anthropometric characteristics, motor abilities, and posture in young judo athletes. *Hum. Mov.* **2019**, *20*, 10–15. [CrossRef]
29. Yaneva, A. Research in judo learning level of 4 to 7 year old children. *Res. Kinesiol.* **2016**, *44*, 178–182.
30. Missawi, K.; Mohamed Zouch, M.; Chaari, H.; Chakroun, Y.; Tabka, Z.; Bouajina, E. Judo practice in early age promotes high level of bone mass acquisition of growing boys' skeleton. *J. Clin. Densitom.* **2018**, *21*, 420–428. [CrossRef] [PubMed]
31. Pereira, M.; Folle, A.; Nascimento Raquel, K.; Cirino, C.; Milan Fabricio, J.; Farias Gelcemar, O. Judo teaching through games: Systematic organisation according to the principles of complex games networks. *Ido Mov. Culture. J. Martial Arts Anthrop.* **2021**, *21*, 1–8. [CrossRef]
32. Lukanova, V. Research of the application of games in teaching judo to children from 7 to 10 years of age. *Trakia J. Sci.* **2019**, *17*, 797–801. [CrossRef]
33. Masenko, L. Discussion of the research results of judo games at the initial stage of long-termtraining. *Cent. Eur. J. Sport Sci. Med.* **2015**, *10*, 109–115.

34. Pocecco, E.; Ruedl, G.; Stankovic, N.; Sterkowicz, S.; Del Vec-chio, F.B.; Gutierrez-Garcia, C.; Rousseau, R.; Wolf, M.; Kopp, M.; Miarka, B.; et al. Injuries in judo: A systematic literature review including suggestions for prevention. *Brit. J. Sport. Med.* **2013**, *47*, 1139–1143. [CrossRef]
35. Demorest, R.A.; Koutures, C. The council on sports medicine and fitness. Youthparticipation and injury risk in martial arts. *Pediatrics* **2016**, *138*, e20163022. [CrossRef]
36. Smaruj, M.; Orkwiszewska, A.; Adam, M.; Jeżyk, D.; Kostrzewa, M.; Laskowski, R. Changes in anthropometric traits and body composition over a four-year period in elite female judoka athletes. *J. Hum. Kinet.* **2019**, *70*, 145–155. [CrossRef]
37. Kostrzewa, M.; Laskowski, R.; Wilk, M.; Błach, W.; Ignatjeva, A.; Nitychoruk, M. Significant predictors of sports performance in elite men judo athletes based on multidimensional regression models. *Int. J. Environ. Res. Public Health* **2020**, *17*, 8192. [CrossRef] [PubMed]

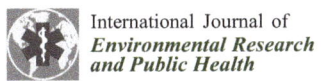

Article

The Effect of 6-Week Combined Balance and Plyometric Training on Dynamic Balance and Quickness Performance of Elite Badminton Players

Zepeng Lu [1,†], Limingfei Zhou [2,†], Wangcheng Gong [3], Samuel Chuang [4], Shixian Wang [5], Zhenxiang Guo [1,6], Dapeng Bao [1,*], Luyu Zhang [2] and Junhong Zhou [7]

[1] China Institute of Sport and Health Science, Beijing Sport University, Beijing 100084, China; luzepeng@bsu.edu.cn (Z.L.); guozhenxiang@nuaa.edu.cn (Z.G.)
[2] School of Strength and Conditioning Training, Beijing Sport University, Beijing 100084, China; zlmf@bsu.edu.cn (L.Z.); luyu_zhang@bsu.edu.cn (L.Z.)
[3] School of Physical Education, Jiujiang University, Jiujiang 332005, China; 6030107@jju.edu.cn
[4] Human Biology Major, University of California San Diego, San Diego, CA 92093, USA; smauelchuang2022@gmail.com
[5] Sports Coaching College, Beijing Sport University, Beijing 100084, China; 2020241004@bsu.edu.cn
[6] Department of Physical Education, Nanjing University of Aeronautics and Astronautics, Nanjing 210016, China
[7] Hebrew SeniorLife Hinda and Arthur Marcus Institute for Aging Research, Harvard Medical School, Boston, MA 02131, USA; junhongzhou@hsl.harvard.edu
* Correspondence: baodp@bsu.edu.cn
† These authors contributed equally to this work.

Citation: Lu, Z.; Zhou, L.; Gong, W.; Chuang, S.; Wang, S.; Guo, Z.; Bao, D.; Zhang, L.; Zhou, J. The Effect of 6-Week Combined Balance and Plyometric Training on Dynamic Balance and Quickness Performance of Elite Badminton Players. *Int. J. Environ. Res. Public Health* **2022**, *19*, 1605. https://doi.org/10.3390/ijerph19031605

Academic Editors: Tadeusz Ambrozy, Mariusz Ozimek, Andrzej Ostrowski, Henryk Duda and Michał Spieszny

Received: 28 December 2021
Accepted: 28 January 2022
Published: 30 January 2022

Publisher's Note: MDPI stays neutral with regard to jurisdictional claims in published maps and institutional affiliations.

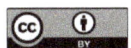

Copyright: © 2022 by the authors. Licensee MDPI, Basel, Switzerland. This article is an open access article distributed under the terms and conditions of the Creative Commons Attribution (CC BY) license (https://creativecommons.org/licenses/by/4.0/).

Abstract: The study aimed to investigate the effect of combined balance and plyometric training on dynamic balance and quickness performance of elite badminton athletes. Sixteen elite male badminton players volunteered to participate and were randomly assigned to a balance-plyometric group (PB: n = 8) and plyometric group (PT: n = 8). The PB group performed balance combined with plyometric training three times a week over 6 weeks (40 min of plyometrics and 20 min of balance training); while the PT group undertook only plyometric training for the same period (3–4 sets × 8–12 reps for each exercise). Both groups were given the same technical training (badminton techniques for 6 days a week). The dynamic stability and quick movement ability were assessed at baseline and after the intervention by measuring the performance of dynamic posture stability test (*DPSI* and COP), T-running test and hexagon jump test. The results showed that compared to PT, PB induced significantly greater improvements in F-DPSI, L-DPSI (p = 0.003, 0.025, respectively), F-COP$_{AP}$, F-COP$_{ML}$, F-COP$_{PL}$, L-COP$_{PL}$ (p = 0.024, 0.002, 0.029, 0.043, respectively), T-running test and hexagon jump test ($p < 0.001$). The change in L-DPSI, L-COP$_{AP}$, L-COP$_{ML}$ did not differ between PB and PT ($p > 0.907$). The findings suggest that combined training holds great promise of improving the dynamic balance and quickness performance in elite badminton athletes.

Keywords: balance training; plyometrics training; dynamic balance; quickness; elite badminton player

1. Introduction

Badminton is one of the fastest racket sports with short intervals and high intensity [1,2]. The badminton players need to make decisions based upon the prediction of the opponent's moving direction and the flight trajectory of the badminton in a very short time [3]. This process is closely associated with the capacity of dynamic balance control, including lunges, landing stability and quick adjustment such as acceleration, deceleration, change of direction (COD) of the body trunk [4,5]. The ability to maintain dynamic balance has been linked to increased speed of COD [6], better control of jumping and running to smash, and making the lunges [7]. Therefore, strategies aiming to improve dynamic balance and quickness hold great promise to improve the match performance of badminton players.

One such strategy is plyometric training (PT), consisting of the motions related to muscle eccentric-concentric contraction cycle, also known as the stretch-shortening cycle (SSC) [8,9] (e.g., depth jump and continuous jump [10,11]). PT is widely used in the training of athletes, it can improve jump performance capabilities and strength. Several studies have used it and examined its effects on strength [12], running economy [10], agility [13] and sprint ability [8]. Recent studies have shown that compared to traditional resistance training (RT), PT can induce comparable or even better effects on enhancing the performance of athletes [14–17] by improving their balance, power, agility and strength. For example, Alikhani et al. [18] observed that a six-week PT could significantly improve dynamic balance and knee proprioception in female badminton players, which can ultimately prevent the injury of participants. Bozdogan et al. [19] also presented that agility and jumping abilities in male badminton athletes were significantly improved after eight-week PT.

More recently, the combined intervention has been developed by implementing two types of training programs at the same time. The combined training can simultaneously improve multiple underlying domains contributing to dynamic balance and quickness, thus inducing greater benefits for the performance compared to the intervention using only one type of training. Studies demonstrated that combined training can significantly improve the strength, balance, and COD ability of basketball and football players [20,21] compared to the intervention using only one type of training. Guo et al., for example, implemented the combined training of balance and PT (PB) in badminton players. This PB training consisted of depth jump and continuous jump with balance exercises on unstable platforms. The results of that study showed that compared to PT only, PB can significantly improve COD performance [22]. However, the effects of this type of combined training of balance and PT on the dynamic balance and quickness in badminton players are not clear.

We here thus in a pilot randomized controlled study aimed to examine the effects of a 6-week combined training on dynamic balance and quickness performance in elite badminton players. Our hypothesis is that a combined training protocol would induce a greater increase in parameters pertaining to dynamic balance and quickness compared to plyometric training.

2. Materials and Methods

2.1. Participants

Sixteen badminton players were recruited (Table 1). The inclusion criteria were: (1) Elite players who had played the quarterfinalists of national youth games, the finals at the provincial games, or higher-level games; (2) The dominant arm or leg is right side; (3) the ability to complete dynamic balance test and plyometric training; and (4) willing to complete the six-week intervention and the tests. The exclusion criteria were: Participants had ACL, hamstring, meniscus, ankle, or any other lower-extremity injuries that are associated with diminished dynamic balance during the last three years. The study protocol was approved by the Research Ethics Committee of Beijing Sport University (Approval number: 2020008H), and all procedures were conducted in accordance with the Declaration of Helsinki. Before the experiment, participants were informed of the benefits and potential risks related to the study, and all signed the informed consent form.

Table 1. The demographic characteristics of the participants.

	Age (Years)	Height (cm)	Weight (kg)	Training Experience (Years)
PB (n = 8)	20.50 ± 1.07	177.75 ± 5.06	68.13 ± 7.22	11.38 ± 1.41
PT (n = 8)	19.13 ± 2.23	179.13 ± 6.06	69.88 ± 8.94	10.63 ± 1.06

No significant difference in the demographic characteristics between PB group and PT group ($p > 0.066$).

2.2. Study Protocol

Sixteen players volunteered for random allocation to combined balance and plyometric training group (PB, n = 8) or a plyometric group (PT, n = 8). All participants from the PB and PT groups conducted the training program three times per week with 24–48 h of recovery between each training session. The PB group practiced a balance training program (Table S1) on the unstable conditions, and the PT group practiced on the floor with the same training plan. Then PB group and PT group conducted the same plyometric training program (Table S2). Before the formal training and test, all participants completed a 2-week practice (3 times/week) to be familiar with balance exercises, plyometric exercises and the procedure of the test. During this period, participants received proper skill instructions from a strength and conditioning coach. All these training programs have been validated and used to help dynamic balance and quickness performance in athletes. In our previous study, we used the same training protocol in badminton athletes [22]. All the protocols were supervised by the study personnel with experience in strength and conditioning training.

2.3. The Assessment of Dynamic Balance and Quickness

The dynamic balance and quickness were assessed at baseline and within three days after the last session of the 6-week training. The tests consisted of Dynamic Posture Stability Test, Modified *t*-test, and Hexagon test. All tests were completed within a day. Before each testing session, participants finished warm-up, including 5-min dynamic stretch, 8-min movement integration, and 2-min neural activation. A 5–10-min rest was given between each test. Each type of test was conducted at the same time and place across different visits, and the participants were asked to wear the same sporting shoes they preferred through all the assessments. The players maintained their normal routine of diet and were prohibited from consuming beverages containing caffeine or alcohol during the whole period. The detailed assessments were as follow:

Dynamic Posture Stability Test

The test was used to assess the dynamic balance of players by dynamic posture stability index and center of pressure [23]. Participants stood on an in-ground force plate (Kistler 9281CA, KISTLER, Winterthur, Switzerland, 1000 Hz) and then jumped front or laterad with a dominant leg standing for 10 s. The distance between the jumping line and the center of the force plate was 40% of the players' height (cm) [23,24]. The fence was placed at the midpoint of the connection between those. The fence height in the jumping front was 30 cm, and that in jumping laterad was 15 cm. All players were asked to complete two kinds of jumps three times, and the average would be taken for data analysis. Matlab software (r2014b, MathWorks, Natick, Massachusetts, USA) was used to calculate dynamic postural stability index (*DPSI*) and center of pressure (COP). The time-series data of ground reaction force (GRF) and center of pressure (COP) were collected within 10 s after players landed on the force plate with a single leg. All data were smoothed through low-pass filtering, and the truncation frequency was set to 13.33 Hz.

DPSI was calculated from the GRF curve within 3 s after touchdown (the time when the GRF value exceeded 5% of body weight) [25]. Where BW is the body weight, GRF_x, GRF_y, and GRF_z are the back and forth, left and right, vertical ground reaction forces. The dynamic posture stability indexes of forward jump (DF-DPSI) and lateral jump (DL-DPSI).

$$DPSI = \frac{\left(\frac{\sqrt{\sum(0-GRF_x)^2 + \sum(0-GRF_y)^2 + \sum(BW-GRF_z)^2}}{\text{number of data points}}\right)}{BW} \quad (1)$$

COP was calculated from the time series within 10 s after landing, and the back and forth displacement difference (COP_{AP}), left-right displacement difference (COP_{ML}) and total displacement distance (COP_{PL}) of forwarding jump (DF) and lateral jump (DL) were calculated [14]. x_t and y_t are the back and forth, left and right displacements at t seconds and the value of t is 1–10 s.

$$COP_{AP} = \sum_{1}^{10}(x_t - \bar{x})^2 \qquad (2)$$

$$COP_{ML} = \sum_{1}^{10}(y_t - \bar{y})^2 \qquad (3)$$

$$COP_{PL} = \sum_{0}^{9}\sqrt{(x_{t+1} - x_t)^2 + (y_{t+1} - y_t)^2} \qquad (4)$$

2.4. Modified t-Test

t-test was widely used for evaluating the quickness of athletes in various sports [26]. To fit the feature of badminton specifically, researchers adjusted the distance to be similar to the badminton court, as shown in Figure S1. Cone bucket A was placed at the starting line, and then cone bucket B was set at 6 m away from A. Cone buckets C and D were placed at 3 m to B side to side. Smart Speed device (Fusion Sport, Coopers Plains, Australia) was set on A. After hearing the order "Ready, go", the players started to forward sprint from A to B with left-hand touching bucket B. Then they made side shuffling from B to C with left-hand touching bucket C. Upon arrival, they did the same side shuffling to D with right-hand touching and made the same shuffling to B. Finally, the players did backpedal to A. Each participant had to perform three times, and the best of results was the final valid score.

2.5. Hexagon Test

The test was applied to assess COD ability for badminton and was verified as an effective method to evaluate the on-court performance of players [27,28]. The participants stood 50 cm behind the No. 1 side of the hexagon (Figure S2), and after hearing the command of "Ready, go", they quickly completed jumping in and out of the line with a circle clockwise from 1 to 6. Smart speed devices would be timed automatically at the beginning and end of the test, with a total of three times, of which the shortest time was recorded for analysis. There was a 2-min passive rest between the two tests.

2.6. Statistical Analysis

Experimental data were processed by IBM SPSS statistical software package (version 25.0, IBM, Chicago, IL, USA). All data were presented as means and SD.

To examine the effects of the combined training on the performance of dynamic balance ability, *t*-test and Hexagon test, we performed two-way repeated-measure ANOVA (group × time), and the Greenhouse-Geisser adjustment was applied. The dependent variable for each model was *DPSI* (front and lateral), COP (AP, ML, PL), the time of *t*-test and Hexagon test. The model effects were group, time and their interaction. When a significant model effect was observed, LSD post-hoc correction was performed to identify significant pairwise differences. Partial η^2 was used to assess the effects size where the significance was observed. The level of significance was set at $p < 0.05$ for all tests.

3. Results

3.1. Dynamic Balance Ability

3.1.1. Dynamic Posture Stability Index

The results of ANOVA models on F-DPSI and L-DPSI showed the significant effects of time (F-DPSI: $p < 0.001$; L-DPSI: $p < 0.001$), that is, compared to baseline, participants in both groups had significantly lower F-DPSI and L-DPSI after the intervention. A significant interaction between group and time (F-DPSI: $p = 0.003$; L-DPSI: $p = 0.025$) was also observed (Table 2). The post-hoc analysis revealed that the participants who received PB had significantly lower F-DPSI and L-DPSI as compared to their baseline performance and those who received PT. [$F_{(1,28)} = 29.661$, $p < 0.001$, partial $\eta^2 = 0.514$]. No significant effects of group were observed (F-DPSI: $p = 0.418$; D-DPSI: $p = 0.593$).

Table 2. The assessment results for PB group and PT group before and after the 6-week training.

		PB (N = 8)			PT (N = 8)		
		Pre	Post	Partial η^2	Pre	Post	Partial η^2
Dynamic balance	F-DPSI	0.386 ± 0.002	0.381 ± 0.003 *#	0.653	0.387 ± 0.002	0.384 ± 0.001 *	0.207
	L-DPSI	0.386 ± 0.003	0.378 ± 0.002 *	0.543	0.384 ± 0.004	0.381 ± 0.003 *	0.175
	F-COP$_{AP}$ (cm)	90.28 ± 16.39	72.20 ± 10.81 *#	0.233	95.15 ± 12.65	88.27 ± 8.28	0.042
	F-COP$_{ML}$ (cm)	72.97 ± 11.99	60.55 ± 6.23 *#	0.192	81.90 ± 10.30	74.81 ± 9.08	0.072
	F-COP$_{PL}$ (cm)	131.60 ± 22.10	109.70 ± 18.56 *#	0.187	137.27 ± 15.39	132.19 ± 11.17	0.012
	L-COP$_{AP}$ (cm)	79.29 ± 12.35	63.37 ± 9.83 *#	0.236	82.44 ± 10.31	74.90 ± 10.68	0.065
	L-COP$_{ML}$ (cm)	90.71 ± 10.32	81.37 ± 10.18 *	0.102	93.64 ± 11.66	85.17 ± 9.65	0.085
	L-COP$_{PL}$ (cm)	131.25 ± 19.38	110.05 ± 16.89 *	0.176	139.82 ± 14.69	127.44 ± 18.14	0.068
Quickness performance	Hexagon test (s)	3.83 ± 0.32	2.95 ± 0.14 *#	0.592	3.95 ± 0.29	3.25 ± 0.33 *	0.472
	t-test (s)	7.38 ± 0.19	6.77 ± 0.11 *#	0.637	7.39 ± 0.24	6.96 ± 0.13 *	0.455

Note: * Statistically significant difference between pre- and post-test, $p < 0.05$. # Statistically significant difference between PB group and PT group, $p < 0.05$. F, forward jump; L, lateral jump; COP, center of pressure.

3.1.2. Center of Pressure

Significant effects of time and group, but non-significant interaction between group and time on F-COP$_{AP}$ [time: $p = 0.008$; group: $p = 0.024$], F-COP$_{ML}$ [time: $p = 0.008$ respectively; group: $p = 0.002$], F-COP$_{PL}$ [time: $p = 0.036$; group: $p = 0.029$] and L-COP$_{PL}$ [time: $p = 0.01$; group: $p = 0.043$] were observed. Specifically, compared to baseline, the F-COP$_{AP}$, F-COP$_{ML}$, F-COP$_{PL}$, and L-COP$_{PL}$ were significantly lower after the intervention, and these outcomes in PT group were significantly greater than those in PB group. Additionally, significant effects of time (L-COP$_{AP}$: $p = 0.005$; L-COP$_{ML}$: $p = 0.023$), but no significant interaction between group and time (L-COP$_{AP}$: $p = 0.283$; L-COP$_{ML}$: $p = 0.907$) on L-COP$_{AP}$ and L-COP$_{ML}$ were observed.

3.2. Quickness Performance

Significant effects of time (*t* test: $p < 0.001$; hexagon test: $p < 0.001$) were observed on the performance of *t* test and hexagon test, while only trends toward significance were presented for the effects of group (*t* test: $p = 0.106$; hexagon test: $p = 0.052$) and the interaction between group and time (*t* test: $p < 0.001$; hexagon test: $p < 0.001$). Specifically, the post-hoc analysis revealed that for both PB and PT group, *t*-test and hexagon test were significantly greater than baseline; and participants who received PB tend to have significant lower *t*-test and hexagon as compared to their baseline performance and those who received PT [*t*-test: $F_{(1,28)} = 5.139$, $p = 0.031$, partial $\eta^2 = 0.155$; hexagon test: $F_{(1,28)} = 4.811$, $p = 0.037$, partial $\eta^2 = 0.147$].

4. Discussion

The results of this pilot study demonstrated that dynamic balance and quickness performance in elite badminton athletes were significantly improved after combined training as compared to those who received PT only, suggesting combined training is thus a promising strategy to improve the functionality of elite badminton athletes and potentially help their on-court performance.

It is observed that compared to the intervention using plyometric training only, 6-week combined training of balance and plyometric training can significantly improve the ability to control dynamic balance and quickness performance in elite professional athletes of badminton as assessed by using the task of dynamic balance ability, *t*-test, and Hexagon test. The performance of *DPSI* and COP reflects the ability of players to maintain landing stability and balance [25,29]. The traditional PT oftentimes focuses only on the musculoskeletal function, while the combined training can simultaneously target multiple aspects pertaining to dynamic balance, such as the integration of the visual, vestibular information and the coordination across those systems [30]. This can thus benefit the capacity of postural control system to appropriately reweight and utilize different types of sensory inputs (e.g., visual, proprioceptive) when receiving the challenges or perturbations. For example, Nepocatych et al. [31] observed that balance training had the potential to induce adaptive responses in the neuromuscular system that enhances postural control, the balance of women, as well as improvement of COP to prevent chronic ankle instability effectively. Additionally, previous studies demonstrated that balance training would lead to spinal reflex during postural movement, which results in less destabilizing movement [32]. Therefore, the combined training is a strategy that would be more appropriate for dynamic balance by simultaneously enhancing multiple underlying elements of dynamic balance control.

Quickness is another important factor for outstanding performance in badminton competitions [33]. Quickness not only requires the power of lower limbs to change body direction but also has good dynamic balance ability to control body posture so as to overcome the inertial effect caused by acceleration and deceleration braking in the process of changing direction [24]. The rounds of multiple rallies occur more frequently in the badminton match [34]. Players thus need to judge the direction and trajectory of the ball quickly before hitting the ball, then quickly change the direction of body, and perform acceleration and deceleration of the movement [2]. Previous studies have shown that combined training improves the performance of change of direction in college-level badminton players [22], as well as in other participant cohorts [20,35,36]. For example, eight weeks of combined training induces significantly greater improvements in the performance of Illinois change of direction in woman basketball players compared to PT intervention [37]. Here we further demonstrate that the combined training can induce significantly greater benefits for quickness in elite badminton players compared to traditional PT. Specifically, the balance training can enhance the adaptive capacity for the rate of force development [38], and increase muscle activation during the landing of jump procedure [39], which might optimize musculotendinous and joint stiffness. The musculotendinous and joint stiffness are critical to the smoothness of action, one critical aspect of quickness [40]. Therefore, the combined training could be considered as a training program in increasing both the performance of dynamic balance and quickness. There are some limitations in this study. First, the sample size of 16 people is relatively small as we focused on only elite athletes, future studies with a larger sample size on other cohorts (e.g., older adults) are thus highly demanded. Second, this study implemented a 6-week intervention with only one follow-up assessment. The optimal intervention intensity and the dose-response relationship between the performance and the "dose" of the intervention are still unknown. Future studies with multiple visits during and after the intervention and longer-term follow-up period are thus needed to determine how long the effects of combined training can sustain and the appropriate intensity, the number of sessions of the combined training that can maximize the benefits of the combined training. This will ultimately help the optimized design of the PB intervention. Additionally, we only included one control group that received PT training. It is worthwhile to include a blank control group so that the elevated benefits from the control group to single-type training to PB can be examined. Future studies implementing more sophisticated measurements of the characteristics of the underlying musculoskeletal system and sensory perception are needed to explore the mechanism through which combined training can induce greater benefits for dynamic balance and quickness compared to single-type training.

5. Conclusions

This pilot study showed that balance training combined with plyometric training can strengthen dynamic balance ability and improve the quickness performance of male elite badminton players. The knowledge obtained from this study will ultimately help inform the design of future larger-scale studies to confirm the findings in this study.

Supplementary Materials: The following supporting information can be downloaded at: https://www.mdpi.com/article/10.3390/ijerph19031605/s1, Figure S1: Modified *t*-test; Figure S2: Hexagon test; Table S1: The balance training program for balance-plyometric (PB) (combined training) group and Table S2: The plyometric training (PT) program for PB and plyometric training group.

Author Contributions: Conceptualization, Z.L., L.Z. (Limingfei Zhou) and D.B.; methodology, Z.L., L.Z. (Limingfei Zhou), W.G. and D.B.; software, L.Z. (Limingfei Zhou) and J.Z.; validation, Z.L., L.Z. (Limingfei Zhou) and S.W.; formal analysis, L.Z. (Limingfei Zhou) and J.Z.; investigation, L.Z. (Limingfei Zhou) and W.G.; resources, Z.L., Z.G. and D.B.; data curation, Z.L. and J.Z.; writing—original draft preparation, Z.L. and W.G.; writing—review and editing, L.Z. (Limingfei Zhou), S.C. and J.Z.; visualization, Z.L. and S.C.; supervision, D.B. and L.Z. (Luyu Zhang); project administration, D.B.; funding acquisition, D.B. and L.Z. (Luyu Zhang). All authors have read and agreed to the published version of the manuscript.

Funding: This research received no external funding.

Institutional Review Board Statement: The study was conducted according to the guidelines of the Declaration of Helsinki, and approved by the Ethics Committee of Beijing Sport University (2020008H, 17 January 2020).

Informed Consent Statement: Informed consent was obtained from all subjects involved in the study.

Conflicts of Interest: The authors declare no conflict of interest.

References

1. Phomsoupha, M.; Laffaye, G. The science of badminton: Game characteristics, anthropometry, physiology, visual fitness and biomechanics. *Sports Med.* **2015**, *45*, 473–495. [CrossRef] [PubMed]
2. Cabello Manrique, D.; González-Badillo, J.J. Analysis of the characteristics of competitive badminton. *Br. J. Sports Med.* **2003**, *37*, 62–66. [CrossRef] [PubMed]
3. Alam, F.; Chowdhury, H.; Theppadungporn, C.; Subic, A.; Khan, M. Aerodynamic properties of badminton shuttlecock. *Int. J. Mech. Mater. Eng.* **2009**, *4*, 266–272.
4. Shariff, A.H.; George, J.; Ramlan, A.A. Musculoskeletal injuries among malaysian badminton players. *Singap. Med. J.* **2009**, *50*, 1095–1097.
5. Hong, Y.; Wang, S.J.; Lam, W.K.; Cheung, J.T.M. Kinetics of badminton lunges in four directions. *J. Appl. Biomech.* **2014**, *30*, 113–118. [CrossRef] [PubMed]
6. Rouissi, M.; Haddad, M.; Bragazzi, N.L.; Owen, A.L.; Moalla, W.; Chtara, M.; Chamari, K. Implication of dynamic balance in change of direction performance in young elite soccer players is angle dependent. *J. Sports Med. Phys. Fit.* **2018**, *58*, 442–449. [CrossRef] [PubMed]
7. Hrysomallis, C. Relationship between balance ability, training and sports injury risk. *Sports Med.* **2007**, *37*, 547–556. [CrossRef]
8. Markovic, G.; Mikulic, P. Neuro-musculoskeletal and performance adaptations to lower-extremity plyometric training. *Sports Med.* **2010**, *40*, 859–895. [CrossRef]
9. Taube, W.; Leukel, C.; Gollhofer, A. How neurons make us jump: The neural control of stretch-shortening cycle movements. *Exerc. Sport Sci. Rev.* **2012**, *40*, 106–115. [CrossRef]
10. Holcomb, W.R.; Lander, J.E.; Rutland, R.M.; Wilson, G.D. The effectiveness of a modified plyometric program on power and the vertical jump. *J. Strength Cond. Res.* **1996**, *10*, 89–92.
11. Stojanović, E.; Ristić, V.; McMaster, D.T.; Milanović, Z. Effect of plyometric training on vertical jump performance in female athletes: A systematic review and meta-analysis. *Sports Med.* **2017**, *47*, 975–986. [CrossRef] [PubMed]
12. Asadi, A. Effects of six weeks depth jump and countermovement jump training on agility performance. *Sport Sci.* **2012**, *5*, 67–70.
13. De Villarreal, E.S.S.; González-Badillo, J.J.; Izquierdo, M. Low and moderate plyometric training frequency produces greater jumping and sprinting gains compared with high frequency. *J. Strength Cond. Res.* **2008**, *22*, 715–725. [CrossRef] [PubMed]
14. Ziv, G.; Lidor, R. Vertical jump in female and male basketball players–a review of observational and experimental studies. *J. Sci. Med. Sport* **2010**, *13*, 332–339. [CrossRef]
15. Asadi, A.; Arazi, H.; Young, W.B.; Sáez de Villarreal, E. The effects of plyometric training on change-of-direction ability: A meta-analysis. *Int. J. Sports Physiol. Perform.* **2016**, *11*, 563–573. [CrossRef]
16. Fischetti, F.; Vilardi, A.; Cataldi, S.; Greco, G. Effects of plyometric training program on speed and explosive strength of lower limbs in young athletes. *J. Phys. Educ. Sport* **2018**, *18*, 2476–2482.
17. Bouguezzi, R.; Chaabene, H.; Negra, Y.; Moran, J.; Sammoud, S.; Ramirez-Campillo, R.; Granacher, U.; Hachana, Y. Effects of jump exercises with and without stretch-shortening cycle actions on components of physical fitness in prepubertal male soccer players. *Sport Sci. Health* **2020**, *16*, 297–304. [CrossRef]

18. Alikhani, R.; Shahrjerdi, S.; Golpaigany, M.; Kazemi, M. The effect of a six-week plyometric training on dynamic balance and knee proprioception in female badminton players. *J. Can. Chiropr. Assoc.* **2019**, *63*, 144–153.
19. Bozdoğan, T.K.; Kizilet, A. The effect of coordination and plyometric exercises on agility, jumping and endurance ability in badminton players. *Int. J. Sport Exerc. Train. Sci.* **2017**, *3*, 178–187. [CrossRef]
20. Makhlouf, I.; Chaouachi, A.; Chaouachi, M.; Ben Othman, A.; Granacher, U.; Behm, D.G. Combination of agility and plyometric training provides similar training benefits as combined balance and plyometric training in young soccer players. *Front. Physiol.* **2018**, *9*, 1611. [CrossRef]
21. Muehlbauer, T.; Wagner, V.; Brueckner, D.; Schedler, S.; Schwiertz, G.; Kiss, R.; Hagen, M. Effects of a blocked versus an alternated sequence of balance and plyometric training on physical performance in youth soccer players. *BMC Sports Sci. Med. Rehabil.* **2019**, *11*, 18. [CrossRef] [PubMed]
22. Guo, Z.; Huang, Y.; Zhou, Z.; Leng, B.; Gong, W.; Cui, Y.; Bao, D. The effect of 6-week combined balance and plyometric training on change of direction performance of elite badminton players. *Front. Psychol.* **2021**, *12*, 684964. [CrossRef] [PubMed]
23. Sell, T.C. An examination, correlation, and comparison of static and dynamic measures of postural stability in healthy, physically active adults. *Phys. Ther. Sport* **2012**, *13*, 80–86. [CrossRef] [PubMed]
24. Bourgeois, F.; McGuigan, M.; Gill, N.; Gamble, G. Physical characteristics and performance in change of direction tasks: A brief review and training considerations. *J. Aust. Strength Cond.* **2017**, *25*, 104–117.
25. Wikstrom, E.A.; Tillman, M.D.; Smith, A.N.; Borsa, P.A. A new force-plate technology measure of dynamic postural stability: The dynamic postural stability index. *J. Athl. Train.* **2005**, *40*, 305. [PubMed]
26. Reiman, M.P.; Manske, R.C. *Functional Testing in Human Performance*; Human Kinetics: Champaign, IL, USA, 2009.
27. Jeyaraman, R.; District, E.; Nadu, T. Prediction of playing ability in badminton from selected anthropometrical physical and physiological characteristics among inter collegiate players. *Int. J. Adv. Innov. Res.* **2012**, *2*, 11.
28. Wong, T.K.K.; Ma, A.W.W.; Liu, K.P.Y.; Chung, L.M.Y.; Bae, Y.-H.; Fong, S.S.M.; Ganesan, B.; Wang, H.-K. Balance control, agility, eye-hand coordination, and sport performance of amateur badminton players: A cross-sectional study. *Medicine* **2019**, *98*, e14134. [CrossRef]
29. Pau, M.; Porta, M.; Arippa, F.; Pilloni, G.; Sorrentino, M.; Carta, M.; Mura, M.; Leban, B. Dynamic postural stability, is associated with competitive level, in youth league soccer players. *Phys. Sport* **2019**, *35*, 36–41. [CrossRef]
30. Wrisley, D.M.; Stephens, M.J. The effects of rotational platform training on balance and adls. *Annu. Int. Conf. IEEE Eng. Med. Biol. Soc.* **2011**, *2011*, 3529–3532.
31. Nepocatych, S.; Ketcham, C.J.; Vallabhajosula, S.; Balilionis, G. The effects of unstable surface balance training on postural sway, stability, functional ability and flexibility in women. *J. Sports Med. Phys. Fit.* **2018**, *58*, 27–34. [CrossRef]
32. Ashton-Miller, J.A.; Wojtys, E.M.; Huston, L.J.; Fry-Welch, D. Can proprioception really be improved by exercises? *Knee Surg. Sports Traumatol. Arthrosc.* **2001**, *9*, 128–136. [CrossRef] [PubMed]
33. Singh, J.; Raza, S.; Mohammad, A. Physical characteristics and level of performance in badminton: A relationship study. *J. Educ. Pract.* **2011**, *2*, 6–9.
34. Gomez, M.-Á.; Rivas, F.; Connor, J.D.; Leicht, A.S. Performance differences of temporal parameters and point outcome between elite men's and women's badminton players according to match-related contexts. *Int. J. Environ. Res. Public Health* **2019**, *16*, 4057. [CrossRef] [PubMed]
35. Chaouachi, A.; Othman, A.B.; Hammami, R.; Drinkwater, E.J.; Behm, D.G. The combination of plyometric and balance training improves sprint and shuttle run performances more often than plyometric-only training with children. *J. Strength Cond. Res.* **2014**, *28*, 401–412. [CrossRef] [PubMed]
36. Chaouachi, M.; Granacher, U.; Makhlouf, I.; Hammami, R.; Behm, D.G.; Chaouachi, A. Within session sequence of balance and plyometric exercises does not affect training adaptations with youth soccer athletes. *J. Sports Sci. Med.* **2017**, *16*, 125–136. [PubMed]
37. Bouteraa, I.; Negra, Y.; Shephard, R.J.; Chelly, M.S. Effects of combined balance and plyometric training on athletic performance in female basketball players. *J. Strength Cond. Res.* **2020**, *34*, 1967–1973. [CrossRef] [PubMed]
38. Hrysomallis, C. Balance ability and athletic performance. *Sports Med.* **2011**, *41*, 221–232. [CrossRef]
39. Kean, C.O.; Behm, D.G.; Young, W.B. Fixed foot balance training increases rectus femoris activation during landing and jump height in recreationally active women. *J. Sports Sci. Med.* **2006**, *5*, 138–148.
40. Sekulic, D.; Spasic, M.; Mirkov, D.; Cavar, M.; Sattler, T. Gender-specific influences of balance, speed, and power on agility performance. *J. Strength Cond. Res.* **2013**, *27*, 802–811. [CrossRef]

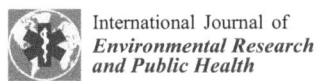

Article

Motor Learning of Complex Tasks with Augmented Feedback: Modality-Dependent Effectiveness

Jarosław Jaszczur-Nowicki [1], Oscar Romero-Ramos [2], Łukasz Rydzik [3,*], Tadeusz Ambroży [3], Michał Biegajło [4], Marta Nogal [4], Waldemar Wiśniowski [4], Dariusz Kruczkowski [5], Iwona Łuszczewska-Sierakowska [6] and Tomasz Niźnikowski [4,*]

[1] Department of Tourism, Recreation and Ecology, University of Warmia and Mazury in Olsztyn, 10-719 Olsztyn, Poland; j.jaszczur-nowicki@uwm.edu.pl
[2] Department of Didactics of Languages, Arts and Sports, University of Malaga, 4, 29017 Málaga, Spain; oromero@uma.es
[3] Institute of Sports Sciences, University of Physical Education, 31-571 Krakow, Poland; tadek@ambrozy.pl
[4] Faculty of Physical Education and Health, Józef Piłsudski University of Physical Education, 21-500 Biala Podlaska, Poland; michal.biegajlo@awf.edu.pl (M.B.); marta.nogal@awf.edu.pl (M.N.); waldemar.wisniowski@awf.edu.pl (W.W.)
[5] Faculty of Health Sciences, Elbląg University of the Humanities and Economics, 82-300 Elbląg, Poland; dyrektor@olimpijczyk.gda.pl
[6] Department of Human Anatomy, Medical University of Lublin, 20-090 Lublin, Poland; iwona.ikona@gmail.com
* Correspondence: lukasz.gne@op.pl (Ł.R.); tomasz.niznikowski@awf.edu.pl (T.N.)

Abstract: Background: This paper aims to evaluate the effectiveness of feedback modalities in the motor learning of complex tasks. Methods: This study examined sixty-one male university students randomised to three groups: group Verbal (VER) = 20 (body height 178.6 ± 4.3 cm, body mass 81.3 ± 3.7 kg, age 20.3 ± 1.2 years), group Visual (VIS) = 21 (body height 179 ± 4.6 cm, body mass 82 ± 3.4 kg, age 20.3 ± 1.2 years), and group Verbal–Visual (VER&VIS) = 20 (body height 178.6 ± 4.3 cm, body mass 81.3 ± 3.7 kg, age 20.3 ± 1.2 years). The duration of the experiment was 6 months. Training sessions were performed three times per week (on Mondays, Wednesdays, and Fridays). The participants were instructed to perform a vertical jump with an arm swing (with forward and upward motion). During the jump, the participants pulled their knees up to their chests and grabbed their lower legs. The jump was completed with a half-squat landing, with arms positioned sideward. The jumping performance was rated by three gymnastic judges on a scale from 1 to 10. Results: A Tukey post hoc test revealed that in the post-test, a significant difference in the quality of performance was found between the Verbal group concerning errors combined with visual feedback on how to correct them (VER&VIS), the Verbal group concerning errors (VER), and the Visual group with visual feedback on the correctness of task performance (VIS). The ratings observed in the post-test were significantly higher in group VER&VIS than in groups VER and VIS (9%; $p < 0.01$ and 15%; $p < 0.001$, respectively). All judges' ratings observed in group VER&VIS and VIS decreased insignificantly, but in group VER the ratings improved insignificantly. Conclusion: Providing verbal feedback combined with visual feedback on how to correct errors made in performing vertical jumps proved more effective than the provision of verbal feedback only or visual feedback only.

Keywords: training sessions; verbal; visual; verbal–visual feedback; vertical jump; complex task

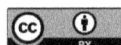

1. Introduction

Numerous researchers have attempted to determine how the process of learning motor tasks is affected by different variables, such as the type of feedback given to the learner (time, type, frequency) [1,2], training organisation (task complexity, context effects) [3,4], training type (physical, mental) and different versions of feedback (verbal, kinaesthetic, visual) [5–9].

So far, simple motor tasks that can be learnt without needing numerous attempts have been used in these studies [3,4]. Numerous advantages of implementing simple tasks (objectivity of measuring effects and time effectiveness) have been emphasised [5,6]. PE teachers, coaches, and physiotherapists should attempt to understand the general guidelines for learning complex motor tasks to improve the breadth of evidence-based practical tips they give during PE lessons or training. This can be accomplished through research using complex motor tasks that are more demanding for learners in terms of cognition and fitness [1,10–16].

In studies on observational learning, it was noted that video demonstration did not lead to an improvement in learning outcomes if it was not combined with verbal instruction. This phenomenon mainly relates to complex motor tasks [17]. Researchers claim that in order to enhance the effects of video demonstration, it needs to be combined with verbal feedback [18,19] or, additionally, light reflective markers or a model with light reflective markers on the most important body segments should be used. Hebert and Landin [20] believe that providing visual feedback combined with verbal feedback makes it possible to draw learners' attention to key elements of a motor task. According to Tzetzis et al. [21], the effectiveness of video demonstration depends on the complexity of a task. When examining the performance of complex motor tasks, Sadowski, Mastalerz, and Niźnikowski [22] noted that giving detailed feedback on key technical elements may exert a more beneficial influence on the process of learning than giving 100% feedback on all task-related errors. The authors claim that more experienced athletes may also make use of intrinsic feedback and in this way they can achieve their goal. In the case of learning complex tasks, determining and providing bandwidth feedback may be more beneficial for experienced learners who possess certain motor skills.

Information regarding effective feedback is particularly important both for PE teachers and coaches [23]. In their study, Nogal and Niźnikowski [16] confirmed that well-adjusted feedback was a key factor in learning complex motor tasks. Lee et al. [24] stated that positive verbal feedback is useful in non-specific tasks. Kernodle and Carlton [25] pointed out providing that verbal feedback on errors and on how to correct them is particularly helpful for beginners who, when given this type of information, can not only improve their skills but also gain self-confidence. Similarly, Smith and Davies [26] noted that receiving feedback on errors and on how to correct them may exert a considerable influence on athletes' mentality and self-confidence.

Coaches, instructors, PE teachers, and physiotherapists ought to know if the effectiveness of learning new motor tasks will increase when the learner practises in conditions that require extra cognitive effort and activity connected with processing information through delaying feedback, limiting cues, or accepting some errors.

The aim of this study is to determine in what way verbal, visual, and verbal–visual feedback influences the effectiveness of learning identical motor tasks. If this problem is not solved, it will not be possible to identify effective rules for learning tasks with different structures of movement. The work of coaches, PE teachers, and physiotherapists will thus continue to be based on intuition rather than scientific knowledge. This problem will hamper the optimisation of the training process (especially in technical training) and discourage students from participating in PE lessons and mastering more and more difficult motor tasks.

2. Materials and Methods

The participants were sixty-one male university students who did not play sports. Participants were randomised into three groups: group Verbal (VER) = 20 (body height 178.6 ± 4.3 cm, body mass 81.3 ± 3.7 kg, age 20.3 ± 1.2 years), group Visual (VIS) = 21 (body height 179 ± 4.6 cm, body mass 82 ± 3.4 kg, age 20.3 ± 1.2 years), and group Verbal–Visual (VER&VIS) = 20 (body height 178.6 ± 4.3 cm, body mass 81.3 ± 3.7 kg, age 20.3 ± 1.2 years).

Research design: The experiment lasted 6 weeks, with training sessions performed 3 times per week (on Mondays, Wednesdays, and Fridays). Each student participated in 18 sessions lasting 60 min, and during the workout each subject performed 20 exercises, which were divided into 4 sets with 5 repetitions each (approximately 3 min per person). The participants learnt how to perform a vertical jump with an arm swing. During the jump, they pulled their knees to their chest and were instructed to grab their lower legs, and then perform a half-squat landing with arms sideways (VJPKL). The participants had not performed similar tasks prior to the experiment. The progressive part method was used, with the task divided into individual parts. The students learnt the preparatory phase during sessions 1 to 4, the main phase during sessions 5 to 8 and the final phase in sessions 9 to 12. Eventually, during sessions 13 to 16, the participants learnt the entire movement task. During each training session, 20 exercises were divided into 4 sets with 5 repetitions. Each set was followed by feedback. Group VER received verbal feedback on errors. Group VIS received visual feedback (concerning the correctness of performance). Group VER&VIS received verbal feedback on errors and visual feedback on how to correct them. Two days prior to the experiment, the participants performed a pre-test (PRET), and a post-test (POST) was conducted one day after it ended. Furthermore, a retention test (RETT) was carried out seven days after the experiment. The participants were instructed to follow a standardised warm-up and to perform a single movement task. Their performance was rated by 3 gymnastic judges on a scale from 1 to 10 based on the rules of the International Gymnastics Federation. During the evaluation, 0 to 0.3 points were deducted from a maximum score of 10 points for each minor error, 0.4 to 0.6 points for medium errors, and 0.7 to 1 points for major errors. The concordance of the experts' ratings was verified using the concordance coefficient (0.94). All the participants were informed in a written and oral manner about the tests that would be carried out in the study and they signed the informed consent form. The consent of the Senate Committee on Research Ethics of the University of Physical Education in Warsaw was obtained.

Statistical analysis: The ANOVA analysis of variance was employed to evaluate the statistical significance of differences between the measurements. The Shapiro–Wilk test was used to test the data for normality of distribution and homogeneity of variances. After the prerequisite was verified, the variables were analysed using a two-way mixed-factor ANOVA, Group (3) × Test Time (3) for judge ratings and Group (3) × Test Time (2) for force measurements. The three experimental groups represented a between-subjects factor, whereas the testing times were considered a within-subjects factor. A probability level was considered critical at $p < 0.05$. The Tukey post-hoc test was used to examine significant differences. The statistical analysis of the results was performed using the Statistica software (StatSoft Inc. (2017), STATISTICA data analysis software system, version 13.3, TIBCO Software Inc., Palo Alto, CA, USA, www.statsoft.com) (accessed on 16 August 2021).

3. Results

The repeated-measures ANOVA revealed significant effects of Group ($F(2,54) = 11.69$; $p = 0.001$) and Group × Test Time interaction ($F(4,108) = 40.52$; $p = 0.001$). Figure 1 presents the means and standard deviations.

Based on a Tukey post-hoc test, the significance of differences between mean ratings of the judges at particular stages of the learning process was determined for groups VER&VIS, VIS and VER (Table 1).

In the study, it was found that in the pre-test, differences in mean scores of the groups for VJPKL performance were not statistically significant $F(2,54) = 1.344$, $p < 0.269$). However, after 6 weeks (post-test), these differences were significant $F(2,54) = 38.651$, $p < 0.001$). The mean score of group VER&VIS was better than the mean scores of groups VIS and VER by 9% ($p < 0.01$) and 15% ($p < 0.001$), respectively. In turn, group VIS had a better mean score than group VER, and the difference was 10% ($p < 0.001$). The retention test revealed that differences in mean scores of the groups were significant $F(2,54) = 15.631$, $p < 0.001$)

in favour of group VER&VIS. This group had a better score than groups VIS and VER by 10% and 7%, respectively.

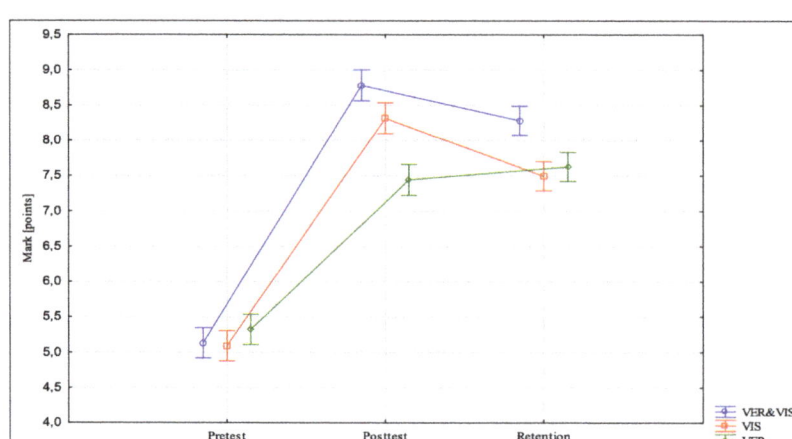

Figure 1. Point-based evaluation of motor task performance in all the groups with regard to time and type of feedback that influences the effectiveness of motor task learning.

Table 1. Significance level of Tukey post-hoc test of experts' ratings (PRET, POST, and RETT) in groups VER, VIS, and VER&VIS.

No.	Groups	VER&VIS (PRET)	VER&VIS (POST)	VER&VIS (RETT)	VIS (PRET)	VIS (POST)	VIS (RETT)	VER (PRET)	VER (POST)	VER (RETT)
1	VER&VIS (PRET)		0.00	0.00	0.99	0.00	0.00	0.94	0.00	0.00
2	VER&VIS (PRET)	0.00		0.00	0.00	0.06	0.00	0.00	0.00	0.00
3	VER&VIS (PRET)	0.00	0.00		0.00	1.00	0.00	0.00	0.00	0.00
4	VIS (PRET)	0.99	0.00	0.00		0.00	0.00	0.83	0.00	0.00
5	VIS (POST)	0.00	0.06	1.00	0.00		0.00	0.00	0.00	0.00
6	VIS (RETT)	0.00	0.00	0.00	0.00	0.00		0.00	0.99	0.99
7	VER (PRET)	0.94	0.00	0.00	0.83	0.00	0.00		0.00	0.00
8	VER (PRET)	0.00	0.00	0.00	0.00	0.00	0.99	0.00		0.59
9	VER (PRET)	0.00	0.00	0.00	0.00	0.00	0.99	0.00	0.59	

4. Discussion

Despite the numerous studies conducted so far, the issue of teaching and learning motor tasks, especially those with a complex structure of movement, needs to be addressed in terms of optimisation. For instance, during a PE lesson or training session, when learners or athletes who try to acquire new motor skills repeat the same error, teachers or coaches may choose not to give any feedback on when the error was made and how to eliminate it. When learners have experience, they will certainly use intrinsic feedback, which helps them acquire technical skills and shorten the learning process. Considerably worse effects will be produced when learners are not experienced enough and they are still incapable of using intrinsic feedback. In such cases, feedback provided by teachers or coaches is particularly meaningful.

Hence, the key question each teacher or coach should ask is 'How can I facilitate the process of teaching and learning motor tasks and how can I optimise PE lessons or training aimed at acquiring technical skills?'. Some of the problems faced are the choice of content and the type and amount of feedback that ought to be provided in the course of the process of learning motor tasks. Should feedback be given in verbal or visual form or as a combination of both? These and other questions cannot be answered unequivocally [1,23,25,27–32]. Despite various studies on this subject, there is no empirical evidence of the influence of different types and content of feedback on the effectiveness of motor learning of complex tasks [9,13–15,29,33–36]. Coaches, teachers, and physiotherapists should always choose feedback adequate for learners' levels of advancement and skills. Feedback should be simple, easy to understand, and concise so that athletes and students can receive, process, and use it when developing motor habits both now and in the future, when more complex and difficult tasks will have to be learnt. This paper attempts to evaluate the effectiveness of feedback modalities in the motor learning of complex tasks.

The team of researchers assumed that providing verbal feedback on errors combined with visual feedback on the correct performance of the task can be more efficient than just verbal feedback on errors or just visual feedback on correctness provided in isolation. The results of the study lead to the conclusion that the use of different strategies to provide feedback to learners can produce different effects. It was found that the three study groups showed statistically significant improvements in the post-test. However, in the retention test, the improvements were reported only in group VIS. The study participants from group VER&VIS, who received verbal feedback on errors and visual feedback on how to correct them, had better scores than those from VIS, who only received visual feedback regarding the correctness of task performance, and the learners from group VER, who only received verbal feedback on errors (the effect size for the post-test was 8.352 in VER&VIS, 3.894 in VIS and 8.147 in VER). Insignificantly improved scores in the retention test were found in group VER. In groups VER&VIS and VIS, the results of the retention test did reveal changes. These findings are partly consistent with data reported by studies that have tested the guidance hypothesis in complex movement skills. The authors of these studies demonstrated that after cessation of 100% feedback, the results of the retention test were worse. In our study, group VIS showed improved performance in the retention test. However, the VER&VIS group, who received more feedback, showed relatively better performance than the participants from groups VIS and VER, who were given less information.

Schmidt and Wrisberg [37] noted that proper feedback produced better effects in the process of learning motor tasks. These results are consistent with the findings of other researchers [19,38,39]. Researchers claim that the combination of verbal feedback with other sources of information increases learning effectiveness. Similarly, Weiss and Klint [40] stated that the presentation of a given task enhanced with verbal feedback improves learning effectiveness. Moreover, numerous studies indicate that there are a lot of relevant factors in the way verbal and visual feedback is provided that impact the learning process [20,39,41–44]. The knowledge of which types of feedback should be combined and in what manner forms the basis of learning process optimisation. This may indicate that providing verbal feedback on errors and visual feedback on task performance is justified when it comes to improving motor skills, while visual feedback combined with verbal feedback proves to be more effective during the learning process. Another important piece of information for both teachers and coaches is that visual feedback on performance correctness, similar to verbal feedback on errors, produces marginal learning outcomes. Considering the above facts, it may seem to be more beneficial to use visual feedback on performance correctness together with verbal feedback on errors.

The type of task performed appears to be a key determinant in the choice of strategy for providing feedback concerning the quality and results in the performance of a task. The results are consistent with those published by Tzetzis and Votsis [30], who argued that during the learning of complex tasks, positive feedback must combine information on errors and ways of correcting the task. In our study, the participants from the group VER&VIS, who received such information, showed significant improvement in the scores ($p < 0.05$). The participants from the groups VIS and VER, who received less information on task performance, obtained worse results. This indicates that the amount of information provided to a learner is the main determinant of the effectiveness of learning a complex movement task. Convincing evidence was provided by Laguna [31], who demonstrated that the effectiveness of learning complex tasks depended on the level of difficulty of the task and specificity of the feedback (task-related information). This is indirectly in line with our findings.

It seems that different types of feedback may be used depending on the type of problem that we want to solve and on the type of the process we will apply when learning. Teachers who provide learners with direct visual feedback on the correctness of task performance as well as verbal feedback on how to correct errors may expect their learners to follow these sources of information, which may considerably enhance the process of learning at an early stage. On the other hand, teachers can select a version of the learning process which, at an early stage, will pose a certain problem or will compel learners to go beyond the feedback received and to discover and develop their own solutions. Although at an early stage this approach does not produce considerable effects, it seems beneficial in the long term. Therefore, the process of learning should focus not only on speed and the ease of acquiring new motor skills, but also on encouraging learners to self-develop internally. Such an approach may be extremely important due to the fact that it will teach learners to be persistent in developing their own skills.

Limitation of the Study

One limitation of our research is that the three learning strategies were used only for one complex movement task. It is recommended that future research should be carried out with consideration of movement tasks with different levels of complexity and different feedback strategies.

5. Conclusions

1. At the early stages of learning, a combination of visual and verbal feedback represents the basis for learning complex movement tasks and most often enhances the learning process.
2. In the post-test, visual feedback on the correctness of task performance combined with verbal feedback on errors in task performance proved to be more effective than visual feedback only on the correctness of task performance or verbal feedback only on errors in performing a vertical jump where the participants pulled their knees up to their chest and grabbed their lower legs. In the retention test, an improvement was only noted in the case of verbal feedback on errors in task performance.
3. Examining such variables can help us to assess the role of feedback and learning complex movement tasks.
4. Future research should focus on verifying whether our results can be applied in learning other more complex movement tasks. For this purpose, modern methods for the verification of research results and experimental programs should be used.

Practical Implication

The results of our research will help coaches to assess the role of feedback in learning complex movement tasks that are commonly taught by personal trainers and physical educators. Providing a lot of information gives good results in the short term, but providing limited information seems to be more effective in the long term.

Author Contributions: Conceptualisation, J.J.-N., T.N., O.R.-R., M.B., W.W.; methodology, J.J.-N., T.N., Ł.R., M.B., T.A., D.K.; software J.J.-N., T.N., M.B., M.N.; validation, J.J.-N., T.N., O.R.-R., M.B. formal analysis, J.J.-N., M.B., T.N., Ł.R., T.A.; investigation, J.J.-N., T.N., I.Ł.-S.; resources, J.J.-N., T.N., M.N., D.K.; data curation, J.J.-N., T.N., O.R.-R.; writing—original draft preparation, J.J.-N., T.N., M.B., W.W.; writing—review and editing, J.J.-N., T.N., Ł.R., T.A., M.B.; visualisation, J.J.-N., T.N., M.N.; supervision, J.J.-N., T.N., Ł.R., T.A.; project administration, J.J.-N., T.N.; funding acquisition, J.J.-N., T.N. All authors have read and agreed to the published version of the manuscript.

Funding: This research received no external funding.

Institutional Review Board Statement: The research was approved by the Bioethics Committee No. SKE 001-101-1/2010.

Informed Consent Statement: Informed consent was obtained from all subjects involved in the study.

Data Availability Statement: The data presented in this study are available on request from the corresponding author.

Conflicts of Interest: The authors declare no conflict of interest.

References

1. Salmoni, A.W.; Schmidt, R.A.; Walter, C.B. Knowledge of results and motor learning: A review and critical reappraisal. *Psychol. Bull.* **1984**, *95*, 355–386. [CrossRef]
2. Winstein, C. Knowledge of results and motor learning—Implications for physical therapy. *Phys. Ther.* **1991**, *71*, 140–149. [CrossRef] [PubMed]
3. Magill, R.A.; Hall, K.G. A review of the contextual interference effect in motor skill acquisition. *Hum. Mov. Sci.* **1990**, *9*, 241–289. [CrossRef]
4. Shapiro, D.; Schmidt, R. The schema theory: Recent evidence and developmental implications. In *The Development of Movement Control and Coordination*; John Wiley & Sons: Hoboken, NJ, USA, 1982.
5. Hagman, J.D. Presentation- and test-trial effects on acquisition and retention of distance and location. *J. Exp. Psychol. Learn. Mem. Cogn.* **1983**, *9*, 334–345. [CrossRef] [PubMed]
6. Winstein, C.J.; Pohl, P.S.; Lewthwaite, R. Effects of physical guidance and knowledge of results on motor learning: Support for the guidance hypothesis. *Res. Q. Exerc. Sport* **1994**, *65*, 316–323. [CrossRef] [PubMed]
7. Jeannerod, M. The representing brain: Neural correlates of motor intention and imagery. *Behav. Brain Sci.* **1994**, *17*, 187–202. [CrossRef]
8. Mccullagh, P.; Weiss, M.R.; Ross, D. Modeling considerations in motor skill acquisition and performance: An integrated approach. *Exerc. Sport Sci. Rev.* **1989**, *17*, 475–514. [PubMed]
9. Wulf, G.; Shea, C.; Lewthwaite, R. Motor skill learning and performance: A review of influential factors. *Med. Educ.* **2010**, *44*, 75–84. [CrossRef]
10. Lee, T.D.; Genovese, E.D. Distribution of practice in motor skill acquisition: Learning and performance effects reconsidered. *Res. Q. Exerc. Sport* **1988**, *59*, 277–287. [CrossRef]
11. Lee, T.D.; Genovese, E.D. Distribution of practice in motor skill acquisition: Different effects for discrete and continuous tasks. *Res. Q. Exerc. Sport* **1989**, *60*, 59–65. [CrossRef]
12. Sadowski, J.; Boloban, W.; Mastalerz, A.; Niznikowski, T. Velocities and joint angles during double backward stretched salto performed with stable landing and in combination with tempo salto. *Biol. Sport* **2009**, *26*, 87–101. [CrossRef]
13. Potdevin, F.; Vors, O.; Huchez, A.; Lamour, M.; Davids, K.; Schnitzler, C. How can video feedback be used in physical education to support novice learning in gymnastics? Effects on motor learning, self-assessment and motivation. *Phys. Educ. Sport Pedagog.* **2018**, *23*, 559–574. [CrossRef]
14. Frikha, M.; Chaâri, N.; ElGhoul, Y.; Mohamed-Ali, H.H.; Zinkovsky, A.V. Effects of combined versus singular verbal or haptic feedback on acquisition, retention, difficulty, and competence perceptions in motor learning. *Percept. Mot. Ski.* **2019**, *126*, 713–732. [CrossRef]
15. Amri-Dardari, A.; Mkaouer, B.; Nassib, S.H.; Amara, S.; Amri, R.; Ben Salah, F.Z. The effects of video modeling and simulation on teaching/learning basic vaulting jump on the vault table. *Sci. Gymnast. J.* **2020**, *12*, 325–344.
16. Nogal, M.; Niźnikowski, T. Effectiveness of verbal feedback on complex motor skill learning. *Theory Pract. Phys. Cult.* **2020**, *8*, 63–66.
17. Hodges, N.J.; Chua, R.; Franks, I.M. The role of video in facilitating perception and action of a novel coordination movement. *J. Mot. Behav.* **2003**, *35*, 247–260. [CrossRef] [PubMed]
18. Carroll, W.R.; Bandura, A. Translating cognition into action. *J. Mot. Behav.* **1987**, *19*, 385–398. [CrossRef] [PubMed]
19. Carroll, W.R.; Bandura, A. Representational guidance of action production in observational learning: A causal analysis. *J. Mot. Behav.* **1990**, *22*, 85–97. [CrossRef]

20. Hebert, E.P.; Landin, D. Effects of a learning model and augmented feedback on tennis skill acquisition. *Res. Q. Exerc. Sport* **1994**, *65*, 250–257. [CrossRef]
21. Tzetzis, G.; Mantis, K.; Zachopoulou, E.; Kioumourtzoglou, E. The effect of modeling and verbal feedback on skill learning. *J. Hum. Mov. Stud.* **1999**, *36*, 137–151.
22. Sadowski, J.; Mastalerz, A.; Niźnikowski, T. Benefits of bandwidth feedback in learning a complex gymnastic skill. *J. Hum. Kinet.* **2013**, *37*, 183–193. [CrossRef]
23. Hodges, N.J.; Franks, I. Learning as a function of coordination bias: Building upon pre-practice behaviours. *Hum. Mov. Sci.* **2002**, *21*, 231–258. [CrossRef]
24. Lee, A.M.; Keh, N.C.; Magill, R.A. Instructional effects of teacher feedback in physical education. *J. Teach. Phys. Educ.* **1993**, *12*, 228–243. [CrossRef]
25. Kernodle, M.W.; Carlton, L.G. Information feedback and the learning of multiple-degree-of-freedom activities. *J. Mot. Behav.* **1992**, *24*, 187–195. [CrossRef] [PubMed]
26. Smith, P.J.; Davies, M. Applying contextual interference to the Pawlata roll. *J. Sports Sci.* **1995**, *13*, 455–462. [CrossRef] [PubMed]
27. Wulf, G.; Shea, C.H.; Matschiner, S. Frequent feedback enhances complex motor skill learning. *J. Mot. Behav.* **1998**, *30*, 180–192. [CrossRef] [PubMed]
28. Scheeler, M.C.; Ruhl, K.L.; McAfee, J.K. Providing performance feedback to teachers: A review. *Teach. Educ. Spec. Educ. J. Teach. Educ. Div. Counc. Except. Child.* **2004**, *27*, 396–407. [CrossRef]
29. Sanchez, X.; Bampouras, M. Augmented feedback over a short period of time: Does it improve netball goal-shooting performance? *Int. J. Sport Psychol.* **2006**, *37*, 349–358.
30. Tzetzis, G.; Votsis, E. Three feedback methods in acquisition and retention of badminton skills. *Percept. Mot. Ski.* **2006**, *102*, 275–284. [CrossRef]
31. Laguna, P.L. Task complexity and sources of task-related information during the observational learning process. *J. Sports Sci.* **2008**, *26*, 1097–1113. [CrossRef] [PubMed]
32. Wulf, G. Attentional focus and motor learning: A review of 15 years. *Int. Rev. Sport Exerc. Psychol.* **2013**, *6*, 77–104. [CrossRef]
33. Shea, J.B.; Titzer, R.C. The influence of reminder trials on contextual interference effects. *J. Mot. Behav.* **1993**, *25*, 264–274. [CrossRef] [PubMed]
34. More, K.G.; Franks, I.M. Analysis and modification of verbal coaching behaviour: The usefulness of a data-driven intervention strategy. *J. Sports Sci.* **1996**, *14*, 523–543. [CrossRef] [PubMed]
35. Hughes, M.; Franks, I. *Notational Analysis of Sport*; E&FN Spon: London, UK, 1997.
36. Horn, R.R.; Williams, A.M.; Hayes, S.J.; Hodges, N.J.; Scott, M.A. Demonstration as a rate enhancer to changes in coordination during early skill acquisition. *J. Sports Sci.* **2007**, *25*, 599–614. [CrossRef] [PubMed]
37. Schmidt, R.; Wrisberg, C. *Motor Learning and Performance. A Problem-Based Learning Approach*; Human Kinetics: Champaign, IL, USA, 2004.
38. Rink, J.E. Teacher education: A focus on action. *Quest* **1993**, *45*, 308–320. [CrossRef]
39. Mccullagh, P.; Stiehl, J.; Weiss, M.R. Developmental modeling effects on the quantitative and qualitative aspects of motor performance. *Res. Q. Exerc. Sport* **1990**, *61*, 344–350. [CrossRef]
40. Weiss, M.R.; Klint, K.A. "Show and tell" in the gymnasium: An investigation of developmental differences in modeling and verbal rehearsal of motor skills. *Res. Q. Exerc. Sport* **1987**, *58*, 234–241. [CrossRef]
41. Adams, J.A. Historical review and appraisal of research on the learning, retention, and transfer of human motor skills. *Psychol. Bull.* **1987**, *101*, 41–74. [CrossRef]
42. Blandin, Y.; Proteau, L.; Alain, C. On the cognitive processes underlying contextual interference and observational learning. *J. Mot. Behav.* **1994**, *26*, 18–26. [CrossRef] [PubMed]
43. Lee, T.D.; White, M.A. Influence of an unskilled model's practice schedule on observational motor learning. *Hum. Mov. Sci.* **1990**, *9*, 349–367. [CrossRef]
44. Pollock, B.J.; Lee, T.D. Effects of the model's skill level on observational motor learning. *Res. Q. Exerc. Sport* **1992**, *63*, 25–29. [CrossRef] [PubMed]

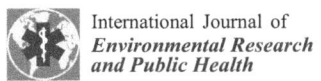

Article

Evaluation of the Level of Technical and Tactical Skills and Its Relationships with Aerobic Capacity and Special Fitness in Elite Ju-Jitsu Athletes

Tadeusz Ambroży [1,*], Łukasz Rydzik [1,*], Michał Spieszny [1], Wiesław Chwała [1], Jarosław Jaszczur-Nowicki [2], Małgorzata Jekiełek [3], Karol Görner [4], Andrzej Ostrowski [1] and Wojciech J. Cynarski [5]

[1] Institute of Sports Sciences, University of Physical Education in Krakow, 31-541 Kraków, Poland; michal.spieszny@awf.krakow.pl (M.S.); wieslaw.chwala@awf.krakow.pl (W.C.); andrzejostrowski@poczta.fm (A.O.)
[2] Department of Tourism, Recreation and Ecology, University of Warmia and Mazury, 10-719 Olsztyn, Poland; j.jaszczur-nowicki@uwm.edu.pl
[3] Department of Ergonomics and Physiological Effort, Institute of Physiotherapy, Jagiellonian University Collegium Medicum, 31-126 Krakow, Poland; malgorzata.jekielek@gmail.com
[4] Department of Physical Education and Sports, Matej Bel University in Banská, 974-01 Banská Bystrica, Slovakia; gornerk@uek.krakow.pl
[5] Institute of Physical Culture Studies, College of Medical Sciences, University of Rzeszow, 35-959 Rzeszów, Poland; ela_cyn@wp.pl
* Correspondence: tadek@ambrozy.pl (T.A.); lukasz.gne@op.pl (Ł.R.); Tel.: +48-730-696-377 (Ł.R.)

Citation: Ambroży, T.; Rydzik, Ł.; Spieszny, M.; Chwała, W.; Jaszczur-Nowicki, J.; Jekiełek, M.; Görner, K.; Ostrowski, A.; Cynarski, W.J. Evaluation of the Level of Technical and Tactical Skills and Its Relationships with Aerobic Capacity and Special Fitness in Elite Ju-Jitsu Athletes. *Int. J. Environ. Res. Public Health* **2021**, *18*, 12286. https://doi.org/10.3390/ijerph182312286

Academic Editors: Paul B. Tchounwou and Richard B. Kreider

Received: 24 September 2021
Accepted: 11 November 2021
Published: 23 November 2021

Publisher's Note: MDPI stays neutral with regard to jurisdictional claims in published maps and institutional affiliations.

Copyright: © 2021 by the authors. Licensee MDPI, Basel, Switzerland. This article is an open access article distributed under the terms and conditions of the Creative Commons Attribution (CC BY) license (https://creativecommons.org/licenses/by/4.0/).

Abstract: Background: Ju-jitsu training has to be comprehensive in terms of training intensity, developing a wide range of physical fitness and learning multiple technical skills. These requirements result from the specificity of the competition characteristic of the sport form of this martial art. The aim of this study was to evaluate the aerobic capacity and special physical fitness of ju-jitsu athletes at the highest sports performance level and to determine the relationships between special fitness and the indices of technical and tactical skills. Methods: In order to determine the current level of special fitness of the athletes, a set of karate fitness tests were used, namely, the Special Judo Fitness Test and the Kickboxer Special Physical Fitness Test. Furthermore, maximal oxygen uptake (VO$_2$peak) was measured using a graded exercise test in a group of 30 sport ju-jitsu athletes at the highest level of sports performance. To evaluate the level of technical and tactical skills, an analysis of recordings of tournament bouts was carried out, and, based on the observations, the indices of effectiveness, efficiency, and activeness of the attack were calculated. Results: Individuals with higher fitness were more active and effective in the attack. The special efficiency indices showed significant correlations with the technical and tactical parameters. Better fighting performance was dependent on the speed of the punches, kicking range, and the results of the special fitness tests. Conclusions: To achieve greater efficiency and effectiveness of sport ju-jitsu, the training process should be based on comprehensive motor development and an optimal level of special fitness.

Keywords: physical fitness; training control: special fitness test; martial arts

1. Introduction

In Poland, modern sport ju-jitsu involves extensive competition in the form of tournaments organized by the Polish Ju-jitsu Association in the following variants: Fighting System, Duo System, and Ne Waza [1]. This makes it necessary to constantly improve physical abilities and to expand the range of techniques used by athletes during sports combat. With such an extensive formula of competition, the training process in sports ju-jitsu must be versatile in terms of training intensity, developing a wide range of motor skills, and mastering multiple technical skills. A review of the literature indicates that during the observation of the course of fights during the Junior Ju-jitsu World Championships (Bucharest 2013) the most frequently used hand techniques in the first phase of the bout were punches and inverted fist techniques, while the kicks included side kick, roundhouse kick, and front kick. In the second phase of the bout (characterized by grappling), hand throws (morote gari and seoi nage), sweep techniques (osoto gari, osoto otoshi, and ouchi gari), and hip throws (goshi guruma and harai goshi) were used most often, while in the third phase, pinning techniques, joint locking, and choking techniques were most frequent [2]. The analysis of the course of the fight conducted by other authors [3,4] suggests that the ju-jitsu bout in the Fighting System resembles karate or kickboxing in the first phase, while in the second and third phase, the fight is similar to judo [5,6]. In sport ju-jitsu, the fight is characterized by acyclic work, and the changing situation requires the athlete to control the situation and respond quickly to the opponent's actions. Physical effort during combat in sport ju-jitsu is based on submaximal and maximal training load [7]. For this reason, energy source is anaerobic glycolysis, while aerobic sources are utilized at the end of the bout. The presented literature analysis indicates that optimal aerobic and anaerobic endurance is necessary in ju-jitsu training [8]. An important objective of the ju-jitsu training is to achieve a high level of anaerobic power (dynamic kicks and throws), strength (throws and ground holds), and limb speed (punches and combinations in the attack, blocks, and dodges in defense) [3,9–13]. The relationships between physical fitness and tournament bouts in ju-jitsu were also established by evaluation of fitness using general and special tests. The research focused on sport ju-jitsu, Brazilian ju-jitsu, and judo [14,15].

Fighting in ju-jitsu is characterized by the use of a wide range of techniques combined into specific sequences. An appropriate level of technical and tactical skills seems to be the most important element of an athlete's success. Technical and tactical actions are used to control the fight and respond to the opponent's attacks, while preventing counterattacks [3,16–18]. As part of the coach's supervision, the analysis of combats is used by determining the indices of the athlete's technical and tactical skills, which allows for the assessment of their potential competitive performance. Such an analysis is a popular indicator used to modify the sports training in martial arts and combat sports. These issues have been studied in detail in judo [19–21] and kickboxing [22,23]. The review of the literature on ju-jitsu shows that, to date, studies have mainly focused on the evaluation of post-training adaptations and a level of the athlete's physical fitness [13,14,24–27], and analysis of morphological [28,29], physiological [30], and biomechanical indices [31,32]. Other studies have focused on the analysis of the ju-jitsu technique [33], the required profiles in ju-jitsu [34,35], the structure of the fight [36], health parameters [29], optimism, and satisfaction with life [37].

A detailed literature review revealed that there is a lack of research on the analysis of the level of technical and tactical skills, especially concerning special physical fitness.

The aim of this study was to evaluate the aerobic capacity and special physical fitness of ju-jitsu athletes at the highest sports performance and to determine the relationships between special fitness and the indices of technical and tactical skills. Evaluation of the correlations will demonstrate whether the level of special physical fitness determines the activeness, effectiveness, and efficiency of the attack and will enable more effective planning of sports training.

2. Materials and Methods

The study was conducted on a group of 30 sport ju-jitsu athletes with the highest level of sports performance who agreed to participate in the study. The selection of the study group was purposeful and the selection criterion was training experience (at least 5 years) and level sports performance (champion level), which was assessed based on the authors' observations and the opinion of coaches. The athletes were included in the ranking list of the Ju-Jitsu International Federation and the Polish Ju-Jitsu Association, and four of them were medalists of the world championships. The mean participants' experience in sport was 7.1 ± 2.26 years. They trained 1.5 to 2 h, 6–10 times a week. The exclusion criterion was a negative opinion of a sports physician and no consent to participate in the study. The mean age of the respondents was 25.43 ± 1.96 years, body weight was 83.74 ± 8.6 kg, and body height was 180.96 ± 4.97 cm. BMI ranged from 21.4 to 29.1 kg/m^2. Body mass was measured using a Tanita BC-601 body composition monitor (Tanita, Tokyo, Japan), whereas the body height was measured using a SECA 2017 body height meter (Seca, Hamburg, Germany).

2.1. Measurement of Physical Fitness and Aerobic Capacity

Aerobic capacity was measured using the aerobic maximal graded treadmill test [38]. The test evaluated maximal oxygen uptake (VO$_2$peak) expressed in milliliters of oxygen per kilogram of body weight per minute (ml/kg/min). During the test, the levels of cardiopulmonary indices were recorded based on the breath-by-breath method using an ergospirometer (Cosmed, Rome, Italy). The test was performed on a treadmill (Saturn 250/100R,h/p/Cosmos, Munich, Germany). The effort began with a 4 min warm-up performed at a speed of 8 km·h^{-1}, with a treadmill inclination angle of 1°. Thereafter, the speed was incremented by 1.0 km*h^{-1} every 2 mins. When the heart rate (bpm) approached the maximum level, the running speed was maintained and the load was increased by changing the angle of the treadmill by 1° every minute. The test was carried out until the participant refused to continue the test due to volitional exhaustion. The heart rate (HR) during the test was measured with a sports tester (S-610i, Polar, Finland). The following indices were analyzed: pulmonary ventilation (VE), oxygen uptake (VO$_2$), carbon dioxide production (VCO$_2$), respiratory-exchange-ratio (RER), expiratory carbon dioxide concentration (%FECO$_2$), the ventilatory equivalent ratio for oxygen and carbon dioxide (VE/VCO$_2$), and heart rate (HR). Data were averaged every 30 s. The highest recorded value of oxygen uptake was considered as peak oxygen uptake [39].

Special physical fitness was assessed based on selected tests taken from special fitness tests in karate, kickboxing, and judo:

1. Evasive action test: In the retreat test, the subject starts from the fighting stance, moving backwards between lines 8 m apart. The track in the shape of a loop between the lines (back and forth) is covered 6 times. Execution time is measured in seconds. Equipment: stopwatch and 2 small cones that are set on lines at a distance of 8 m [40].
2. Hip turning speed test: In the test of the speed (frequency) of the hip turns, each subject should be tied with a belt over his or her right hip (unless they usually fight in the reverse position), take a fighting stance, and twists the hips to the left. This movement will tighten the belt held by the coach at the back (control). Then the subject retracts with his or her hips. On the command "Hajime!" ("Forward!"), the participant makes 30 hip turns as quickly as possible (belt pulls are counted). The time taken to execute 30 pulls is recorded. Equipment: stopwatch and ju-jitsu belt [40].
3. Speed punches test: Punches by the fighter performed from the fighting stance. Each participant performs a combination of two punches: left, straight to the head (Oi seiken jodan tsuki) and right, straight to the torso (Gyaku seiken chudan tsuki), without changing the designated distance. The targets to which the participant performs 30 such combinations (60 punches in total) are held by a second person at a constant height. The time to complete 30 full punches is measured in seconds with an accuracy of 0.1 s. Two assistants need a stopwatch and 2 targets [40].
4. Flexibility test using Mawashi Geri kick: The flexibility index = maximum range of kick/body height (cm/cm) was calculated. In the flexibility test, the maximum range (foot hit height) of the Jodan Mawashi Geri roundhouse kick was evaluated. Five measurements were taken for the preferred limb by recording the maximum score (cm) [40].
5. Special Judo Fitness Test (SJFT):

Before the first test, the participant performs a warm-up consisting of 5 min of jogging (moderate intensity) and a few Ippon-seoi-nage throws at a slow pace to familiarize themselves with the distance and exercise partners [41,42].

This test consists of three periods of effort (A = 15 s; B and C after 30 s) separated by 10 s breaks. In each period/series of throws, the thrower's (tori) score is based on the maximum number of Ippon-seoi-nage throws on two partners (uke A and B) standing 6 m apart on the mat. Both uke A and B should have a similar body height and weight to the tori. Heart rate is measured one minute after the test. The Index in SJFT was also counted as

$$SJFT\ Index = \frac{Final\ HR(bpm)\ +\ HR1\ min\ (bpm)}{Throws\ (N)}$$

where:

Final HR—heart rate recorded immediately after the test
HR1 min—heart rate recorded 1 min after the test
Throws—number of throws completed during the test

The body's response to exercise was recorded using the heart rate monitor S-610i (Polar, Finland).

6. Kickboxer Special Physical Fitness Test (KSPFT):

Before performing the test, the participant performs a warm-up consisting of approximately 10 min of a general warm-up, followed by stretching exercises. Then the participant performs left and right straight punches on the partner's shield from the fighting position to the head continuously for 30 s. After completing this part of the test, the participant runs 10 m in a straight line to the next station, where they perform left and right roundhouse kicks from the fighting position to the partner's shields for 30 s to the head level. Then the participant runs back to the first shield and performs techniques for 30 s in a sequence consisting of the left straight punch, followed by the right hook to the head. After completing this part of the test, the participant runs 10 m to the target mate and performs a roundhouse kick (left and right feet, alternately) to the torso for 30 s. The total time of special effort during the test is 2 min (4 × 30 s), which corresponds to the duration of one round of a kickboxing bout. Figure 1 shows a diagram of individual test components and the direction of the athlete's movement. Correctly performed hits are counted for each of the four parts. The sum of strikes (punches and kicks) is recorded as the score [43,44].

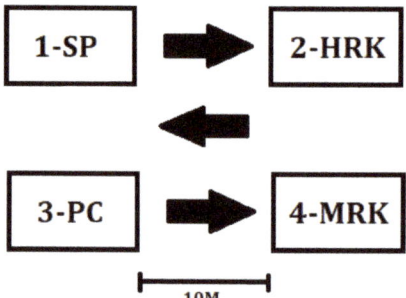

Figure 1. Graphical diagram of the Kickboxer Special Physical Fitness Test. Source: own study. SP—straight punches/jabs, punches; HRK—high roundhouse kick; PC—a combination of straight punches and hooks (punch combinations); MRK—middle roundhouse kick.

The tests were supervised by the authors of the present study for 3 days, two weeks before the competition, after the completion of the direct pre-competition training period. On the first day, the maximal graded exercise test was carried out. On the second day, the special fitness tests (tests 1–5 given above) were performed, whereas the KSPFT test was scheduled for the third day. Two days before the test, the training intensity was reduced to 30–40%.

2.2. Measurement of Indices of Technical and Tactical Skills

Analysis of bouts was performed based on digital recordings of selected tournament fights of the athletes in 2020. Three fights of each athlete were analyzed and semifinal, or final fights, were taken into consideration. The recordings were made using three cameras (Sony HDR-CX115, Manufacturer, Tokyo, Japan). The video editing program Movavi Video Editor 14 was used to process the images. The setting of the cameras allowed for continuous observation of the fighting athletes, judges, and the scoreboard. A single spreadsheet was developed as a primary research tool. The data from the spreadsheets were entered into Excel software. Then, the values of indices of technical and tactical skills were calculated for all three stages of the bout. The formulas for calculating the indices were developed based on the formulas used for judo and kickboxing [23,45].

Efficiency of the attack (S_a)

$$S_a = \frac{(n1 \times 1) + (n2 \times 2) + (n3 \times 3)}{N}$$

n1—number of attacks assessed in waza-ari as 1 point
n2—number of attacks assessed in ippon as 2 points
n3—number of attacks assessed in ippon as 3 points
1,2,3—point values of successful attacks
N—sum of observed bouts

Effectiveness of the attack (E_a)

$$E_a = \frac{number\ of\ effective\ attacks}{total\ number\ of\ attacks} \times 100$$

* An effective attack is a technical action awarded a point
* Number of all attacks is the number of all offensive actions

Activeness of the attack (A_a)

$$A_a = \frac{number\ of\ attacks\ recorded\ for\ the\ athlete}{number\ of\ bouts\ performed\ by\ the\ athlete} \tag{1}$$

2.3. Bioethics Committee

Prior to participation in the tests, the participants were informed about the research procedures, which were in accordance with the ethical principles of the Declaration of Helsinki WMADH (2000). The participant's written consent was the inclusion criterion. The research was approved by the Bioethics Committee at the Regional Medical Chamber (No. 287/KBL/OIL/2020).

2.4. Statistical Analysis

The statistical analysis of the collected material was performed using the Statistica 13.1 package by StatSoft. Basic descriptive statistics were calculated: arithmetic means, 95% confidence intervals, median, minimum and maximum, first and third quartiles, and standard deviations. The consistency of the distribution with the normal distribution was verified using the Shapiro–Wilk test, whereas the relationships between individual variables were calculated using the Pearson linear correlation. The following ranges of correlation coefficient r were adopted: low up to 0.2, mild for 0.2 to 0.5, moderate for 0.5 to 0.8, and high for >0.8. The level of statistical significance was set at $p < 0.05$ [46].

3. Results

Tables 1 and 2 present the means, standard deviations, medians, and basic statistical analysis of the physical capacity and special performance parameters of the ju-jitsu athletes studied. Table 3 presents the indices of activeness, efficiency, and effectiveness of the attack. Table 4 shows the statistical relationships between the indices of technical and tactical skills and the physical fitness of the athletes. Aerobic capacity results ranged from 42.29 to 59.21 mL/kg/min, with a mean of 51.83 mL/kg/min (Table 1).

Table 1. Fitness level of athletes studied expressed by VO_2peak and maximum heart rate.

Variables	No	m	−95%CI	+95%CI	Me	Min	Max	Q1	Q3	SD
VO_2peak [ml/kg/min]	30	51.83	50.54	53.11	51.05	45.29	59.21	49.63	55.32	3.37
HR max [bpm]	30	190.48	187.99	192.96	189.00	180.00	208.00	186.00	195.00	6.53

No—number, m—mean, 95%CI—confidence interval, Me—median, Min—minimum, Max—maximum, Q1—first quartile, Q3—third quartile, SD—standard deviation.

Table 2. Special physical fitness of the respondents.

Variables	No	m	−95%CI	+95%CI	Me	Min	Max	Q1	Q3	SD
Evasive action test [s]	30	42.74	42.26	43.22	42.60	40.33	45.95	41.80	43.29	1.25
Hip turning speed test [s]	30	11.97	11.58	12.35	11.76	10.06	14.15	11.40	12.70	1.00
Speed punches test [s]	30	11.83	11.42	12.25	11.82	10.02	13.90	11.03	12.71	1.08
1/Flexibility Ind	30	0.99	0.96	1.03	0.98	0.87	1.32	0.94	1.02	0.09
SJFT	30	14.56	14.18	14.94	14.63	12.59	16.61	14.02	15.24	1.00
KSPFT	30	288.68	276.70	300.67	290.00	239.00	349.00	263.00	312.00	31.51

1/Flexibility Ind—flexibility index for the test using Mawashi Geri kick [m] SJFT—Special Judo Fitness Test, KSPFT—Kickboxer Special Physical Fitness Test.

Table 3. Activeness, efficiency, and effectiveness of the attack in the group of athletes studied.

Variables	No	m	−95%CI	+95%CI	Me	Min	Max	Q1	Q3	SD
Activeness	30	15.49	13.60	17.38	14.60	13.11	41.12	14.20	15.09	4.97
Effectiveness	30	48.93	48.33	49.54	49.13	45.12	51.23	48.55	49.97	1.58
Efficiency	30	18.15	17.79	18.50	18.32	16.32	19.82	17.43	18.86	0.93

The activeness of the attack was calculated at a mean level of 15.49 and ranged from 13.11 to 41.12. The mean effectiveness s of the attack was 48.93, and it ranged from 45.12 to 51.23. The efficiency of the attack was at a mean level of 18.15, ranging from 16.32 to 19.82 (Table 3).

People with a greater kicking range were more active (r = 0.55), efficient (r = 0.67), and effective in the attack (r = 0.73) (moderate correlation). In all three categories of the indices, higher values were achieved in the special throwing fitness test in terms of the number of completed throws. The activeness and effectiveness of the attack correlated significantly with the speed of punches. The activeness and efficiency of the attack depend on the accuracy, precision, and speed of kicks and punches, which is illustrated by the significant moderate correlations between these indices and the Kickboxer Special Physical Fitness Test. The activeness, effectiveness, and efficiency of athletes expressed by the indices of technical and tactical skills showed a strong dependence on the level of maximum oxygen uptake (VO_2peak) (Table 4).

Table 4. Effect of selected variables on the results of special fitness tests.

Pearson Correlation (r)	Activeness	Efficiency	Effectiveness
VO$_2$peak	0.79	0.57	0.73
	$p < 0.05$	$p < 0.05$	$p < 0.05$
Evasive action test [s]	0.05	0.07	−0.04
	$p > 0.05$	$p > 0.05$	$p > 0.05$
Hip turning speed test [s]	0.18	0.19	0.25
	$p > 0.05$	$p > 0.05$	$p > 0.05$
Speed punches test [s]	0.83	0.46	0.34
	$p < 0.05$	$p < 0.05$	$p > 0.05$
1/Flexibility Ind	0.55	0.67	0.73
	$p < 0.05$	$p < 0.05$	$p < 0.05$
SJFT (Index)	0.64	0.62	0.59
	$p < 0.05$	$p < 0.05$	$p < 0.05$
SJFT (number of throws)	0.78	0.73	0.69
	$p < 0.05$	$p < 0.05$	$p < 0.05$
KSPFT	0.78	0.35	0.44
	$p < 0.05$	$p > 0.05$	$p < 0.05$

There were no statistically significant correlations between the maximal oxygen uptake (VO$_2$peak) and the results of special fitness tests (Table 5).

Table 5. Correlation coefficient between aerobic capacity and the results of special fitness tests.

Pearson Correlation (r)	VO$_2$peak
SJFT	0.36
	$p > 0.05$
KSPFT	−0.11
	$p > 0.05$
Evasive action test [s]	−0.038
	$p > 0.05$
Hip turning speed test [s]	−0.14
	$p > 0.05$
Speed punches test [s]	0.27
	$p > 0.05$

4. Discussion

In the present study, we performed an innovative analysis of the bouts in sport ju-jitsu by measuring indices of technical and tactical skills and determining their correlations with special fitness. Based on the literature review concerning the relationships of physical fitness with technical patterns in sport ju-jitsu, the correlations occur with a high-level of hand-eye coordination, maximum anaerobic power, arm strength, endurance, speed of movement, and flexibility [13,25,47,48]. The results of special fitness tests of athletes studied were similar to those achieved by elite ju-jitsu athletes in previous studies [13]. When competing at the elite level, the appropriate aerobic capacity is important [30,49]. In this study, the mean VO$_2$peak reached the value of 51.83 ± 3.37 mL/kg/min, which is considered a high level [8,50,51]. In other similar sports, the average level of maximum minute oxygen uptake in Polish athletes was 40.8 mL/kg/min (judo athletes),

50.3 mL/kg/min (boxers), 58.4 mL/kg/min (MMA fighters), and 47.65 mL/kg/min (kickboxers) [22,52–54]. Therefore, the athletes were characterized by a level of aerobic capacity similar to judo athletes, kickboxers, boxers, and MMA athletes. The technical structure of MMA combats is similar to those in ju-jitsu [55], but their duration is much longer, ranging from 15 to 25 min. Therefore, a higher level of aerobic endurance is needed. Other studies have indicated that the mean VO_2peak in elite kickboxers ranged from 54 to 69 mL/kg/min [56,57], while in the judo athletes, it was 53.75 mL/kg/min [58]. Comparison of the results of our research to these findings reveals that in the present study, ju-jitsu athletes had a lower level of aerobic capacity than the world's elite kickboxers and judo athletes. However, it seems that aerobic capacity is an important element of the physiological fitness of ju-jitsu athletes, which results from the course of the fight. It is worth noting that the bout in sport ju-jitsu consists of periods of intense exercise in standing position, ground fighting, and breaks. The average time of a bout with breaks is 193.6 s [3]. Given the duration of the bout, it can be assumed that the athletes use aerobic metabolism. This analysis shows that aerobic capacity is essential for achieving the optimal level of special strength. Analysis of combats seems to be the best tool for a reliable assessment of a competitive activity of an athlete. For this reason, special fitness tests are used in combat sports, with their contents corresponding to the temporal and material structure of the fight [13,44]. In this study, we used the most effective tests for assessing the special fitness of athletes based on elements of judo and kickboxing. The results of our research showed differences between the ju-jitsu athletes and judo athletes in the results of the special throwing test of the SJFT (index) in favor of judo practitioners [59]. As the SJFT provides comprehensive information on the performance requirements necessary to take up a fight [60], the development of special throwing endurance can also be used to improve the activeness of the sport ju-jitsu athletes during tournaments. In terms of the total number of kicks and punches performed during the KSPFT test (288.68 ± 31.51), the athletes studied here were better than kickboxers (275.3 ± 31.1), karatekas (271.5 ± 47.7), and non-elite ju-jitsu athletes (269.1 ± 47.2) [43]. These results indicate an adequate level of technical preparation for tournament efforts during the first stage of the bout. The KSPFT used in our research allows for the assessment of the level of technical skills in athletes in terms of the most frequently used upper limb strikes (punches) and lower limb strikes (kicks), speed (number of punches and kicks per unit of time), and special endurance (number of strikes), coordination (combination of strikes), and flexibility (kicking range) [44]. The most important factors influencing the success include an appropriate level of technical and tactical skills and the potential and ability to use them effectively during a tournament fight. The level of technical-tactical skills has an impact on the course of the fight. Therefore, when describing a fight in sport ju-jitsu, one should bear in mind such elements as actual fighting time, work and rest time, and number and types of technical and tactical activities performed by athletes (activeness, efficiency, and effectiveness of the attack) [4,61]. Performing actions in both attack and defense affects the final result of the fight and helps the athlete score points [62]. When planning an optimal training program to ensure that the athlete reaches the champion level, the information obtained from the monitoring of the fights that determines the so-called ju-jitsu combat model should be used. The most popular form of the evaluation of sports performance of an athlete are the indices of technical and tactical skills, which can be used by coaches to adjust training programs and determine the current level of skills for an athlete [61].

The most important aspect of this study was to demonstrate the potential relationships of the indices of technical and tactical skills and physiological parameters with the general and special fitness of ju-jitsu athletes. To control the sports combats in ju-jitsu, a detailed analysis of the temporal and material structure was performed [3,4]. In this study, indices of technical and tactical skills were used for the first time to characterize the athletes' performance. They were illustrated using the data collected during the ju-jitsu tournaments, calculated according to the author's formulas, and prepared based on well-established and popular indices used to evaluate the performance of judo [45,63] and kickboxing athletes [23].

Ju-jitsu athletes with greater kicking ranges were more active, efficient, and effective in the attack, as indicated by high positive correlations of indices of activeness, efficiency, and effectiveness of the attack with the flexibility index. Athletes fighting in the Fighting System variant of sport ju-jitsu often use kicks to the body trunk and head in the first phase of the fight [4]. These actions make it possible to keep the opponent at an appropriate distance without giving them the opportunity to attack. This way of fighting may indicate the need for a high-level of flexibility, which may also, in some situations, partially compensate for the poorer performance in the second and third phases of the bout. It is also worth noting that Ambroży et al. demonstrated that the high roundhouse kick is the most effective leg technique [64]. No significant correlations were found between VO_2peak and special fitness tests. This may be due to the fact that the duration of the tests is relatively short and takes place at the level of anaerobic exercise, while the duration of the entire bout, especially during tournaments, requires optimal levels of aerobic endurance [4].

One of the most important results of the present research is the assessment of correlations between special fitness test scores and activeness, efficiency, and effectiveness of attack. The results showed positive correlations between the three indices and the results in the special throwing fitness test. Therefore, it can be concluded that the throwing skills used in the second phase of the bout determine the effectiveness of the attack, which is proved by the positive correlations in the number of throws completed in the test, in relation to the indices of technical and tactical skills. The positive correlation between SJFT (Index) and the indices of technical and tactical skills can be explained by the fact of a high heart rate observed in the athletes, which could be genetically or emotionally determined, and affected the final value of the index. It is also worth identifying other elements related to the level of technical and tactical skills, e.g., searching for the dependency of special efficiency on individual techniques and determining the value of the elements that were not examined (overthrows and grappling).

The activeness and efficiency of the attack also depend on the accuracy, precision, and speed of kicks and punches, which is illustrated by the significant correlations between these indices and the Kickboxer Special Physical Fitness Test (KSPFT). According to Ouergui et al., a high level of combat activity directly translates into its result fight [65]. The results of our research clearly indicate that the most important element of the high level of technical and tactical skills of sport ju-jitsu athletes (Fighting System) during tournaments is an adequate level of special fitness (especially endurance and special speed) and technical skills (in terms of all striking techniques and throws) used in the first, second, and third phases of the bout.

5. Conclusions

The activeness, effectiveness, and efficiency of the attack, expressed in terms of the level of the athlete's technical and tactical skills, show a dependence on the level of maximum oxygen uptake (VO_2peak), in the range of $r = 0.57$–0.59.

It follows that ju-jitsu athletes should develop in the preparation period, and then maintain in the competitive season, an optimal level of aerobic capacity, which should have a direct effect on their competitive performance.

The most important element of the high level of technical and tactical skills in sport ju-jitsu athletes competing in the Fighting System variant is an adequate level of special fitness (especially endurance) and technical skills (in terms of all striking techniques and throws) demonstrated in all combat phases.

5.1. Practical Implication

The training programs for ju-jitsu athletes competing in the Fighting System variant during tournaments should be focused on the development of an optimal level of special fitness. Improvements in the competitive performance of ju-jitsu athletes can be achieved by increasing the level of special endurance and quality of technique in performing throws, kicks, and strikes.

5.2. Limitation of the Study

Only the results of fitness tests based on the same testing methodology as in the present study were analyzed as comparative material. The literature review was made only in the field of the sport studied, i.e., sport ju-jitsu (Fighting System). Other forms of sport ju-jitsu (Duo, Brazilian ju-jitsu, Ne-Waza) were not taken into account.

Author Contributions: Conceptualization, T.A., Ł.R. and M.S.; methodology, T.A., Ł.R., J.J.-N. and M.J.; validation, T.A. and Ł.R.; formal analysis, T.A., Ł.R. and J.J.-N.; resources, T.A., Ł.R., W.C. and A.O.; data curation, T.A., Ł.R., J.J.-N. and W.C.; writing—original draft preparation, Ł.R., T.A., J.J.-N. and M.S.; writing—review and editing, Ł.R., T.A., W.J.C. and W.C.; supervision, T.A., Ł.R., W.J.C., J.J.-N. and M.S.; project administration, T.A., Ł.R. and K.G.; funding acquisition, T.A., Ł.R. and A.O. All authors have read and agreed to the published version of the manuscript.

Funding: The study was carried out as part of the international research project No. 02/MIS-iSW/2019, carried out by the Academy of Physical Education in Krakow and the International Institute for the Development of Martial Arts and Sports in cooperation with the Matej Bel University in Banska Bystrica, Slovakia, the Faculty of Philosophy, Department of Physical Education and Sports.

Institutional Review Board Statement: The research was approved by the Bioethics Committee at the Regional Medical Chamber (No. 287/KBL/OIL/2020).

Informed Consent Statement: Informed consent was obtained from all subjects involved in the study.

Data Availability Statement: The data presented in this study are available on request from the corresponding author.

Conflicts of Interest: The authors declare no conflict of interest.

References

1. Available online: http://jujitsu.pl (accessed on 27 May 2021).
2. Galan, D.; Rata, G. Study of the frequency of fighting system techniques in Ju-jitsu. *Discobolul–Phys. Educ. Sport Kinetother. J.* **2016**, *12*, 42–47.
3. Ambroży, T. *Struktura Treningu Ju-Jitsu*; Biblioteka Trenera, Centralny Ośrodek Sportu: Warszawa, Poland, 2008.
4. Sterkowicz, S.; Ambroży, T. *Struktura Walki Sportowej Ju-Jitsu*. W: *Czynności Zawodowe Trenera i Problemy Badawcze w Sportach Walki*; Zeszyty Naukowe Kraków: Kraków, Poland, 2001; pp. 187–200.
5. Sterkowicz, S. *Ju-Jitsu: Wybrane Aspekty Sztuki Walki Obronnej*; Studia i Monografie, Akademia Wychowania Fizycznego Kraków: Kraków, Poland, 1998.
6. Sterkowicz-Przybycień, K.; Ambrozy, T.; Jasiński, M.; Kędra, A. Body build, body composition and special fitness of female top ju-jitsu contestants. *Arch. Budo* **2014**, *10*, 117–125.
7. Sozański, H. *Podstawy Teorii Treningu Sportowego*; Blblioteka Trenera: Warszawa, Poland, 1999; ISBN 83-86504-67-7.
8. Górski, J. *Fizjologia Wysiłku i Treningu Fizycznego*; PZWL Wydawnictwo Lekarskie: Warszawa, Poland, 2019; ISBN 978-83-200-5676-1.
9. Franchini, E.; Nunes, A.V.; Moraes, J.M.; Del Vecchio, F.B. Physical Fitness and Anthropometrical Profile of the Brazilian Male Judo Team. *J. Physiol. Anthropol.* **2007**, *26*, 59–67. [CrossRef]
10. Franchini, E.; Branco, B.M.; Agostinho, M.F.; Calmet, M.; Candau, R. Influence of Linear and Undulating Strength Periodization on Physical Fitness, Physiological, and Performance Responses to Simulated Judo Matches. *J. Strength Cond. Res.* **2015**, *29*, 358–367. [CrossRef]
11. Kim, J.; Cho, H.-C.; Jung, H.-S.; Yoon, J.-D. Influence of Performance Level on Anaerobic Power and Body Composition in Elite Male Judoists. *J. Strength Cond. Res.* **2011**, *25*, 1346–1354. [CrossRef]
12. Drapšin, M.; Drid, P.; Grujić, N.; Trivić, T. Fitness level of male competitive judo players. *J. Combat Sport. Martial Arts* **2010**, *1*, 27–29.
13. Ambroży, T.; Sterkowicz-Przybycień, K.; Sterkowicz, S.; Kędra, A.; Mucha, D.; Ozimek, M.; Mucha, D. Differentiation of Physical Fitness in Polish Elite Sports Ju-Jitsu Athletes Physical Fitness in Elite Ju-Jitsu Athletes. *J. Kinesiol. Exerc. Sci.* **2017**, *27*, 57–70. [CrossRef]
14. Zaggelidis, G.; Zaggelidis, C.; Malkogeorgos, A. Evaluation of Elite Ju-Jitsu Athletes' Physical Fitness Using the JMG Test. *Stud. Univ. Babeş-Bolyai Educ. Artis Gymnast.* **2019**, *64*, 17–22. [CrossRef]
15. Mishyn, M.; Petrenko, I.; Kiyko, A. Optimization of physical training process of 10–11 years old athletes with hearing impairment ingaged in ju-jitsu. *Slobozhanskyi Her. Sci. Sport* **2020**, *8*, 27–39.

16. Brito, C.J.; Miarka, B.; de Durana, A.L.D.; Fukuda, D.H. Home Advantage in Judo: Analysis by the Combat Phase, Penalties and the Type of Attack. *J. Hum. Kinet.* **2017**, *57*, 213–220. [CrossRef]
17. Sterkowicz, S.; Lech, G.; Blecharz, J. Effects of laterality on the technical/tactical behavior in view of the results of judo fights. *Arch. Budo* **2010**, *6*, 173–177.
18. Lees, A. Technique analysis in sports: A critical review. *J. Sports Sci.* **2002**, *20*, 813–828. [CrossRef] [PubMed]
19. Kłys, A.; Sterkowicz-przybycień, K.; Adam, M.; Casals, C. Performance analysis considering the technical-tactical variables in female judo athletes at different sport skill levels: Optimization of predictors. *J. Phys. Educ. Sport* **2020**, *20*, 1775–1782. [CrossRef]
20. Coswig, V.S.; Gentil, P.; Bueno, J.C.A.; Follmer, B.; Marques, V.A.; Del Vecchio, F.B. Physical fitness predicts technical-tactical and time-motion profile in simulated Judo and Brazilian Jiu-Jitsu matches. *PeerJ* **2018**, *6*, e4851. [CrossRef] [PubMed]
21. Miarka, B.; Pérez, D.I.V.; Aedo-Muñoz, E.; da Costa, L.O.F.; Brito, C.J. Technical-Tactical Behaviors Analysis of Male and Female Judo Cadets' Combats. *Front. Psychol.* **2020**, *11*, 1389. [CrossRef]
22. Rydzik, Ł.; Ambroży, T. Physical Fitness and the Level of Technical and Tactical Training of Kickboxers. *Int. J. Environ. Res. Public Health* **2021**, *18*, 3088. [CrossRef]
23. Rydzik, Ł.; Niewczas, M.; Kędra, A.; Grymanowski, J.; Czarny, W.; Ambroży, T. Relation of indicators of technical and tactical training to demerits of kickboxers fighting in K1 formula. *Arch. Budo Sci. Martial Arts Extrem. Sports* **2020**, *16*, 1–5.
24. Vidal Andreato, L.; Franzói de Moraes, S.M.; Lopes de Moraes Gomes, T.; Del Conti Esteves, J.V.; Vidal Andreato, T.; Franchini, E. Estimated aerobic power, muscular strength and flexibility in elite Brazilian Jiu-Jitsu athletes. *Sci. Sports* **2011**, *26*, 329–337. [CrossRef]
25. Sterkowicz, S.; Ambroży, T. The fitness profile of the men who train ju-jitsu. *Antropomotoryka* **1992**, *7*, 135–141.
26. Menz, V.; Marterer, N.; Amin, S.B.; Faulhaber, M.; Hansen, A.B.; Lawley, J.S. Functional vs. Running Low-Volume High-Intensity Interval Training: Effects on VO2max and Muscular Endurance. *J. Sports Sci. Med.* **2019**, *18*, 497–504.
27. Ambroży, T.; Nowak, M.; Mucha, D.; Chwała, W.; Piwowarski, J.; Sieber, L. The influence of an original training programme on the general physical fitness of ju-jitsu trainees. *Ido Mov. Cult. J. Martial Arts Anthropol.* **2014**, *14*, 69–76.
28. Sterkowicz-Przybycień, K. Technical diversification, body composition and somatotype of both heavy and light Polish ju-jitsukas of high level. *Sci. Sports* **2010**, *25*, 194–200. [CrossRef]
29. Pitirkin, F.Y.; Kolomiets, O.I.; Petrushkina, N.P.; Sazanova, E.A. Optimization technologies of spine muscular-ligamentous apparatus functional state in young athletes, who go in for jiu-jitsu. *Pedagog.-Psychol. Med.-Biol. Probl. Phys. Cult. Sports* **2020**, *15*, 93–99. [CrossRef]
30. Ambroży, T.; Klimek, A.T.; Pilch, W. Wydolność anaerobowa reprezentantów Polski w Ju-Jitsu. *Med. Sport. Pract.* **2007**, *8*, 5–7.
31. Chwała, W.; Ambroży, T.; Sterkowicz, S. Three-dimensional analysis of the ju-jitsu competitors' motion during the performance of the ippon-seoi-nage throw. *Arch. Budo Sci. Martial Arts Extrem. Sports* **2013**, *9*, 41–53.
32. Ambroży, T.; Piwowarski, J.; Badeński, S. *Polski Związek Ju-Jitsu A Bezpieczeństwo: Sprawność, Skuteczność, Organizacja*; WSBPI Apeiron: Kraków, Poland, 2013.
33. Staller, M. The analysis of successfully applied techniques in part 1 in ju-jitsu fighting. *LASE J. Sport Sci.* **2013**, *4*, 14.
34. Heckele, S. Anforderungsprofile im Ju-Jutsu [Requirement profiles in ju-jitsu]. *Ju-Jutsu J.* **2002**, *10*, 3–4.
35. Litwiniuk, A.; Daniluk, A.; Cynarski, W.J.; Jespersen, E. Structure of personality of person training ju-jitsu and wrestling. *Arch. Budo* **2009**, *5*, 139–141.
36. Staller, M. The structure of ju-jitsu fighting fights and its relevance for elite athletes and coaches. *J. Teach. Educ.* **2013**, *2*, 241–247.
37. Wojdat, M.; Kanupriya, R.; Janowska, P.; Wolska, B.; Stępniak, R.; Adam, M. Comparative analysis of optimism and life satisfaction in Brazilian male and female Ju-Jitsu society. *J. Educ. Health Sport* **2017**, *7*, 139–154.
38. Lech, G.; Tyka, A.; Pałka, T.; Krawczyk, R. Effect of physical endurance on fighting and the level of sports per formance in junior judokas. *Arch. Budo* **2010**, *6*, 1–6.
39. Ambroży, T.; Maciejczyk, M.; Klimek, A.T.; Wiecha, S.; Stanula, A.; Snopkowski, P.; Pałka, T.; Jaworski, J.; Ambroży, D.; Rydzik, Ł.; et al. The effects of intermittent hypoxic training on anaerobic and aerobic power in boxers. *Int. J. Environ. Res. Public Health* **2020**, *17*, 9361. [CrossRef] [PubMed]
40. Story, G. Fitness testing for karate. *Sport* **1989**, 35–38.
41. Sterkowicz, S.; Zuchowicz, A.; Kubica, R. Levels of anaerobic and aerobic capacity indices and results for the special fitness test in judo competitors. *J. Hum. Kinet.* **1999**, *2*, 115–135.
42. Sterkowicz, S. Test specjalnej sprawnosci ruchowej w judo. Special Judo Fitness Test. *Antropomotoryka* **1995**, *12*, 13.
43. Ambroży, T.; Andrzej, K.; Krzysztof, W.; Kwiatkowski, A.; Sebastian, K.; Mucha, D. Propozycja Wykorzystania Autorskiego Testu Specjalnej Sprawności Fizycznej W Różnych Sportach Walki. *Secur. Econ. Law* **2017**, *3/2017*, 139–154. [CrossRef]
44. Ambroży, T.; Omorczyk, J.; Stanula, A.; Kwiatkowski, A.; Błach, W.; Mucha, D.; Andrzej, K. A Proposal for Special Kickboxing Fitness Test. *Secur. Dimens. Int. Natl. Stud.* **2016**, *20*, 96–110. [CrossRef]
45. Adam, M.; Smaruj, M.; Pujszo, R. Charakterystyka indywidualnego przygotowania techniczno-taktycznego zawodników judo, zwycięzców Mistrzostw Świata z Paryża w 2011 oraz z Tokio w 2010 roku. *IDO Mov. Cult. J. Martial Arts Anthropol.* **2012**, *12*, 60–69.
46. Arska-Kotlińska, M.; Bartz, J.; Wieliński, D. *Wybrane Zagadnienia Statystyki dla Studiujących Wychowanie Fizyczne*; AWF: Poznań, Poland, 2002.

47. Chwała, W.; Ambroży, T.; Ambroży, D. Poziom sprawności motorycznej warunkujący uzyskiwanie wysokich wyników w teście oceny podstawowej umiejętności samoobrony. In *R.M.Kalina (Red.): Wychowawcze i Utylitarne Aspekty Sportów Walki*; AWF Warszawa: Warszawa, Poland, 2000; pp. 53–57.
48. Sterkowicz, S.; Ambroży, T. *Ju-Jitsu Sportowe: Proces Szkolenia (Podręcznik Trenera)*; Europan Association for Security: Kraków, Poland, 2003.
49. Zoladz, J.A. *Muscle and Exercise Physiology*; Academic Pressa is an imprint of Elsevier: London, UK, 2019; ISBN 978-0-12-814593-7.
50. Myers, J.; Kaminsky, L.A.; Lima, R.; Christle, J.W.; Ashley, E.; Arena, R. A Reference Equation for Normal Standards for VO 2 Max: Analysis from the Fitness Registry and the Importance of Exercise National Database (FRIEND Registry). *Prog. Cardiovasc. Dis.* **2017**, *60*, 21–29. [CrossRef] [PubMed]
51. Silva, G.; Oliveira, N.L.; Aires, L.; Mota, J.; Oliveira, J.; Ribeiro, J.C. Calculation and validation of models for estimating VO 2max from the 20 -m shuttle run test in children and adolescents. *Arch. Exerc. Health Dis.* **2012**, *3*, 145–152. [CrossRef]
52. Pałka, T.; Lech, G.; Tyka, A.; Tyka, A.; Sterkowicz-Przybycień, K.; Sterkowicz, S.; Cebula, A.; Stawiarska, A. Differences in the level of anaerobic and aerobic components of physical capacity in judoists at different age. *Arch. Budo* **2013**, *9*, 195–203.
53. Ambroży, T.; Snopkowski, P.; Mucha, D.; Tota, Ł. Observation and analysis of a boxing fight. *Secur. Econ. Law* **2015**, *4*, 58–71.
54. Tota, Ł.; Drwal, T.; Maciejczyk, M.; Szyguła, Z.; Pilch, W.; Pałka, T.; Lech, G. Effects of original physical training program on changes in body composition, upper limb peak power and aerobic performance of a mixed martial arts fighter. *Med. Sport.* **2014**, *18*, 78–83. [CrossRef]
55. Ambroży, T.; Drwal, T.; Lech, G. Mixed Martial Arts fight analysis as an element of the trainer's control. In *Hiznayova K, Tonkovicova A. Športovy Trening. Vedecké Poznatky zo Športového Tréningu v Gymnastických Športoch, Tancoch, Úpoloch, Kulturistike a Fitness*; Katedra Gymnastiky FTVS UK: Bratisława, Slovakia, 2010; pp. 15–20.
56. Ouergui, I.; Hssin, N.; Haddad, M.; Padulo, J.; Franchini, E.; Gmada, N.; Bouhlel, E. The effects of five weeks of kickboxing training on physical fitness. *Muscles Ligaments Tendons J.* **2014**, *4*, 106–113. [CrossRef] [PubMed]
57. Ouergui, I.; Benyoussef, A.; Houcine, N.; Abedelmalek, S.; Franchini, E.; Gmada, N.; Bouhlel, E.; Bouassida, A. Physiological Responses and Time-Motion Analysis of Kickboxing: Differences Between Full Contact, Light Contact, and Point Fighting Contests. *J. Strength Cond. Res.* **2021**, *35*, 2558–2563. [CrossRef]
58. Little, N.G. Physical performance attributes of junior and senior women, juvenile, junior, and senior men judokas. *J. Sports Med. Phys. Fit.* **1991**, *31*, 510–520.
59. Drid, P.; Trivić, T.; Tabakov, S. Special Judo Fitness Test—A Review. *Serb. J. Sports Sci.* **2012**, *6*, 117–125.
60. Franchini, E.; Sterkowicz, S.; Szmatlan-Gabrys, U.; Gabrys, T.; Garnys, M. Energy System Contributions to the Special Judo Fitness Test. *Int. J. Sports Physiol. Perform.* **2011**, *6*, 334–343. [CrossRef] [PubMed]
61. Błach, W.; Rydzik, Ł.; Błach, Ł.; Cynarski, W.J.; Kostrzewa, M.; Ambroży, T. Characteristics of Technical and Tactical Preparation of Elite Judokas during the World Championships and Olympic Games. *Int. J. Environ. Res. Public Health* **2021**, *18*, 5841. [CrossRef]
62. Sertić, H.; Segedi, I. Structure of importance of techniques of throws in different age groups in men judo. *J. Combat Sport Martial Arts* **2012**, *3*, 59–62. [CrossRef]
63. Cynarski, W.J.; Słopecki, J.; Dziadek, B.; Böschen, P.; Piepiora, P. Indicators of Targeted Physical Fitness in Judo and Jujutsu—Preliminary Results of Research. *Int. J. Environ. Res. Public Health* **2021**, *18*, 4347. [CrossRef] [PubMed]
64. Ambroży, T.; Rydzik, Ł.; Kędra, A.; Ambroży, D.; Niewczas, M.; Sobiło, E.; Czarny, W. The effectiveness of kickboxing techniques and its relation to fights won by knockout. *Arch. Budo* **2020**, *16*, 11–17.
65. Ouergui, I.; Hssin, N.; Franchini, E.; Gmada, N.; Bouhlel, E. Technical and tactical analysis of high level kickboxing matches. *Int. J. Perform. Anal. Sport* **2013**, *13*, 294–309. [CrossRef]

Article

Is 20 Hz Whole-Body Vibration Training Better for Older Individuals than 40 Hz?

Shiuan-Yu Tseng [1], Chung-Po Ko [2], Chin-Yen Tseng [3], Wei-Ching Huang [4], Chung-Liang Lai [5,6] and Chun-Hou Wang [7,8,*]

1. Graduate Institute of Service Industries and Management, Minghsin University of Science and Technology, Hsinchu 30401, Taiwan; sytseng@must.edu.tw
2. Department of Neurosurgery, Tungs' Taichung MetroHarbor Hospital, Taichung 43503, Taiwan; cbko1218@gmail.com
3. Department of Physical Therapy, Upright Come Scoliosis Clinic, Hsinchu 30286, Taiwan; uprightcome@gmail.com
4. Department of Physical Medicine and Rehabilitation, Taichung Hospital, Ministry of Health and Welfare, Taichung 40343, Taiwan; fredaex@gmail.com
5. Department of Occupational Therapy, College of Medical and Health Science, Asia University, Taichung 41354, Taiwan; laipeter57@yahoo.com.tw
6. Department of Physical Medicine and Rehabilitation, Puzi Hospital, Ministry of Health and Welfare, Chiayi County 61347, Taiwan
7. Department of Physical Therapy, Chung Shan Medical University, Taichung 40201, Taiwan
8. Physical Therapy Room, Chung Shan Medical University Hospital, Taichung 40201, Taiwan
* Correspondence: chwang@csmu.edu.tw

Abstract: In recent years, whole-body vibration (WBV) training has been used as a training method in health promotion. This study attempted to use WBV at three different frequencies (20, 30, and 40 Hz) with subjects from different age groups to analyze the activation of the rectus femoris muscle. The subjects included 47 females and 51 males with an average age of 45.1 ± 15.2 years. Results indicated significant differences in subjects from different age groups at 20 Hz WBV. Muscle contraction was greater in the subjects who were older ($F_{(4,93)}$ = 82.448, $p < 0.001$). However, at 30 Hz WBV, the difference was not significant ($F_{(4,93)}$ = 2.373, $p = 0.058$). At 40 Hz WBV, muscle contraction was less in the older subjects than in the younger subjects ($F_{(4,93)}$ = 18.025, $p < 0.001$). The spectrum analysis also indicated that at 40 Hz there was less muscle activity during WBV in the older subjects than in the younger ones. Therefore, age was found to have a significant effect on muscle activation during WBV at different frequencies. If the training is offered to elderly subjects, their neuromuscular responses to 20 Hz WBV will be more suitable than to 40 Hz WBV.

Keywords: exercise; age groups; electromyography; rectus femoris

1. Introduction

Whole-body vibration (WBV) training is a neuromuscular training method. In recent years it has become popular in health promotion centers and gyms as an alternative training method or as a supplement to traditional training and treatment [1]. In addition, WBV has been comprehensively applied to various populations, such as young adults, middle-aged adults, and older adults [2,3], to achieve positive effects on neuromuscular performance, such as increased muscle strength [4], increased muscle endurance [5], and increased electromyography (EMG) activities [6].

It has been verified that the WBV training process can increase the neuromuscular activity recorded by surface EMG [7]. Although no consensus has been reached on the mechanism of the effect of WBV training on the neuromuscular system, many studies suggest that WBV training triggers the mechanism of the stretch reflex. This causes an excitatory response in the muscle spindles to induce a large amount of activity in the motor units [8]. Many studies have confirmed that the vibration frequency parameters of a body structure subjected to WBV training have an important effect on neurophysiological responses [9]. In an analysis of the effects of WBV characteristics on neuromuscular performance, Luo et al. (2005) suggested that the most effective frequency for generating greater muscle activity is between 30 and 50 Hz [10]. However, some studies have indicated that the maximum acceleration of the knee and hip occurs at approximately 15 Hz, and then decreases as the vibration frequency is increased [11].

Although WBV training has been comprehensively used in sports training and rehabilitation, no consensus has been reached on how WBV training induces neurophysiological responses in skeletal muscle [12]. Some studies have suggested that increased muscle activity during WBV training is associated with higher vibration frequencies and a greater vibration machine amplitude [13]. On the contrary, a study by Cardinale and Lim showed that compared with 40 and 50 Hz, a WBV frequency of 30 Hz provided the largest EMG activities of the vastus lateralis muscle [6].

A previous study showed that the median frequency (MF) and mean power frequency (MPF) slopes in the electromyography activities of elderly males during muscle endurance tests consisting of back stretching were significantly lower than those of young males [14]. This suggests that the corresponding muscle fibers in older adults are different from those in young people. Therefore, it would indeed be worthwhile to investigate whether WBV training may cause different neuromuscular responses in young people and in older adults. Previous studies have seldom investigated or tested the neuromuscular signal performances of all age groups during WBV training at different frequencies. Therefore, this study recorded the electromyography activities on the rectus femoris muscle of different age groups using WBV at 20, 30, and 40 Hz. These frequencies are often selected for WBV training and were analyzed to determine whether any responses were different.

2. Materials and Methods

2.1. Subjects

This study was one part of a research project titled "Effects of Vibration Training on Physiology in the Human Body". The research project was conducted according to the Declaration of Helsinki and was approved by the hospital's Institutional Review Board for research involving human subjects (Taichung Hospital, Ministry of Health and Welfare, Taiwan, I980021). All of the participants were fully informed of the study's content policy before they participated, and all signed informed consent forms. The registered clinical trial number is ChiCTR-ICR-15006239. The subjects enrolled in the study were hospital volunteers and community members. All the subjects were healthy. None of the subjects had a history of neuromuscular disease, and none of the subjects were diagnosed with illness at the time of the investigation. The subjects were divided into groups according to their age: 20–29 years old; 30–39 years old; 40–49 years old; 50–59 years old; and 60–69 years old. There were a total of 5 groups.

2.2. WBV Training

The instrument used in this study was a whole-body vibration training machine (Commercial Grade Vibration Machine LV-1000; X-Trend, Taiwan). The vibration patterns had a peak-to-peak amplitude of 4 mm with a synchronous vibration platform. The frequencies were 20 Hz, 30 Hz, and 40 Hz. Participants received training for five minutes each time. Each frequency of whole-body vibration was randomly executed on different days. The subjects stood barefoot and without any support on the vibration platform with the knees in slight flexion position (10–15°).

2.3. Measurement of the EMG Signals of Rectus Femoris Muscle

The surface EMG signals were recorded from the rectus femoris muscle of the dominant leg to represent the knee extension muscle by a Noraxon EMG system (Noraxon Telemyo 2400T G2, Scottsdale, AZ, USA). Bipolar surface electrodes (Ag/AgCl) were applied over the belly muscle (interelectrode distance 25 mm) in accordance with SENIAM recommendations [15]. The pre-amplified EMG signals were amplified (×1000), band-pass filtered at 10–500 Hz ± 2% cut-off (Butterworth/Bessels), and sampled at 1500 Hz. MyoResearch software (Noraxon, Scottsdale, AZ, USA) was used to collect and store the data for analysis.

2.3.1. Measurement of the EMG Signals of Maximal Voluntary Isometric Contraction (MVIC)

A Biodex dynamometer (Biodex System 4 Pro, Biodex Medical Systems Inc., Shirley, NY, USA) was used to provide appropriate resistance against the MVIC; subjects were in a sitting position with knee flexion of 30 degrees [16]. The Noraxon EMG system was used to record the muscle activity of the rectus femoris muscle during MVIC [17]. Each subject performed the MVIC three times consecutively for five seconds each time, with three-minute rests between trials. The average value was recorded as EMG_{MVIC}.

2.3.2. Measurement of the Muscle Activity during Static Standing and WBV

The EMG signals were recorded once the subjects had taken up the correct position on the vibration platform (trunk erect with hip and knee in slight flexion). In the first 6–8 s, muscle activity was recorded without a WBV stimulus (static standing). Then WBV was applied at the frequency the participant was randomized to, and the EMG was recorded for the next 5 min. The root mean square (RMS) value was determined based on the EMG signal during the period of static standing and WBV, which represented the amplitude of muscle activity. Neuromuscular activation during the exercises was defined as the RMS EMG signal normalized to the peak RMS EMG signal of a MVIC [18], recorded as percentage of EMG_{MVIC}.

2.3.3. Frequency Spectrum Analysis of the EMG Signals

The EMG activities of the subjects at 20, 30, and 40 Hz of WBV during standing with slight knee flexion were recorded, and then a spectral analysis of the EMG signal was performed using fast Fourier transformation (FFT). After the frequency spectrum was obtained, a band-stop filter was used to block the interference signal generated by the vibration of the WBV machine. It was also used to block artifacts caused by harmonic vibration at 60 Hz that would coincide with any interference from nearby electrical equipment and power lines. Then, the frequency spectrum of the voluntary muscle contraction during WBV at different frequencies was obtained [19].

2.4. Statistical Analysis

All statistical analyses were conducted with SPSS v17.0 software (IBM Corp., Armonk, NY, USA). This study used the chi-square test and one-way ANOVA to analyze whether there were any differences in the basic attributes of the subjects in different age groups. Two-way mixed repeated-measure ANOVA was used to analyze the differences in EMG signals among the subjects of different age groups at 20, 30, and 40 Hz WBV. Then the Scheffe post hoc test was used to compare the differences among various age groups. All tests were two-sided, and the significance level was defined as $\alpha = 0.05$.

3. Results

The basic characteristics of the subjects (including age, sex, and BMI), the RMS of the MVIC, and the static standing of the rectus femoris muscle are shown in Table 1. The subjects included 47 females and 51 males with an average age of 45.1 ± 15.2 years and an average BMI of 23.5 ± 3.3 kg/m^2, respectively. The average EMG_{MVIC} was 260.6 ± 109.5 μV. The static standing EMGRMS normalized by EMG_{MVIC} was 12.1 ± 7.6%. The data in Table 1 shows statistically significant differences in age, height, and BMI between different groups ($p < 0.05$). Young people had higher EMG_{MVIC} than older people ($p < 0.001$), while SS_EMG_{MVIC} was much higher for older people than for young people ($p < 0.001$).

Table 1. The basic characteristics of the participants ($n = 98$).

	20–29 Years Old Group ($n = 21$)	30–39 Years Old Group ($n = 18$)	40–49 Years Old Group ($n = 18$)	50–59 Years Old Group ($n = 20$)	60–69 Years Old Group ($n = 21$)	p-Value
Age (years)	24.2 (22.9–25.5)	34.7 (33.3–36.1)	46.1 (44.9–47.3)	54.0 (52.6–55.4)	65.7 (64.7–66.7)	<0.001 *
Sex (Male/Female)	12/9	9/9	11/7	10/10	9/12	0.811
Height (cm)	168.6 (164.0–173.3)	162.3 (157.5–167.0)	164.1 (160.4–167.9)	164.0 (160.8–167.2)	160.2 (157.2–163.2)	0.024 *
Body Mass (kg)	62.0 (56.4–67.7)	61.2 (54.5–67.9)	68.2 (62.8–73.6)	64.8 (58.9–70.6)	61.9 (57.3–66.5)	0.357
Body Mass Index	21.6 (20.5–22.7)	23.0 (21.4–24.6)	25.3 (23.6–27.0)	23.9 (22.3–25.6)	23.6 (22.7–25.3)	0.007 *
EMG_{MVIC} (µV)	321.4 (289.5–353.4)	296.4 (273.5–369.6)	275.0 (226.0–324.0)	210.8 (167.8–253.8)	182.8 (156.2–209.4)	<0.001 *
SS_EMG_{MVIC} (%)	7.6 (6.0–9.24)	8.5 (6.6–10.4)	8.1 (6.2–9.9)	15.3 (11.8–18.9)	19.0 (15.8–22.1)	<0.001 *

* $p < 0.05$; the values are given as mean (95% confidence interval). EMG_{MVIC}: the root mean square EMG of the rectus femoris muscle during maximum voluntary isometric contraction; SS_EMG_{MVIC}: the root mean square EMG of the rectus femoris muscle during static standing normalized by the EMG_{MVIC}.

3.1. Comparison between Different Age Groups during Same Frequency WBV

This study found a significant difference in the neuromuscular activation of the rectus femoris muscle (normalized by EMG_{MVIC}) among the various age groups at 20 Hz WBV. Muscle contraction was greater in the subjects who were older than in those who were younger ($F_{(4,93)} = 82.448$, $p < 0.001$). However, at 30 Hz WBV, the difference among the various age groups was not significant ($F_{(4,93)} = 2.373$, $p = 0.058$). At 40 Hz WBV, there was also a significant difference among the various age groups. Muscle contraction was less in the subjects who were older than in those who were younger ($F_{(4,93)} = 18.025$, $p < 0.001$) (Table 2).

Table 2. The neuromuscular activation of the rectus femoris muscle during whole-body vibration training at different frequencies in different age groups.

WBV Frequency	20–29 Years Old Group ($n = 21$)	30–39 Years Old Group ($n = 18$)	40–49 Years Old Group ($n = 18$)	50–59 Years Old Group ($n = 20$)	60–69 Years Old Group ($n = 21$)	p-Value
20 Hz	21.4 [d,e] (18.0–24.7)	22.2 [d,e] (17.1–27.3)	22.7 [d,e] (18.3–27.1)	49.7 [a,b,c,e] (44.4–54.9)	69.2 [a,b,c,d] (62.8–75.7)	<0.001 *
30 Hz	43.7 (38.0–49.4)	40.3 (34.1–46.6)	50.0 (40.4–59.7)	53.3 (44.2–62.3)	39.9 (30.8–49.0)	0.058
40 Hz	64.7 [d,e] (58.9–70.6)	60.6 [d,e] (54.4–66.8)	60.4 [d,e] (51.7–69.1)	35.6 [a,b,c] (26.8–44.4)	34.4 [a,b,c] (27.2–41.6)	<0.001 *
p-Value	<0.001 *	<0.001 *	<0.001 *	0.006 *	<0.001 *	

* $p < 0.05$; the values are given as mean (95% confidence interval); WBV: whole-body vibration. Using the Scheffe test, [a]: showed a significant difference in the 20–29 years old age group ($p < 0.001$); [b]: showed a significant difference in the 30–39 years old age group ($p < 0.001$); [c]: showed a significant difference in the 40–49 years old age group ($p < 0.001$); [d]: showed a significant difference in the 50–59 years old age group ($p < 0.001$); [e]: showed a significant difference in the 60–69 years old age group ($p < 0.001$).

3.2. Interactions of Different Age Groups during WBV at Different Frequencies

Comparisons of the three frequencies (20, 30, and 40 Hz) showed significant differences in the 20–29 years old, 30–39 years old and 40–49 years old age groups: higher frequencies of WBV were related to greater neuromuscular activation ($p < 0.001$), and rectus femoris muscle activity was greater at 30 and 40 Hz than at 20 Hz. In the 50–59 years old age group, there was a significant difference ($p = 0.006$). The between-group comparisons of the three frequencies showed that unlike the muscle activity at 20 and 30 Hz, there was a significant difference at 40 Hz (p was 0.018 and 0.005, respectively). The muscle activity was also greater at 20 and 30 Hz than at 40 Hz. In the 60–69 years old age group, there was a significant difference (F = 29.026, $p < 0.001$). The between-group comparisons of the three frequencies showed a significant difference at 20 Hz ($p < 0.001$); the muscle activity at 20 Hz WBV was greater than that at 30 and 40 Hz. However, the between-group comparison of 30 and 40 Hz showed no significant difference ($p > 0.999$), as shown in Figure 1.

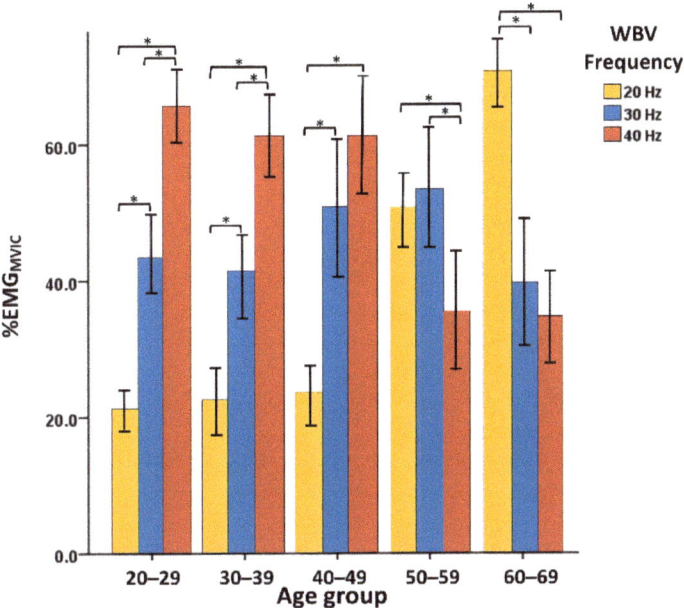

Figure 1. The neuromuscular activation of rectus femoris muscle during 20, 30, and 40 Hz whole-body vibration normalized by EMG_{MVIC}. * $p < 0.05$; the values are presented as mean ± 1.96 SE (standard error).

3.3. Frequency Spectrum Analysis

The spectrum analysis also indicated that there was no significant difference between older subjects and younger subjects during WBV at 20 Hz. However, during WBV at 30 and 40 Hz, the muscle activity patterns of older subjects were different from those of younger subjects. The 50–59 and 60–69 years old age groups had more muscle firing at 20 Hz WBV than 30 Hz or 40 Hz, as shown in Figure 2.

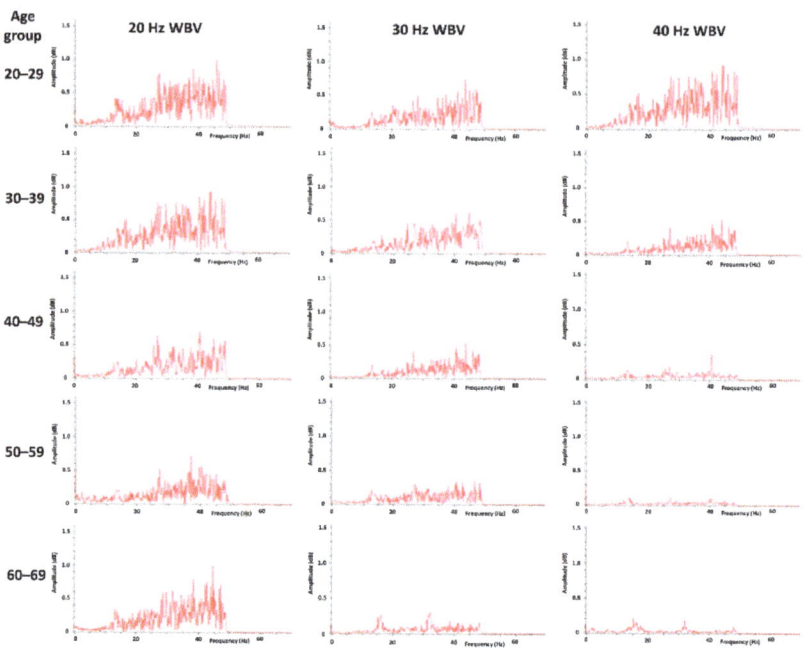

Figure 2. The frequency spectrum of a typical case of rectus femoris muscle EMG signals of different age groups during whole-body vibration at different frequencies.

4. Discussion

The aim of this study was to investigate the lower limb electromyography activities of different age groups during training with WBV at different frequencies. The results showed that age had a significant effect on rectus femoris EMG activity with WBV at different frequencies. Therefore, it is advised that age be considered in the setting of the frequency parameters of WBV training. Macadam and Feser (2019) recommend a high level of activation (41 to 60% of MVIC) [20], and a very high level of activation (greater than 60% of MVIC). This study found that 20 Hz WBV should be used in older subjects (>50 years old) at a high and very high level of muscle activation, while 40 Hz WBV should be used in younger subjects (<50 years old) at a very high level of activation to strengthen the muscle of the knee extension. Boren et al. (2011) pointed out the exercises that produced greater than 70% of MVIC. These exercises were deemed acceptable for the enhancement of strength [21]. This study found that 20 Hz WBV could induce about 70% of MVIC in the 60–69 years old age group, which might be a good choice as a muscle-strengthening program for older persons. The mixed use of WBV at different frequencies in training programs should be reviewed and possibly changed.

When the WBV training frequency was set at 20 Hz, there was a significant increase in the EMG signals of muscle activations for all age groups as compared with static standing (F = 627.834, $p < 0.001$). This result is consistent with those of other studies [13,22]. Although there is a lack of consistent evidence, it has been generally perceived that during WBV training, the displacement changes generated by the vibration platform cause a sensory reflex and muscle contraction of the Ia muscle spindle. This is considered to be the main cause of motor unit changes [23]. Similar results have been reported in previous studies, reflecting the increase in muscle activity during vibration stimulation [19]. Vibration is an external disturbance to the body's standing balance. When it is in contact with the body structure, it is sensed by the central nervous system, which in turn regulates the stiffness of the stimulated muscle groups. According to the study of Cardinale and Lim (2003), the muscle activity of the stretch reflex can be considered as a neuromuscular regulatory response that minimizes the effect on soft tissues caused by vibration [6].

The percentage of MVIC values in ages above 50 years old were significantly larger than in age groups below 50 years old at 20 Hz WBV ($p < 0.001$). Previous research results have shown that the balance ability and lower-limb knee extensor muscle strength performance in the elderly are significantly higher after WBV training at 20 Hz than after WBV training at 40 Hz [24]. This study also found that during WBV training at frequencies of 30 Hz and 40 Hz, there was a trend of smaller muscle activity in the older subjects. At the vibration frequency of 40 Hz, the percentage of MVIC values in two groups (the 60–69 age group and the 50–59 age group) were significantly smaller than those in the 40–49, 30–39, and 20–29 age groups ($p < 0.001$). The spectrum analysis figures also showed less EMG activity in the older subjects than in the younger subjects during WBV training at 40 Hz. This result is similar to those of previous studies, suggesting that the training frequency amplitude is unlikely to cause muscle strengthening in healthy young people at a frequency greater than 15 Hz. However, this frequency may be sufficient to cause muscle strengthening in physically weak individuals [11]. Jakobsson (1990) and Verdijk et al. (1990) indicated that the proportion of Type I muscle fibers in the lower-limb muscles is higher in the elderly than in young people, which may be the reason why there is no neuromuscular signal response in the elderly receiving high-frequency WBV training [25,26].

One limitation of this study is that the intensity of WBV (frequency and amplitude) was not investigated. In this study, only the frequency was changed. The amplitude of the WBV was not. However, other studies have verified that there is no dose–response relationship between the intensity of WBV and the optimization of neuromuscular activation and muscle strength [13,27]. In consideration of the research limitations, future studies may lengthen the WBV training time to two or three months, or expand the vibration training to different amplitudes to understand the relative neuromuscular changes in the WBV training of different age groups.

The results of this study are consistent with those of previous studies in that electromyography activity in the elderly did not increase with increases in WBV frequency to 30 Hz and 40 Hz. Previous literature has suggested that studies on surface EMG analysis should be done cautiously during WBV training [19]. The alternating current signal interference (60 Hz) and the vibration frequencies (20, 30, and 40 Hz) of the WBV machine will degrade the quality and reliability of the analysis data [28]. The above signal can be removed using spectrum analysis filtered by a band-stop filter. As proven by Fratini et al. (2009), a relatively correct EMG signal can be obtained after a specific filter is used for proper signal processing [29]. This study also dealt with EMG signals in accordance with this recommendation.

5. Conclusions

The research results showed that the muscle activities of the rectus femoris in the 60–69 years old age group at 20 Hz WBV were significantly greater than those in the 20–29, 30–39, 40–49, and 50–59 years old age groups. However, opposite results were obtained at 30 and 40 Hz WBV. As a result, age was found to have a significant effect on the EMG activity during WBV at different frequencies. Therefore, during WBV training, it is necessary to prioritize age when setting the training parameters. It is advised that WBV at 20 Hz be provided in the training of older adults (>60 years old), which may result in more significant neuromuscular responses.

Author Contributions: Conceptualization, S.-Y.T. and C.-H.W.; methodology, S.-Y.T., C.-H.W., C.-L.L. and C.-P.K.; validation, C.-Y.T. and W.-C.H.; formal analysis, S.-Y.T. and. C.-H.W.; investigation, S.-Y.T., C.-L.L. and C.-P.K.; resources, C.-L.L. and C.-P.K.; data curation, C.-Y.T. and W.-C.H.; writing—original draft preparation, S.-Y.T. and C.-H.W.; writing—review and editing, S.-Y.T., C.-H.W., C.-L.L., C.-Y.T., W.-C.H. and C.-P.K.; visualization, C.-L.L.; supervision, C.-P.K.; project administration, C.-

H.W.; funding acquisition, C.-H.W., C.-L.L. and C.-P.K. All authors have read and agreed to the published version of the manuscript.

Funding: This work was supported by a research grant from Taichung Hospital, Ministry of Health and Welfare, Taiwan (No. 9914). The funder had no role in study design, data collection and analysis, decision to publish, or preparation of the manuscript. No commercial party having a direct financial interest in the results of the research supporting this article has or will confer a benefit upon the authors or upon any organization with which the authors are associated.

Institutional Review Board Statement: The research project was conducted according to the Declaration of Helsinki and was approved by the hospital Institutional Review Board for research involving human subjects (Taichung Hospital, Ministry of Health and Welfare, Taiwan, I980021). The registered clinical trial number is ChiCTR-ICR-15006239.

Informed Consent Statement: Informed consent was obtained from all subjects involved in the study.

Data Availability Statement: The datasets used and/or analyzed during the current study are available from the study group on reasonable request. Please contact the corresponding author.

Acknowledgments: The authors would like to thank Ing-Shiou Hwang, who assisted with processing the EMG signals in this study.

Conflicts of Interest: The authors declare no conflict of interest.

References

1. Alam, M.M.; Khan, A.A.; Farooq, M. Effect of whole-body vibration on neuromuscular performance: A literature review. *Work* **2018**, *59*, 571–583. [CrossRef]
2. Cochrane, D.J.; Sartor, F.; Winwood, K.; Stannard, S.R.; Narici, M.V.; Rittweger, J. A Comparison of the Physiologic Effects of Acute Whole-Body Vibration Exercise in Young and Older People. *Arch. Phys. Med. Rehabil.* **2008**, *89*, 815–821. [CrossRef]
3. Nam, S.-S.; Sunoo, S.; Park, H.-Y.; Moon, H.-W. The effects of long-term whole-body vibration and aerobic exercise on body composition and bone mineral density in obese middle-aged women. *J. Exerc. Nutr. Biochem.* **2016**, *20*, 19–27. [CrossRef] [PubMed]
4. Lai, C.-C.; Tu, Y.-K.; Wang, T.-G.; Huang, Y.-T.; Chien, K.-L. Effects of resistance training, endurance training and whole-body vibration on lean body mass, muscle strength and physical performance in older people: A systematic review and network meta-analysis. *Age Ageing* **2018**, *47*, 367–373. [CrossRef]
5. Ritzmann, R.; Krämer, A.; Bernhardt, S.; Gollhofer, A. Whole Body Vibration Training—Improving Balance Control and Muscle Endurance. *PLoS ONE* **2014**, *9*, e89905. [CrossRef] [PubMed]
6. Cardinale, M.; Lim, J. Electromyography Activity of Vastus Lateralis Muscle During Whole-Body Vibrations of Different Frequencies. *J. Strength Cond. Res.* **2003**, *17*, 621–624. [CrossRef] [PubMed]
7. Wirth, B.; Zurfluh, S.; Müller, R. Acute effects of whole-body vibration on trunk muscles in young healthy adults. *J. Electromyogr. Kinesiol.* **2011**, *21*, 450–457. [CrossRef]
8. Bosco, C.; Cardinale, M.; Tsarpela, O. Influence of vibration on mechanical power and electromyogram activity in human arm flexor muscles. *Graefe's Arch. Clin. Exp. Ophthalmol.* **1999**, *79*, 306–311. [CrossRef]
9. Bazett-Jones, D.M.; Finch, H.W.; Dugan, E.L. Comparing the Effects of Various Whole-Body Vibration Accelerations on Counter-Movement Jump Performance. *J. Sports Sci. Med.* **2008**, *7*, 144–150.
10. Luo, J.; McNamara, B.; Moran, K. The Use of Vibration Training to Enhance Muscle Strength and Power. *Sports Med.* **2005**, *35*, 23–41. [CrossRef]
11. Pollock, R.D.; Woledge, R.; Mills, K.R.; Martin, F.C.; Newham, D. Muscle activity and acceleration during whole body vibration: Effect of frequency and amplitude. *Clin. Biomech.* **2010**, *25*, 840–846. [CrossRef] [PubMed]
12. Borges, D.T.; Macedo, L.; Lins, C.A.A.; Sousa, C.; Brasileiro, J.S. Effects of Whole Body Vibration on the Neuromuscular Amplitude of Vastus Lateralis Muscle. *J. Sports Sci. Med.* **2017**, *16*, 414–420. [PubMed]
13. Hazell, T.J.; Jakobi, J.M.; Kenno, K.A. The effects of whole-body vibration on upper- and lower-body EMG during static and dynamic contractions. *Appl. Physiol. Nutr. Metab.* **2007**, *32*, 1156–1163. [CrossRef] [PubMed]
14. Süüden, E.; Ereline, J.; Gapeyeva, H.; Pääsuke, M. Low back muscle fatigue during Sørensen endurance test in patients with chronic low back pain: Relationship between electromyographic spectral compression and anthropometric characteristics. *Electromyogr. Clin. Neurophysiol.* **2008**, *48*, 185–192.
15. Hermens, H.J.; Freriks, B.; Disselhorst-Klug, C.; Rau, G. Development of recommendations for SEMG sensors and sensor placement procedures. *J. Electromyogr. Kinesiol.* **2000**, *10*, 361–374. [CrossRef]
16. Krishnan, C.; Allen, E.J.; Ms, P.E.J.A. Effect of knee position on quadriceps muscle force steadiness and activation strategies. *Muscle Nerve* **2011**, *43*, 563–573. [CrossRef]

17. Girard, O.; Brocherie, F.; Millet, G.P. High Altitude Increases Alteration in Maximal Torque but Not in Rapid Torque Development in Knee Extensors after Repeated Treadmill Sprinting. *Front. Physiol.* **2016**, *7*, 97. [CrossRef]
18. Andersen, L.L.; Magnusson, S.P.; Nielsen, M.; Haleem, J.; Poulsen, K.; Aagaard, P. Neuromuscular Activation in Conventional Therapeutic Exercises and Heavy Resistance Exercises: Implications for Rehabilitation. *Phys. Ther.* **2006**, *86*, 683–697. [CrossRef]
19. Abercromby, A.F.J.; Amonette, W.E.; Layne, C.S.; Mcfarlin, B.K.; Hinman, M.R.; Paloski, W.H. Variation in Neuromuscular Responses during Acute Whole-Body Vibration Exercise. *Med. Sci. Sports Exerc.* **2007**, *39*, 1642–1650. [CrossRef]
20. Macadam, P.; Feser, E.H. Examination of Gluteus Maximus Electromyographic Excitation Associated with Dynamic Hip Extension During Body Weight Exercise: A Systematic Review. *Int. J. Sports Phys. Ther.* **2019**, *14*, 14–31. [CrossRef]
21. Boren, K.; Conrey, C.; Le Coguic, J.; Paprocki, L.; Voight, M.; Robinson, T.K. Electromyographic Analysis of Gluteus Medius And Gluteus Maximus During Rehabilitation Exercises. *Int. J. Sports Phys. Ther.* **2011**, *6*, 206–223. [PubMed]
22. Ritzmann, R.; Kramer, A.; Gruber, M.; Gollhofer, A.; Taube, W. EMG activity during whole body vibration: Motion artifacts or stretch reflexes? *Graefe's Arch. Clin. Exp. Ophthalmol.* **2010**, *110*, 143–151. [CrossRef] [PubMed]
23. Pollock, R.D.; Woledge, R.; Martin, F.C.; Newham, D. Effects of whole body vibration on motor unit recruitment and threshold. *J. Appl. Physiol.* **2012**, *112*, 388–395. [CrossRef] [PubMed]
24. Tseng, S.Y.; Hsu, P.S.; Lai, C.L.; Liao, W.C.; Lee, M.C.; Wang, C.H. Effect of Two Frequencies of Whole-Body Vibration Training on Balance and Flexibility of the Elderly: A Randomized Controlled Trial. *Am. J. Phys. Med. Rehabil.* **2016**, *95*, 730–737. [CrossRef]
25. Jakobsson, F.; Borg, K. Fibre-type composition, structure and cytoskeletal protein location of fibres in anterior tibial muscle. Comparison between young adults and physically active aged humans. *Acta Neuropathol.* **1990**, *80*, 459–468. [CrossRef]
26. Verdijk, L.B.; Koopman, R.; Schaart, G.; Meijer, K.; Savelberg, H.H.C.M.; van Loon, L.J.C. Satellite cell content is specifically reduced in type II skeletal muscle fibers in the elderly. *Am. J. Physiol. Metab.* **2007**, *292*, E151–E157. [CrossRef]
27. Marín, P.J.; Herrero, A.J.; García-López, D.; Rhea, M.R.; López-Chicharro, J.; González-Gallego, J.; Garatachea, N. Acute Effects of Whole-Body Vibration on Neuromuscular Responses in Older Individuals: Implications for Prescription of Vibratory Stimulation. *J. Strength Cond. Res.* **2012**, *26*, 232–239. [CrossRef]
28. Lienhard, K.; Cabasson, A.; Meste, O.; Colson, S.S. Comparison of sEMG processing methods during whole-body vibration exercise. *J. Electromyogr. Kinesiol.* **2015**, *25*, 833–840. [CrossRef]
29. Fratini, A.; Cesarelli, M.; Bifulco, P.; Romano, M. Relevance of motion artifact in electromyography recordings during vibration treatment. *J. Electromyogr. Kinesiol.* **2009**, *19*, 710–718. [CrossRef]

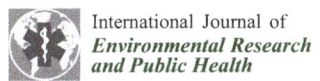

Review

Physical Characteristics and Physical Fitness Profiles of Korean Taekwondo Athletes: A Systematic Review

Jeong-Weon Kim [1] and Sang-Seok Nam [2,*]

1. Graduate School of Professional Therapy, Gachon University, 1342 Seongnam-daero, Sujeong-gu, Seongnam-si 13120, Korea; zeezone@gachon.ac.kr
2. Taekwondo Research Institute, Kukkiwon, 32 Teheran 7-gil, Gangnam-gu, Seoul 06130, Korea
* Correspondence: playdata.n@gmail.com; Tel.: +82-2-3469-0181

Abstract: This study aimed to present a standard and normal distribution of Taekwondo athletes' physical characteristics and physical fitness profiles using a systematic review. A systematic search was conducted using four Korean databases (Research Information Sharing Service, National Digital Science Library, DBpia, and Korean Studies Information Service System). From 2010 to 2020, we reviewed 838 papers on Taekwondo athletes' physical characteristics and physical fitness factors (e.g., body composition, muscle strength, muscular endurance, flexibility, cardiorespiratory fitness, power, agility, balance, speed, and reaction time). Of them, 24 papers were selected and analyzed. The criteria for selecting the physical characteristics and physical fitness factors for data extraction were set to have a total sample size of more than 30 individuals and included two or more studies. The sample size and average and standard deviation of physical characteristics and physical fitness factors were extracted from each selected study. In this study, the estimation error of all variables, except for the eyes-closed single-leg stance (15.71%), was less than 8%. Therefore, it was confirmed that there was no problem with the validity of the estimated values. These results could be used as an essential objective basis for evaluating the physical characteristics and physical fitness profiles of Taekwondo athletes in most countries worldwide and setting training goals.

Keywords: taekwondo; physical characteristics; physical fitness; systematic review; normal distribution

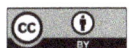

1. Introduction

Taekwondo is an international martial arts sport conducted in 210 countries worldwide as an official Olympic sport. A Taekwondo competition occurs in three rounds, with a duration of 2 min per round and a rest duration of 1 min between rounds [1]. Athletes who score more points or knock out their opponent win. During a competition, athletes use powerful and fast kicks and punches on their opponent's trunk and sometimes kicks to the face [2]. These movements are high-intensity anaerobic or aerobic exercises that induce powerful lower-extremity movements [3]. In addition, agility, flexibility, and muscular endurance are required to maintain an excellent performance among Taekwondo athletes [4–6]. Therefore, it is necessary to manage physical fitness factors to improve their performance [7]. This can be achieved by accurately evaluating the level of fitness of athletes and setting goals. Athletes need to know their physical characteristics and physical fitness profiles for effective training because high levels of physical fitness can affect their exercise performance [8]. Suppose there is a basis for the standard distribution of physical fitness profiles necessary for the characteristics of sports events. In this case, it can be used to evaluate athletes' fitness levels and set training goals. Although the physical fitness profiles of taekwondo athletes have been well described in the previous studies, no studies have examined the standard distribution of physical fitness [9–11].

Heller et al. [9] compared the physical fitness factors of 23 national Taekwondo athletes from the Czech Republic to those of the general public. Meanwhile, Marković [10] divided

13 women from the Croatian national Taekwondo team into medal-winning and non-medal-winning athletes at World Championships or Olympic Games, comparing the physical fitness profiles between them. In addition, Mathunjwa et al. [11] studied the physical characteristics of 36 internationally ranked junior Taekwondo athletes; the physical fitness test results were standardized in z-scores, which were then compared among the athletes. Furthermore, Bridge et al. [12] and da Silva Santos et al. [13] reported the physical characteristics and physical fitness of Taekwondo athletes using a systematic review but did not present any quantitative results.

Previous studies have provided information on the physical characteristics and physical fitness of Taekwondo athletes [12,13]. However, it is difficult to use them as a specific indicator because there is no standard distribution to evaluate the level of physical fitness of Taekwondo athletes. Standard distribution data are needed to determine the mean and percentile values of Taekwondo athletes' physical characteristics and physical fitness parameters. In general, a standard distribution is meaningful when the measurement results of a large sample form a normal distribution [14]. However, it can be analyzed via a systematic review using the measured variables in a previous study [15]. In other words, the results could be interpreted as a normal distribution when the sum of sample sizes is sufficiently large by integrating each previous study [15]. Nevertheless, the validity and reliability of the resulting values can be questioned if different prior studies have different measurement tools. However, the measurement of physical characteristics and physical fitness variables has become common worldwide. Furthermore, the systematic review method can resolve the concerns about reliability and validity by eliminating extreme values when integrating the results of variables [15]. Thus, the standard distribution of physical characteristics and physical fitness factors can be estimated using the pooled mean and pooled standard deviation from previous studies.

The purpose of this study was to present a standard and normal distribution of Taekwondo athletes' physical characteristics and physical fitness profiles using a systematic review.

2. Materials and Methods

2.1. Search Strategy

A systematic search was conducted using four Korean databases. Korean taekwondo athletes were selected as the research subjects because they have the best performance in the world. We searched the Research Information Sharing Service (RISS), National Digital Science Library (NDSL), DBpia, and Korean Studies Information Service System (KISS), using the following terms: "Taekwon", "athlete", "physical fitness", and Korean terms. Data were collected up to December 2020 and regularly updated manually. At the initial stage of screening, articles published before 31 December 2009 were excluded. The study was conducted in accordance with the guidelines of the Declaration of Helsinki and was approved by the Institutional Review Board of Konkuk University (7001355-201804-E-077).

2.2. Inclusion and Exclusion Criteria

In the first step we input the database search results to Microsoft Excel 2019 and performed duplicate elimination. This study focused on describing the physical characteristics and physical fitness profiles of Korean Taekwondo athletes. For this reason, all papers on the physical characteristics and physical fitness of Korean Taekwondo athletes were included in this study. Articles were excluded for the following reasons: (1) data aside from physical characteristics; (2) data aside from physical fitness; (3) irrelevant data for analysis; (4) non-competition Taekwondo athletes; (5) unavailable full-text; (6) duplicates; and (7) conference presentations, case reports, commentaries, and review articles. Two independent authors evaluated the eligibility of each item. In addition, qualified articles were collected for data extraction steps via reading and evaluation of the full text of each paper. Finally, an article suitable for the data extraction process was included.

2.3. Data Extraction

Two independent authors performed the data extraction. The criteria for selecting the physical characteristics and physical fitness factors for data extraction were set to have a total sample size of more than 30 individuals and included two or more studies. The sample size and average and standard deviation of the physical characteristics and physical fitness factors were extracted from each selected study.

2.4. Data Calculation and Statistical Analysis

2.4.1. Pooled Mean Calculation

Two independent authors performed the data extraction. The pooled mean was calculated using the mean and sample size from the final selected study using Formula (1).

$$\text{Mean}_{\text{pooled}} = \frac{(m_1 \times n_1) + (m_2 \times n_2) + (m_3 \times n_3) + \ldots + (m_i \times n_i)}{n_1 + n_2 + n_3 + \ldots + n_i} \quad (1)$$

Formula (1). Calculation formula for the pooled mean. Note. m: mean of each study; n: sample size of each study; and i: number of studies.

2.4.2. Pooled Standard Deviation Calculation

The pooled standard deviation was calculated using the standard deviation and sample size from the final selected study using Formula (2).

$$\text{SD}_{\text{pooled}} = \sqrt{\frac{(n_1 - 1) \times S_1^2 + (n_2 - 1) \times S_2^2 + \ldots + (n_i - 1) \times S_i^2}{n_1 + n_2 + \ldots + n_i - i}} \quad (2)$$

Formula (2). Calculation formula for the pooled standard deviation. Note. SD: standard deviation; n: sample size of each study; S: standard deviation of each study; and i: number of studies.

2.4.3. Estimated Physical Characteristic and Physical Fitness Value Calculation

The estimated values were calculated using the pooled mean, pooled standard deviation, and Z-score in the cumulative normal distribution (Table 1) using Formula (3).

$$\text{Estimated Value}_{p\%} = \text{Mean}_{\text{pooled}} + Z_{p\%} \times \text{SD}_{\text{pooled}} \quad (3)$$

Formula (3). Calculation formula for the estimated values$_{p\%}$. Note. $p\%$: cumulative probability in the normal distribution, $Z_{p\%}$: Z-score of cumulative $p\%$.

Table 1. Z-score in the cumulative normal distribution.

p(%)	1%	5%	10%	20%	30%	40%	50%	60%	70%	80%	90%	95%	99%
Z	−2.33	−1.64	−1.28	−0.84	−0.52	−0.25	0.00	0.25	0.52	0.84	1.28	1.64	2.33

2.4.4. Estimation Error Calculation

The estimation error was calculated using the sample size, standard deviation, and Z-score for a confidence level of 95% using Formula (4).

$$\text{Error}_{\text{estimation}} = \pm 1.96 \times \frac{\sigma}{\sqrt{n}} \quad (4)$$

Formula (4). Calculation formula for the estimation error. Note. n: sample size, σ: standard deviation.

3. Results

3.1. Study Selection

After a systematic search that selectively focused on clinical trials and cross-sectional studies, we retrieved 130, 66, 279, and 363 articles from DBpia, KISS, NDSL, and RISS, respectively. During the screening phase, 389 duplicate records and 29 conference presentations were excluded from the 838 articles. In addition, 327 not presenting physical characteristics and physical fitness data, 10 focusing on non-competition Taekwondo athletes, and 23 reporting irrelevant data for analysis were excluded from the 420 articles. Finally, 19 not including adults, 1 with unavailable full-text, 2 with unclear physical fitness data, and 14 with unclear patient sex were excluded from the 60 remaining articles. Twenty-four articles were then included after the screening and selection processes. The screening and selection processes are shown in Figure 1.

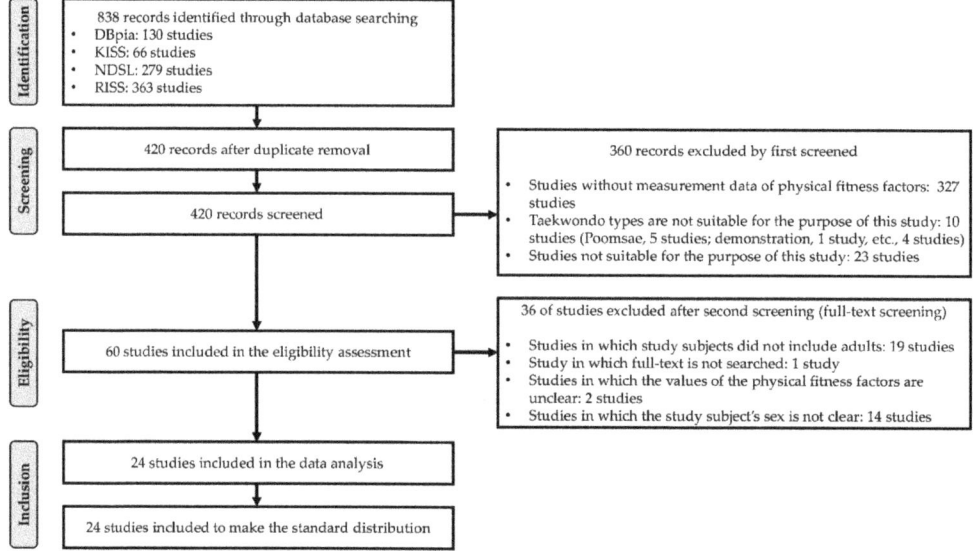

Figure 1. Flow diagram of the study screening and selection processes.

3.2. Study Characteristics

The study characteristics of the selected literature are listed in Table 2. Data were extracted from 22 studies on male Taekwondo athletes (n = 430, age: 20.10 ± 1.00 years, career: 5–15 years) and 7 studies on female Taekwondo athletes (n = 99, age: 19.40 ± 1.18 years, career: approximately 7.7 years). The variables involving a total sample size of more than 30 were extracted for each physical characteristic and physical fitness factor. As a result, 37 variables were extracted from studies on male Taekwondo athletes and 28 from studies on female Taekwondo athletes. We reviewed whether the final selected literature could allow an analysis of the physical characteristics and physical fitness factors by weight class; however, no weight class information was described. We attempted to classify the weight classes by the weight values from previous studies, although errors can occur because of the mean values. Therefore, weight classification was not analyzed, considering the validity of the resulting values. In addition, the side-step variables were excluded from the analysis owing to a lack of reliability because each study had different metrics. We then considered separating the excellent Taekwondo athletes from the non-excellent Taekwondo athletes. However, we failed to analyze them because the number of studies was very small.

Table 2. Study characteristics and extracted outcome variables.

Sex	Study	Sample Size	Age (y)	Career (y)	Weight (kg)	Outcome Variables
Male	Cho et al., 2011 [16]	40	20.56 ± 1.25	>5	75.33 ± 8.68	Physiques (height, body fat); Cardiorespiratory endurance (VO$_2$max, HRmax); Isokinetic muscular strength (left knee joint flexion at 60°/s, left knee joint extension at 60°/s, right knee joint flexion at 60°/s, right knee joint extension at 60°/s)
	Cho, 2020 [17]	67	19.69 ± 1.13	NR	70.48 ± 7.56	Physiques (height, BMI)
	Feng et al., 2020 [18]	27	19.7 ± 1.03	NR	70.5 ± 8.73	Physiques (height, BMI); Cardiorespiratory endurance (VO$_2$max); Isokinetic muscular strength (peak anaerobic power)
	Hong et al., 2020 [19]	28	20.18 ± 10.8	9.61 ± 2.27	74.01 ± 8.29	Physiques (height, BMI, body fat, fat mass, LBM, thigh circumference); Muscular strength (back strength); Muscular endurance (sit-up per 60 s); Muscular power (standing long jump, vertical jump); Flexibility (backward flexion, sit and reach); Balance (eyes-closed single-leg stance); Agility (whole-body reaction time to light, whole-body reaction time to sound); Isokinetic muscular strength (average power, relative peak anaerobic power, absolute peak anaerobic, peak drop, total energy, left knee joint flexion at 60°/s, left knee joint extension at 60°/s, right knee joint flexion at 60°/s, right knee joint extension at 60°/s)
	Jang and Park, 2020 [20]	10	20.7 ± 0.95	NR	69.8 ± 1.17	Physiques (height, BMI, body fat); Muscular endurance (sit-up per 30 s, sit-up per 60 s); Muscular power (standing long jump); Flexibility (sit and reach); Isokinetic muscular strength (average power, relative peak anaerobic power, absolute peak anaerobic power, peak drop)
	Jang, 2020 [21]	10	20.7 ± 0.95	NR	69.8 ± 4.93	Physiques (height, BMI, body fat); Muscular endurance (sit-up per 30 s, sit-up per 60 s); Muscular power (standing long jump); Flexibility (sit and reach); Isokinetic muscular strength (average power, relative peak anaerobic power, absolute peak anaerobic power, peak drop)
	Jung, 2015 [22]	16	22.44 ± 0.96	NR	70.23 ± 6.28	Physiques (height); Muscular strength (back strength, hand grip); Muscular endurance (push-up per 60 s, sit-up per 60 s); Muscular power (vertical jump); Flexibility (sit and reach); Isokinetic muscular strength (left knee joint flexion at 60°/s, left knee joint extension at 60°/s, right knee joint flexion at 60°/s, right knee joint extension at 180°/s, left knee joint flexion at 180°/s, right knee joint extension at 180°/s, right knee joint flexion at 180°/s, left hip joint extension at 60°/s, left hip joint flexion at 60°/s, right hip joint extension at 60°/s, right hip joint flexion at 60°/s, left hip joint extension at 180°/s, left hip joint flexion at 180°/s, right hip joint extension at 180°/s, right hip joint flexion at 180°/s, trunk joint flexion at 60°/s, and trunk joint extension at 60°/s

Table 2. *Cont.*

Sex	Study	Sample Size	Age (y)	Career (y)	Weight (kg)	Outcome Variables
Male	Kim and Lee, 2011 [23]	14	NR	≥10	71.01 ± 11.15	Physiques (height, BMI, body fat, LBM, and thigh circumference); muscular strength (back strength, left hand grip, and right hand grip); muscular power (vertical jump); flexibility (backward flexion, sit and reach); agility (whole-body reaction time to light, whole-body reaction time to sound); and isokinetic muscular strength (relative peak anaerobic power, peak drop)
	Kim et al., 2012 [24]	20	NR	NR	68.80 ± 8.29	Physiques (height, body fat); muscular strength (back strength); muscular endurance (sit-up per 30 s); muscular power (vertical jump); flexibility (sit and reach); and cardiorespiratory endurance (VO$_2$max)
	Kwon and Cho, 2017 [25]	8	21.70 ± 1.50	≥10	66.50 ± 3.15	Physiques (height, body fat, and thigh circumference); muscular strength (hand grip); muscular endurance (sit-up per 60 s); muscular power (standing long jump, vertical jump); cardiorespiratory endurance (Harvard step test); flexibility (sit and reach); and balance (eyes-closed single-leg stance)
	Kwon and Cho, 2019 [26]	14	22.50 ± 1.56	10.45 ± 2.63	72.57 ± 2.20	Physiques (height); agility (eyes-closed single-leg stance); muscular strength (left hand grip, right hand grip); muscular endurance (sit-up per 30 s); muscular power (standing long jump, vertical jump); flexibility (sit and reach); and agility (whole-body reaction time to sound)
	Lee and Ham, 2018 [27]	13	20.00 ± 1.08	6.23 ± 1.23	72.57 ± 11.12	Physiques (height)
	Monks, 2016 [28]	17	19.78 ± 0.58	7.98 ± 2.13	74.46 ± 10.47	Physiques (height, body fat, and LBM); muscular endurance (sit-up per 60 s); muscular power (vertical jump); cardiorespiratory endurance (VO$_2$max, HRmax, and all-out duration time); flexibility (sit and reach); and isokinetic muscular strength (average power, relative peak anaerobic power, absolute peak anaerobic power, peak drop, left knee joint flexion at 60°/s, left knee joint extension at 60°/s, right knee joint flexion at 60°/s, right knee joint extension at 60°/s, left knee joint flexion at 180°/s, left knee joint extension at 180°/s, right knee joint flexion at 180°/s, and right knee joint extension at 180°/s)
	Moon et al., 2016 [29]	11	19.64 ± 0.92	NR	74.29 ± 10.56	Physiques (height)
	Noh, 2015 [30]	31	19.60 ± 0.20	7.80 ± 0.30	72.50 ± 1.70	Physiques (height, BMI)
	Park & Yang, 2020 [31]	8	20.9 ± 1.06	NR	69.65 ± 2.35	Physiques (height, BMI, body fat); muscular endurance (sit-up per 30 s, sit-up per 60 s); muscular power (standing long jump); isokinetic muscular strength (average power, relative peak anaerobic power, absolute peak anaerobic power, and peak drop)

Table 2. Cont.

Sex	Study	Sample Size	Age (y)	Career (y)	Weight (kg)	Outcome Variables
Male	Park, 2016 [32]	29	18.87 ± 0.24	NR	70.09 ± 4.11	Physiques (height, BMI, body fat, fat mass, and LBM); muscular strength (hand grip); muscular endurance (sit-up per 60 s); muscular power (standing long jump); cardiorespiratory endurance (20-m MST); flexibility (sit and reach); and agility (10-m two repeated run test)
	Seo et al., 2015 [7]	22	19.40 ± 0.95	9.50 ± 1.91	69.80 ± 9.46	Physiques (height, body fat, fat mass, and LBM); muscular power (standing long jump); cardiorespiratory endurance (20-m MST); flexibility (sit and reach); and isokinetic muscular strength (relative peak anaerobic power, and peak drop)
	Song et al., 2010 [33]	10	19.40 ± 1.20	NR	69.30 ± 3.80	Physiques (height, body fat, and fat mass); cardiorespiratory endurance (VO$_2$max, HRmax); isokinetic muscular strength (relative peak anaerobic power, peak drop, left knee joint flexion at 60°/s, left knee joint extension at 60°/s, right knee joint flexion at 60°/s, right knee joint extension at 60°/s, left knee joint flexion at 180°/s, left knee joint extension at 180°/s, right knee joint flexion at 180°/s, and right knee joint extension at 180°/s)
	Tak et al., 2019 [34]	15	19.20 ± 0.78	>6	74.87 ± 10.28	Physiques (height); muscular strength (left hand grip, right hand grip); muscular endurance (sit-up per 60 s); muscular power (standing long jump); cardiorespiratory endurance (VO$_2$max); flexibility (sit and reach); and agility (eyes-closed single-leg stance)
	Yoo et al., 2015 [35]	12	20.58 ± 0.79	11.08 ± 2.27	72.42 ± 9.96	Physiques (height, body fat, and muscle mass); muscular power (standing long jump)
	Yoo et al., 2011 [36]	8	21.87 ± 1.12	NR	78.03 ± 8.80	Physiques (height, body fat, and muscle mass); muscular power (standing long jump)
	Feng et al., 2020 [18]	7	20.00 ± 0.82	NR	62.67 ± 6.35	Physiques (height, BMI); cardiorespiratory endurance (VO$_2$max); and isokinetic muscular strength (relative peak anaerobic power)
Female	Monks, 2016 [28]	16	20.00 ± 0.83	8.16 ± 1.91	64.15 ± 8.49	Physiques (height, body fat, and LBM); muscular endurance (sit-up per 60 s); muscular power (vertical jump); cardiorespiratory endurance (VO$_2$max, HRmax, and all-out duration time); flexibility (sit and reach); and isokinetic muscular strength (average power, peak anaerobic power, peak drop, left knee joint flexion at 60°/s, left knee joint extension at 60°/s, right knee joint flexion at 60°/s, right knee joint extension at 60°/s, left knee joint flexion at 180°/s, left knee joint extension at 180°/s, right knee joint flexion at 180°/s, and right knee joint extension at 180°/s)

Table 2. Cont.

Sex	Study	Sample Size	Age (y)	Career (y)	Weight (kg)	Outcome Variables
	Han, 2014 [37]	22	19.13 ± 1.29	6.81 ± 1.78	59.86 ± 3.27	Physiques (height, body fat, fat mass, and LBM); muscular endurance (sit-up per 60 s); muscular power (standing long jump); cardiorespiratory endurance (20-m MST); flexibility (sit and reach); isokinetic muscular strength (left knee joint flexion at 60°/s, left knee joint extension at 60°/s, right knee joint flexion at 60°/s, right knee joint extension at 120°/s, left knee joint flexion at 120°/s, left knee joint extension at 120°/s, right knee joint flexion at 120°/s, right knee joint extension at 120°/s, left knee joint flexion at 240°/s, left knee joint extension at 240°/s, right knee joint flexion at 240°/s, right knee joint extension at 240°/s, left hip joint flexion at 30°/s, left hip joint extension at 30°/s, right hip joint flexion at 30°/s, right hip joint extension at 30°/s, left hip joint flexion at 60°/s, left hip joint extension at 60°/s, right hip joint flexion at 60°/s, right hip joint extension at 60°/s, trunk joint flexion at 120°/s, and trunk joint extension at 120°/s)
	Moon et al., 2016 [29]	10	19.50 ± 1.10	NR	61.95 ± 8.73	Physiques (height)
	Seo et al., 2015 [7]	12	18.90 ± 1.24	8.90 ± 2.23	59.80 ± 6.56	Physiques (height, body fat, fat mass, and LBM); muscular power (standing long jump); cardiorespiratory endurance (20-m MST); flexibility (sit and reach); and isokinetic muscular strength (relative peak anaerobic power, peak drop)
	Song et al., 2010 [33]	10	19.60 ± 1.30	NR	62.50 ± 7.20	Physiques (height, body fat, and fat mass); cardiorespiratory endurance (VO$_2$max, HRmax); and isokinetic muscular strength (relative peak anaerobic power, peak drop, left knee joint flexion at 60°/s, left knee joint extension at 60°/s, right knee joint flexion at 60°/s, right knee joint extension at 60°/s, left knee joint flexion at 180°/s, left knee joint extension at 180°/s, right knee joint flexion at 180°/s, and right knee joint extension at 180°/s)
Female	Song et al., 2015 [38]	22	19.16 ± 1.33	NR	55.96 ± NR	Physiques (height, body fat, fat mass, LBM); muscular strength (hand grip); muscular endurance (sit-up per 60 s); muscular power (standing long jump); cardiorespiratory endurance (20-m MST); flexibility (sit and reach); and isokinetic muscular strength (left knee joint flexion at 60°/s, left knee joint extension at 60°/s, right knee joint flexion at 60°/s, right knee joint extension at 60°/s, left knee joint flexion at 120°/s, left knee joint extension at 120°/s, right knee joint flexion at 120°/s, right knee joint extension at 120°/s, left knee joint flexion at 240°/s, left knee joint extension at 240°/s, right knee joint flexion at 240°/s, right knee joint extension at 240°/s, trunk joint flexion at 60°/s, trunk joint extension at 60°/s, trunk joint flexion at 120°/s, trunk joint extension at 120°/s, trunk joint flexion at 240°/s, and trunk joint extension at 240°/s)

NR, not reported; MST, multistage shuttle-run test; BMI, body mass index; LBM, lean body mass; VO$_2$max, maximal oxygen consumption per minute; and HRmax, maximal heart rate per minute.

3.3. Pooled Mean Value and Estimated Error
3.3.1. Physical Characteristics

For the male Taekwondo athletes, the total sample size in relation to the physical characteristics was 224–430, and the estimated error was ±0.28–2.79%. The estimated error was the smallest height and the largest percentage of body fat. In addition, the estimated error of body mass index (BMI) (n = 224, ±0.89%) was smaller than that of the percentage of body fat (n = 236, ±2.79%).

For the female Taekwondo athletes, the total sample size in relation to the physical characteristics was 82–99, and the estimated error was ±0.64–3.05%. The estimated error was the smallest height and the largest percentage of body fat. The pooled and estimated error statistics for each variable are listed in Table 3.

Table 3. Pooled and estimated statistics for the Taekwondo athletes' physical characteristics.

Sex	Variables	Total Sample Size	Pooled Mean ± SD	Estimated Error (%)
Male	Height	430	178.00 ± 5.27 (cm)	±0.28
	Weight	430	71.76 ± 11.84 (kg)	±1.56
	Percentage of body fat	236	12.67 ± 2.77 (%)	±2.79
	BMI	224	22.16 ± 1.51 (kg/m^2)	±0.89
Female	Height	99	168.49 ± 5.48 (cm)	±0.64
	Weight	99	60.30 ± 5.88 (kg)	±1.92
	Percentage of body fat	82	23.25 ± 3.28 (%)	±3.05

SD: standard deviation; BMI: body mass index.

3.3.2. Physical Fitness Variables

For the male Taekwondo athletes, the total sample size in relation to the physical fitness variables was 42–203, and the estimated error was ±0.01–0.71%. The estimated error for all fitness variables was less than 8% without the eyes-closed single-leg stance (n = 65, ±15.71%). In addition, the estimated error of the maximal heart rate per minute (n = 67, ±1.26%) was smaller than that of the maximal oxygen consumption per minute (VO$_2$max) (n = 129, ±2.49%).

The pooled and estimated error statistics of the physical fitness variables of the male Taekwondo athletes are shown in Table 4.

For the female Taekwondo athletes, the total sample size in relation to the physical fitness variables was 33–72, and the estimated error was ±1.94–7.44%. The estimated error for all fitness variables was less than 8%. The pooled and estimated error statistics of the physical fitness variables of the female Taekwondo athletes are shown in Table 5.

Table 4. Pooled and estimated statistics for the male Taekwondo athletes' physical fitness.

Sex	Variables	Total Sample Size	Pooled Mean ± SD	Estimated Error (%)
Male	Hand-grip strength	53	44.68 ± 4.38 (kg)	±2.64
	Back strength	78	120.13 ± 19.59 (kg)	±3.62
	Sit-up per 30 s	62	30.52 ± 4.50 (times)	±3.67
	Sit-up per 60 s	141	57.41 ± 6.09 (times)	±1.75
	Sit and reach	203	15.95 ± 6.52 (cm)	±5.63
	Backward flexion	42	58.61 ± 6.87 (cm)	±3.54
	VO$_2$max	129	52.71 ± 7.62 (mL/kg/min)	±2.49
	HRmax	67	179.95 ± 9.51 (bpm)	±1.26
	20-m MST	51	97.75 ± 6.63 (times)	±1.86
	Standing long jump	164	242.97 ± 13.90 (cm)	±0.88
	Vertical jump	117	54.54 ± 5.23 (cm)	±1.74
	Whole-body reaction time (light)	42	0.283 ± 0.027 (ms)	±2.89
	Whole-body reaction time (sound)	56	0.280 ± 0.032 (ms)	±3.01

Table 4. *Cont.*

Sex	Variables	Total Sample Size	Pooled Mean ± SD	Estimated Error (%)
Male	Eyes-closed single leg stance	65	35.70 ± 23.06 (s)	±15.71
	Anaerobic average power	73	534.70 ± 76.09 (watt)	±3.26
	Peak anaerobic power (relative value)	146	11.07 ± 1.31 (watt/kg)	±1.92
	Peak anaerobic power (absolute value)	73	720.08 ± 115.17 (watt)	±3.67
	Peak drop	119	48.71 ± 7.78 (%)	±2.87
	Isokinetic flexion muscle strength of the left knee joint (60°/s)	94	127.30 ± 23.66 (Nm)	±3.76
	Isokinetic extension muscle strength of the left knee joint (60°/s)	94	208.27 ± 33.26 (Nm)	±3.23
	Isokinetic flexion muscle strength of the right knee joint (60°/s)	94	131.13 ± 24.35 (Nm)	±3.75
	Isokinetic extension muscle strength of the right knee joint (60°/s)	94	214.13 ± 32.24 (Nm)	±3.04

SD, standard deviation; VO$_2$max, maximal oxygen consumption per minute; HRmax, maximal heart rate per minute; and MST, multistage shuttle run test.

Table 5. Pooled and estimated statistics for the female Taekwondo athletes' physical fitness.

Sex	Variables	Total Sample Size	Pooled Mean ± SD	Estimated Error (%)
Female	Sit-up per 60 s	60	54.20 ± 6.84 (times)	±3.19
	Sit and reach	72	21.33 ± 6.87 (cm)	±7.44
	VO$_2$max	33	48.28 ± 5.68 (mL/km/min)	±4.01
	20-m MST	56	81.04 ± 12.32 (times)	±3.98
	Standing long jump	56	192.47 ± 14.25 (cm)	±1.94
	Peak anaerobic power (relative value)	45	9.22 ± 1.08 (watt/kg)	±3.43
	Peak drop	38	52.16 ± 6.14 (%)	±3.74
	Isokinetic flexion muscle strength of the left knee joint (60°/s)	70	97.77 ± 14.84 (Nm)	±3.56
	Isokinetic extension muscle strength of the left knee joint (60°/s)	70	172.82 ± 24.80 (Nm)	±3.36
	Isokinetic flexion muscle strength of the right knee joint (60°/s)	70	97.38 ± 15.93 (Nm)	±3.83
	Isokinetic extension muscle strength of the right knee joint (60°/s)	70	167.01 ± 25.70 (Nm)	±3.61
	Isokinetic flexion muscle endurance of the left knee joint (120°/s)	44	75.77 ± 6.95 (Nm/s)	±2.71
	Isokinetic extension muscle endurance of the left knee joint (120°/s)	44	125.80 ± 15.84 (Nm)	±3.72
	Isokinetic flexion muscle endurance of the right knee joint (120°/s)	44	73.62 ± 8.79 (Nm)	±3.53
	Isokinetic extension muscle endurance of the right knee joint (120°/s)	44	125.12 ± 15.65 (Nm)	±3.70
	Isokinetic flexion muscle power of the left knee joint (240°/s)	44	58.30 ± 7.41 (Nm)	±3.76
	Isokinetic extension muscle power of the left knee joint (240°/s)	44	90.90 ± 11.91 (Nm)	±3.87
	Isokinetic flexion muscle power of the right knee joint (240°/s)	44	56.36 ± 6.32 (Nm)	±3.31
	Isokinetic extension muscle power of the right knee joint (240°/s)	44	90.53 ± 11.42 (Nm)	±3.73
	Isokinetic flexion muscle strength of the trunk joint (60°/s)	44	143.45 ± 23.46 (Nm)	±4.83
	Isokinetic extension muscle strength of the trunk joint (60°/s)	44	154.62 ± 30.41 (Nm)	±5.81
	Isokinetic flexion muscle endurance of the trunk joint (120°/s)	44	143.08 ± 29.51 (Nm)	±6.09
	Isokinetic extension muscle endurance of the trunk joint (120°/s)	44	140.91 ± 27.78 (Nm)	±5.83

SD, standard deviation; VO$_2$max, maximal oxygen consumption per minute; and MST, multistage shuttle-run test.

3.4. Estimated Normal Distribution and 95% Confidence Interval

3.4.1. Physical Characteristics

The estimated values of each grade were calculated by applying the pooled mean and pooled standard deviation for each physical characteristic to the normal distribution and setting the grade at 10% intervals of cumulative probability. Examples of the estimated values corresponding to the top 10% of each physical characteristic in the study results were as follows: (1) the top 10% for the BMI of the male Taekwondo athletes was 20.0–20.4 kg/m^2; and (2) the top 10% for the percentage of body fat of the female Taekwondo athletes was 18.3–19.8%. The estimated normal distribution and 95% confidence interval of each physical characteristic are listed in Table 6.

Table 6. Ninety-five percent confidence intervals for the Taekwondo athletes' physical characteristics.

Sex	Variables	95% CI	1%	5%	10%	20%	30%	40%	50%	60%	70%	80%	90%	95%	99%
Male	Height (cm)	95% LV	165.2	168.8	170.7	173.1	174.7	176.2	177.5	178.8	180.3	181.9	184.3	186.2	189.8
		95% UV	166.2	169.8	171.7	174.1	175.7	177.2	178.5	179.8	181.3	182.9	185.3	187.2	190.8
	Weight (kg)	95% LV	43.1	51.2	55.5	60.7	64.4	67.6	70.6	73.6	76.9	80.6	85.8	90.1	98.2
		95% UV	45.3	53.4	57.7	62.9	66.7	69.9	72.9	75.9	79.1	82.8	88.1	92.4	100.4
	Percentage of body fat (%)	95% LV	18.8	16.9	15.9	14.7	13.8	13.0	12.3	11.6	10.9	10.0	8.8	7.8	5.9
		95% UV	19.5	17.6	16.6	15.4	14.5	13.7	13.0	12.3	11.6	10.7	9.5	8.5	6.6
	BMI (kg/m^2)	95% LV	25.5	24.5	23.9	23.2	22.8	22.3	22.0	21.6	21.2	20.7	20.0	19.5	18.5
		95% UV	25.9	24.8	24.3	23.6	23.2	22.7	22.4	22.0	21.6	21.1	20.4	19.9	18.8
Female	Height (cm)	95% LV	154.7	158.4	160.4	162.8	164.5	166.0	167.4	168.8	170.3	172.0	174.4	176.4	180.2
		95% UV	156.8	160.6	162.5	165.0	166.7	168.2	169.6	171.0	172.4	174.2	176.6	178.6	182.3
	Weight (kg)	95% LV	45.5	49.5	51.6	54.2	56.1	57.7	59.1	60.6	62.2	64.1	66.7	68.8	72.8
		95% UV	47.8	51.8	53.9	56.5	58.4	60.0	61.5	63.0	64.5	66.4	69.0	71.1	75.2
	Percentage of body fat (%)	95% LV	30.2	27.9	26.7	25.3	24.3	23.4	22.5	21.7	20.8	19.8	18.3	17.1	14.9
		95% UV	31.6	29.4	28.2	26.7	25.7	24.8	24.0	23.1	22.2	21.2	19.8	18.6	16.3

BMI, body mass index; CI, confidence interval; LV, lower value; and UV, upper value.

3.4.2. Physical Fitness Variables

The estimated values of each grade were calculated by applying the pooled mean and pooled standard deviation for each physical fitness variable to the normal distribution and setting the grade at 10% intervals of cumulative probability.

Examples of the estimated values corresponding to the top 10% of each physical fitness variable in the study results were as follows: (1) the top 10% for the hand-grip strength of the male Taekwondo athletes was 49.1–51.5 kg; and (2) the top 10% for the VO$_2$max of the female Taekwondo athletes was 61.2–63.8 mL/kg/min. The estimated normal distribution and 95% confidence interval of each physical fitness variable are listed in Table 7.

Table 7. Ninety-five percent confidence intervals for the Taekwondo athletes' physical fitness.

Sex	Variables	95% CI	1%	5%	10%	20%	30%	40%	50%	60%	70%	80%	90%	95%	99%
Male	Hand-grip strength (kg)	95% LV	33.3	36.3	37.9	39.8	41.2	42.4	43.5	44.6	45.8	47.2	49.1	50.7	53.7
		95% UV	35.7	38.7	40.3	42.2	43.6	44.8	45.9	47.0	48.2	49.5	51.5	53.1	56.0
	Back strength (kg)	95% LV	70.2	83.5	90.7	99.3	105.5	110.8	115.8	120.7	126.1	132.3	140.9	148.0	161.4
		95% UV	78.9	92.2	99.4	108.0	114.2	119.5	124.5	129.4	134.8	141.0	149.6	156.7	170.1
	Sit-up per 30 s (times)	95% LV	18.9	22.0	23.6	25.6	27.0	28.3	29.4	30.5	31.8	33.2	35.2	36.8	39.9
		95% UV	21.2	24.2	25.9	27.8	29.3	30.5	31.6	32.8	34.0	35.4	37.4	39.0	42.1
	Sit-up per 60 s (times)	95% LV	42.2	46.4	48.6	51.3	53.2	54.9	56.4	57.9	59.6	61.5	64.2	66.4	70.6
		95% UV	44.2	48.4	50.6	53.3	55.2	56.9	58.4	60.0	61.6	63.5	66.2	68.4	72.6
	Sit and reach (cm)	95% LV	−0.1	4.3	6.7	9.6	11.6	13.4	15.1	16.7	18.5	20.5	23.4	25.8	30.2
		95% UV	1.7	6.1	8.5	11.4	13.4	15.2	16.8	18.5	20.3	22.3	25.2	27.6	32.0
	Backward flexion (cm)	95% LV	40.6	45.2	47.7	50.8	52.9	54.8	56.5	58.3	60.1	62.3	65.3	67.8	72.5
		95% UV	44.7	49.4	51.9	54.9	57.1	59.0	60.7	62.4	64.3	66.5	69.5	72.0	76.7
	VO$_2$max (mL/kg/min)	95% LV	33.7	38.9	41.6	45.0	47.4	49.5	51.4	53.3	55.4	57.8	61.2	63.9	69.1
		95% UV	36.3	41.5	44.3	47.6	50.0	52.1	54.0	56.0	58.0	60.4	63.8	66.6	71.8
	HRmax (bpm)	95% LV	155.6	162.0	165.5	169.7	172.7	175.3	177.7	180.1	182.7	185.7	189.9	193.3	199.8
		95% UV	160.1	166.6	170.0	174.2	177.2	179.8	182.2	184.6	187.2	190.2	194.4	197.9	204.3
	20-m MST (times)	95% LV	80.5	85.0	87.4	90.4	92.5	94.3	95.9	97.6	99.4	101.5	104.4	106.8	111.4
		95% UV	84.1	88.7	91.1	94.0	96.1	97.9	99.6	101.3	103.0	105.2	108.1	110.5	115.0
	Standing long jump (cm)	95% LV	208.5	218.0	223.0	229.1	233.6	237.3	240.8	244.4	248.1	252.5	258.7	263.7	273.2
		95% UV	212.8	222.2	227.3	233.4	237.8	241.6	245.1	248.6	252.4	256.8	262.9	268.0	277.4
	Vertical jump (cm)	95% LV	41.4	45.0	46.9	49.2	50.8	52.3	53.6	54.9	56.3	58.0	60.3	62.2	65.8
		95% UV	43.3	46.9	48.8	51.1	52.7	54.2	55.5	56.8	58.2	59.9	62.2	64.1	67.7
	Whole-body reaction time (light, ms)	95% LV	0.338	0.320	0.310	0.298	0.289	0.282	0.275	0.268	0.261	0.252	0.240	0.231	0.212
		95% UV	0.355	0.336	0.326	0.314	0.306	0.298	0.292	0.285	0.277	0.269	0.257	0.247	0.229
	Whole-body reaction time (sound, ms)	95% LV	0.346	0.324	0.313	0.299	0.288	0.280	0.272	0.263	0.255	0.245	0.230	0.219	0.197
		95% UV	0.363	0.341	0.330	0.315	0.305	0.297	0.288	0.280	0.272	0.261	0.247	0.236	0.214
	Eyes-closed single-leg stance (s)	95% LV	−23.6	−7.8	0.5	10.7	18.0	24.2	30.1	35.9	42.2	49.5	59.6	68.0	83.7
		95% UV	−12.3	3.4	11.7	21.9	29.2	35.5	41.3	47.1	53.4	60.7	70.9	79.2	95.0

Table 7. Cont.

Male	Anaerobic average power (watt)	95% LV	340.2	392.1	419.7	453.2	477.3	498.0	517.2	536.5	557.1	581.3	614.8	642.4	694.3
		95% UV	375.1	427.0	454.6	488.1	512.3	532.9	552.2	571.4	592.1	616.2	649.7	677.3	729.2
	Peak anaerobic power (relative value, watt/kg)	95% LV	7.8	8.7	9.2	9.8	10.2	10.5	10.9	11.2	11.5	12.0	12.5	13.0	13.9
		95% UV	8.2	9.1	9.6	10.2	10.6	11.0	11.3	11.6	12.0	12.4	13.0	13.4	14.3
	Peak anaerobic power (absolute value, watt)	95% LV	425.7	504.2	546.1	596.7	633.3	664.5	693.7	722.8	754.1	790.6	841.3	883.1	961.6
		95% UV	478.6	557.1	598.9	649.6	686.1	717.3	746.5	775.7	806.9	843.4	894.1	935.9	1014.4
	Peak drop (%)	95% LV	29.2	34.5	37.3	40.8	43.2	45.3	47.3	49.3	51.4	53.9	57.3	60.1	65.4
		95% UV	32.0	37.3	40.1	43.6	46.0	48.1	50.1	52.1	54.2	56.7	60.1	62.9	68.2
	Left knee joint flexion (60°/s, Nm) [a]	95% LV	67.5	83.6	92.2	102.6	110.1	116.5	122.5	128.5	134.9	142.4	152.8	161.4	177.6
		95% UV	77.0	93.2	101.8	112.2	119.7	126.1	132.1	138.1	144.5	152.0	162.4	171.0	187.1
	Left knee joint extension (60°/s, Nm) [a]	95% LV	124.2	146.8	158.9	173.5	184.1	193.1	201.5	210.0	219.0	229.5	244.2	256.3	278.9
		95% UV	137.6	160.3	172.4	187.0	197.5	206.6	215.0	223.4	232.4	243.0	257.6	269.7	292.4
	Right knee joint flexion (60°/s, Nm) [a]	95% LV	69.5	86.1	95.0	105.7	113.4	120.0	126.2	132.4	139.0	146.7	157.4	166.3	182.9
		95% UV	79.4	96.0	104.8	115.6	123.3	129.9	136.1	142.2	148.8	156.6	167.3	176.1	192.7
	Right knee joint extension (60°/s, Nm) [a]	95% LV	132.6	154.6	166.3	180.5	190.7	199.4	207.6	215.8	224.5	234.8	248.9	260.6	282.6
		95% UV	145.6	167.6	179.3	193.5	203.7	212.5	220.7	228.8	237.6	247.8	262.0	273.7	295.7
Female	Sit-up per 60 s (times)	95% LV	36.6	41.2	43.7	46.7	48.9	50.7	52.5	54.2	56.1	58.2	61.2	63.7	68.4
		95% UV	40.0	44.7	47.2	50.2	52.3	54.2	55.9	57.7	59.5	61.7	64.7	67.2	71.8
	Sit and reach (cm)	95% LV	3.8	8.4	10.9	14.0	16.1	18.0	19.7	21.5	23.3	25.5	28.5	31.0	35.7
		95% UV	6.9	11.6	14.1	17.1	19.3	21.2	22.9	24.7	26.5	28.7	31.7	34.2	38.9
	VO$_2$max (mL/kg/min)	95% LV	33.1	37.0	39.1	41.6	43.4	44.9	46.3	47.8	49.3	51.1	53.6	55.7	59.5
		95% UV	37.0	40.9	42.9	45.4	47.2	48.8	50.2	51.7	53.2	55.0	57.5	59.6	63.4
	20-m MST (times)	95% LV	49.2	57.6	62.0	67.4	71.4	74.7	77.8	80.9	84.3	88.2	93.6	98.1	106.5
		95% UV	55.6	64.0	68.5	73.9	77.8	81.1	84.3	87.4	90.7	94.6	100.1	104.5	112.9
	Standing long jump (cm)	95% LV	155.6	165.3	170.5	176.7	181.3	185.1	188.7	192.3	196.2	200.7	207.0	212.2	221.9
		95% UV	163.1	172.8	177.9	184.2	188.7	192.6	196.2	199.8	203.7	208.2	214.5	219.6	229.4
	Peak anaerobic power (relative value, watt/kg)	95% LV	6.4	7.1	7.5	8.0	8.3	8.6	8.9	9.2	9.5	9.8	10.3	10.7	11.4
		95% UV	7.0	7.8	8.2	8.6	9.0	9.3	9.5	9.8	10.1	10.4	10.9	11.3	12.1

Table 7. Cont.

	Peak drop (%)	95% LV	35.9	40.1	42.3	45.0	47.0	48.7	50.2	51.8	53.4	55.4	58.1	60.3	64.5
		95% UV	39.8	44.0	46.2	48.9	50.9	52.6	54.1	55.7	57.3	59.3	62.0	64.2	68.4
	Left knee joint flexion (60°/s, Nm) [a]	95% LV	59.8	69.9	75.3	81.8	86.5	90.5	94.3	98.1	102.1	106.8	113.3	118.7	128.8
		95% UV	66.7	76.8	82.2	88.8	93.5	97.5	101.2	105.0	109.0	113.7	120.3	125.7	135.8
	Left knee joint extension (60°/s, Nm) [a]	95% LV	109.3	126.2	135.2	146.1	154.0	160.7	167.0	173.3	180.0	187.9	198.8	207.8	224.7
		95% UV	120.9	137.8	146.8	157.8	165.6	172.3	178.6	184.9	191.6	199.5	210.4	219.4	236.3
	Right knee joint flexion (60°/s, Nm) [a]	95% LV	56.6	67.4	73.2	80.2	85.3	89.6	93.6	97.7	102.0	107.0	114.1	119.8	130.7
		95% UV	64.1	74.9	80.7	87.7	92.8	97.1	101.1	105.1	109.5	114.5	121.5	127.3	138.2
	Right knee joint extension (60°/s, Nm) [a]	95% LV	101.2	118.7	128.0	139.4	147.5	154.5	161.0	167.5	174.5	182.6	193.9	203.3	220.8
		95% UV	113.2	130.8	140.1	151.4	159.6	166.5	173.0	179.5	186.5	194.7	206.0	215.3	232.8
	Left knee joint flexion (120°/s, Nm) [a]	95% LV	57.5	62.3	64.8	67.9	70.1	72.0	73.7	75.5	77.4	79.6	82.6	85.1	89.9
		95% UV	61.7	66.4	68.9	72.0	74.2	76.1	77.8	79.6	81.5	83.7	86.7	89.3	94.0
Female	Left knee joint extension (120°/s, Nm) [a]	95% LV	84.3	95.1	100.8	107.8	112.8	117.1	121.1	125.1	129.4	134.5	141.4	147.2	158.0
		95% UV	93.6	104.4	110.2	117.2	122.2	126.5	130.5	134.5	138.8	143.8	150.8	156.5	167.3
	Right knee joint flexion (120°/s, Nm) [a]	95% LV	50.6	56.6	59.8	63.6	66.4	68.8	71.0	73.3	75.6	78.4	82.3	85.5	91.5
		95% UV	55.8	61.8	65.0	68.8	71.6	74.0	76.2	78.4	80.8	83.6	87.5	90.7	96.7
	Right knee joint extension (120°/s, Nm) [a]	95% LV	84.1	94.8	100.4	107.3	112.3	116.5	120.5	124.5	128.7	133.7	140.5	146.2	156.9
		95% UV	93.3	104.0	109.7	116.6	121.5	125.8	129.7	133.7	137.9	142.9	149.8	155.5	166.1
	Left knee joint flexion (240°/s, Nm) [a]	95% LV	38.9	43.9	46.6	49.9	52.2	54.2	56.1	58.0	60.0	62.4	65.6	68.3	73.4
		95% UV	43.3	48.3	51.0	54.3	56.6	58.6	60.5	62.4	64.4	66.7	70.0	72.7	77.7
	Left knee joint extension (240°/s, Nm) [a]	95% LV	59.7	67.8	72.1	77.4	81.1	84.4	87.4	90.4	93.6	97.4	102.6	107.0	115.1
		95% UV	66.7	74.8	79.2	84.4	88.2	91.4	94.4	97.4	100.7	104.4	109.7	114.0	122.1
	Right knee joint flexion (240°/s, Nm) [a]	95% LV	39.8	44.1	46.4	49.2	51.2	52.9	54.5	56.1	57.8	59.8	62.6	64.9	69.2
		95% UV	43.5	47.8	50.1	52.9	54.9	56.6	58.2	59.8	61.5	63.5	66.3	68.6	72.9
	Right knee joint extension (240°/s, Nm) [a]	95% LV	60.6	68.4	72.5	77.5	81.2	84.3	87.2	90.0	93.1	96.8	101.8	105.9	113.7
		95% UV	67.3	75.1	79.3	84.3	87.9	91.0	93.9	96.8	99.9	103.5	108.5	112.7	120.5
	Trunk joint flexion (60°/s, Nm) [a]	95% LV	81.9	97.9	106.4	116.8	124.2	130.6	136.5	142.5	148.8	156.3	166.6	175.1	191.1
		95% UV	95.8	111.8	120.3	130.6	138.1	144.4	150.4	156.3	162.7	170.1	180.4	189.0	205.0
	Trunk joint extension (60°/s, Nm) [a]	95% LV	74.9	95.6	106.7	120.0	129.7	137.9	145.6	153.3	161.6	171.2	184.6	195.7	216.4
		95% UV	92.8	113.6	124.6	138.0	147.7	155.9	163.6	171.3	179.6	189.2	202.6	213.6	234.4
Female	Trunk joint flexion (120°/s, Nm) [a]	95% LV	65.7	85.8	96.5	109.5	118.9	126.9	134.4	141.8	149.8	159.2	172.2	182.9	203.0
		95% UV	83.2	103.3	114.0	127.0	136.3	144.3	151.8	159.3	167.3	176.6	189.6	200.3	220.4
	Trunk joint extension (120°/s, Nm) [a]	95% LV	68.1	87.0	97.1	109.3	118.1	125.7	132.7	139.7	147.3	156.1	168.3	178.4	197.3
		95% UV	84.5	103.4	113.5	125.7	134.6	142.1	149.1	156.2	163.7	172.5	184.7	194.8	213.7

VO$_2$max, maximal oxygen consumption per minute; HRmax, maximal heart rate per minute; MST, multistage shuttle-run test; CI, confidence interval; LV, lower value; UV, upper value; [a], isokinetic muscular strength.

4. Discussion

For Taekwondo competitions, athletes must have excellent physical fitness, including aerobic capacity, anaerobic capacity, muscle strength, muscle endurance, flexibility, speed, and agility [9,10,39,40]. In addition, data-based exercise science information is helpful in improving Taekwondo athletes' physical fitness and weakness [6]. Therefore, this study aimed to provide a profile of physical characteristics and physical fitness for Taekwondo competitors. To increase the value of this study's data-based exercise science information, we secured the validity of the estimation results. In a previous study that developed an estimation model of the physical fitness level, the validity of the estimation results was recognized when the estimated error was within 8–10% [41–43]. In this study, the estimation error of all variables, except for the eyes-closed single-leg stance (15.71%), was less than 8%. Therefore, it was confirmed that there was no problem with the validity of the estimated values.

The following can be interpreted as the causes of the higher estimation error in the eyes-closed single-leg stance than in the other variables. First, the sample size in relation to the variable was small. The estimation error was calculated by dividing the standard deviation by the square root of the sample size; therefore, the smaller the sample size, the larger the estimation error. However, the total sample size for the eyes-closed single-leg stance was 65, so the sample size was not small compared to that of the other variables. Therefore, this problem is hardly attributable to the increase in the estimation error. Second, there was a large deviation between individuals in the measurement of the variables. The eyes-closed single-leg stance is a variable that shows a large individual difference in measurement. Therefore, the estimation error was calculated based on the eyes-closed single-leg stance data presented in a previous study.

Based on the results of the previous study, the estimated error of the eyes-closed single-leg stance was calculated to be 40.7% for 16 college soccer players (34.0 ± 28.21 s) [44] and 54.6% for 10 high school female volleyball players (59.5 ± 52.4 s) [45]. Therefore, the estimation error increases proportionally because the individual difference between the measurements is large in the eyes-closed single-leg stance test. However, the results of our study have general validity because the estimation error of all variables, except for the eyes-closed single-leg stance, was less than 8%.

The utilization of different measurements that evaluate the same physical fitness factors favoring indicators with small estimation errors may be preferred. However, they should be carefully selected considering the inherent reliability of the measurement methods. For example, selecting BMI should be avoided because it has a smaller estimation error than the percentage of body fat when measuring obesity. The percentage of body fat directly tested using the bioelectrical impedance method was more accurate in obesity assessment than BMI calculated based on height and weight [46,47]. Nevertheless, BMI is being used to assess obesity in the public health and sports fields. The results of this study may be fully utilized for evaluation because the error in the estimated BMI distribution was not significant. For sit-up tests, it is recommended to conduct such for 60 s with a lower estimation error than that for 30 s. Measurements via the same test method and reliability should utilize a distribution with a smaller estimation error. Nevertheless, sit-up tests for 30 s are also available in public health and sports because of the low estimation error.

Combat sports, such as Taekwondo, require high levels of physical fitness and physical characteristics [48]. Exercise program plans are important for improving and maintaining a high level of physical fitness suitable for the characteristics of Taekwondo events [49]. Taekwondo athletes should be conditioned to effectively manage and improve their physical fitness through systematic exercise programs [50]. Conditioning management requires detailed knowledge of the physiological and physical abilities required for competition [51,52]. Therefore, sports scientists and Taekwondo coaches should organize long-term and short-term training programs and provide objective feedback to motivate athletes. As in this study, objective collection and presentation of information on an athlete's physical ability are important for feedback to the athlete [53]. The results of this study can help identify the physical profiles favorable to Taekwondo competitions and provide indicators of physical fitness standards for Taekwondo athletes [9,10]. This study had limitations. In the study, Korean Taekwondo athletes were considered the study subjects for the systematic search because they have the best performance in the world. However, Taekwondo athlete's skills and performance are becoming similar around the world. Therefore, future studies need to analyze the physical characteristics and physical fitness factors of Taekwondo elite athletes worldwide.

5. Conclusions

This study estimated the standard distribution of each factor by aggregating previous studies measuring the physical characteristics and physical fitness variables of Taekwondo athletes in South Korea through a systematic literature review. This study found that almost all physical characteristics and the estimated distribution of the physical fitness variables were generally applicable (estimated error of less than 8%). These results could be an essential objective basis for evaluating Taekwondo athletes' physical characteristics and physical fitness factors and setting training goals.

Author Contributions: Conceptualization, S.-S.N. and J.-W.K.; methodology, S.-S.N. and J.-W.K.; software, S.-S.N.; validation, S.-S.N. and J.-W.K.; formal analysis, S.-S.N.; investigation, S.-S.N. and J.-W.K.; resources, J.-W.K.; data curation, S.-S.N. and J.-W.K.; writing-original draft preparation, S.-S.N.; writing-review and editing, J.-W.K.; visualization, S.-S.N.; supervision, S.-S.N.; project administration, J.-W.K.; funding acquisition, S.-S.N. and J.-W.K. Both authors have read and agreed to the published version of the manuscript.

Funding: This research received no external funding.

Institutional Review Board Statement: This study was reviewed and approved by the Institutional Review Board of Konkuk University (7001355-201804-E-077).

Informed Consent Statement: Not applicable.

Data Availability Statement: No new data were created or analyzed in this study. Data sharing is not applicable to this study.

Conflicts of Interest: The authors declare no conflict of interest.

References

1. Janiszewska, K.; Przybyłowicz, K. Pre-competition weight loss among Polish taekwondo competitors–occurrence, methods and health consequences. *Arch. Budo* **2015**, *11*, 41–45.
2. Kazemi, M.; Waalen, J.; Morgan, C.; White, A.R. A profile of olympic taekwondo competitors. *J. Sports Sci. Med.* **2006**, *5*, 114–121.
3. Kim, H.-B.; Jung, H.-C.; Song, J.-K.; Chai, J.-H.; Lee, E.-J. A follow-up study on the physique, body composition, physical fitness, and isokinetic strength of female collegiate Taekwondo athletes. *J. Exerc. Rehabil.* **2015**, *11*, 57–64. [CrossRef]
4. Campos, F.A.; Bertuzzi, R.; Dourado, A.C.; Santos, V.G.; Franchini, E. Energy demands in taekwondo athletes during combat simulation. *Graefe's Arch. Clin. Exp. Ophthalmol.* **2011**, *112*, 1221–1228. [CrossRef] [PubMed]
5. Ball, N.; Nolan, E.; Wheeler, K. Anthropometrical, Physiological, and Tracked Power Profiles of Elite Taekwondo Athletes 9 Weeks before the Olympic Competition Phase. *J. Strength Cond. Res.* **2011**, *25*, 2752–2763. [CrossRef] [PubMed]
6. Zar, A.; Gilani, A.; Ebrahim, K.; Gorbani, M. A survey of the physical fitness of the male taekwondo athletes of the Iranian national team. *Facta Univ. Ser. Phys. Educ. Sport* **2008**, *6*, 21–29.
7. Seo, M.-W.; Jung, H.-C.; Song, J.-K.; Kim, H.-B. Effect of 8 weeks of pre-season training on body composition, physical fitness, anaerobic capacity, and isokinetic muscle strength in male and female collegiate taekwondo athletes. *J. Exerc. Rehabil.* **2015**, *11*, 101–107. [CrossRef]
8. Andreato, L.V.; Lara, F.J.D.; Andrade, A.; Branco, B.H.M. Physical and Physiological Profiles of Brazilian Jiu-Jitsu Athletes: A Systematic Review. *Sports Med. Open* **2017**, *3*, 9. [CrossRef]
9. Heller, J.; Peric, T.; Dlouha, R.; Kohlikova, E.; Melichna, J.; Nováková, H. Physiological profiles of male and female taekwon-do (ITF) black belts. *J. Sports Sci.* **1998**, *16*, 243–249. [CrossRef]
10. Marković, G.; Misigoj-Duraković, M.; Trninić, S. Fitness profile of elite Croatian female taekwondo athletes. *Coll. Antropol.* **2005**, *29*, 93–99. [PubMed]

11. Mathunjwa, M.; Mugandani, S.; Djarova-Daniels, T.; Ngcobo, M.; Ivanov, S. Physical, anthropometric and physiological profiles of experienced junior male and female South African Taekwondo athletes. *Afr. J. Phys. Health Educ. Recreat. Danc.* **2015**, *21*, 1402–1416.
12. Bridge, C.A.; da Silva Santos, J.F.; Chaabene, H.; Pieter, W.; Franchini, E. Physical and Physiological Profiles of Taekwondo Athletes. *Sports Med.* **2014**, *44*, 713–733. [CrossRef]
13. da Silva Santos, J.F.; Wilson, V.D.; Herrera-Valenzuela, T.; Machado, F.S.M. Time-Motion Analysis and Physiological Responses to Taekwondo Combat in Juvenile and Adult Athletes: A Systematic Review. *Strength Cond. J.* **2020**, *42*, 103–121. [CrossRef]
14. Krithikadatta, J. Normal distribution. *J. Conserv. Dent.* **2014**, *17*, 96–97. [CrossRef]
15. Impellizzeri, F.M.; Bizzini, M. SYSTEMATIC REVIEW AND META-ANALYSIS: A PRIMER. *Int. J. Sports Phys. Ther.* **2012**, *7*, 493–503. [PubMed]
16. Cho, C.-H.; Choi, C.-Y.; Lee, S.-E.; Shin, K.-C.; Song, E.-K.; Hyun, S.-J.; Lee, C.-Y.; Park, M.-S. Respiratory Circulatory Function and Knee Joint Equi-Speed Kinetic Capacity of College Taekwondo Athletes. *J. World Soc. Taekwondo Cult.* **2011**, *2*, 1–11.
17. Cho, H.-C. The Characteristics and Correlations of ACE and ACTN-3 Gene Polymorphism between Aerobic and Anaerobic Power, and Bone Density in Martial Arts Athletic. *J. Korean Alliance Martial Arts* **2020**, *22*, 191–203.
18. Feng, H.W.; Wang, J.-M.; Qian, C.; Cho, I.-H.; Cho, H.-C. The Relations between ACE Gene Polymorphism and Aerobic, Anaerobic Performance as Well as BMD of Taekwondo Athletes in Different Competition Types. *Taekwondo J. Kukkiwon* **2020**, *11*, 255–272. [CrossRef]
19. Hong, C.-B.; Lee, S.-J.; Park, J.-S. Comparative Analysis of Physical Fitness Factors, Anaerobic Exercise Capacity, and Isokinetic Muscle Function of Male College Taekwondo Excellent Players and Non-excellent Players. *J. Coach. Dev.* **2020**, *22*, 123–131. [CrossRef]
20. Jang, J.-E.; Park, E.H. Comparison of Anaerobic Capacity and Physical Ability of Athletes by Specific Events in Taekwondo. *Taekwondo J. Kukkiwon* **2020**, *11*, 91–102. [CrossRef]
21. Jang, J.-E. Comparison of Anaerobic Exercise Performance, Fatigue Factors and Physical Capacity of Taekwondo Kyorugi and Poomsae Athletes. Graduate School of Sungshin Women's University. 2020. Available online: http://dcollection.sungshin.ac.kr/public_resource/pdf/000000013822_20210910091946.pdf (accessed on 10 September 2021).
22. Jung, J.-S. Isokinetic Strength Capacity between Elite Athletes and Taekwondo Player. *J. Learn. Curric. Instr.* **2015**, *15*, 649–664.
23. Kim, S.-J.; Lee, H.-S. A Comparative Analysis of Body Types, Strength Traits between Excellent Players and Non-excellent Players: Centering on Boxing Players and Taekwon-do Players. *Yongln Unlverslty J. Martlal Arts Instltute* **2011**, *22*, 125–137.
24. Kim, A.-N.; Yoon, O.-N.; Cho, W.-J. The Effects of Plyometric Training on Physical Fitness and Isokinetic Muscular Strength in Male Taekwondo Players. *Korean J. Sport* **2012**, *10*, 201–211.
25. Kwon, T.-W.; Cho, H.-S. A Study on the Way of Training for physical fitness for players of Tae Kwon Do Demonstration and Gyurugi(Competition). *Korean J. Sports Sci.* **2017**, *26*, 1217–1225. [CrossRef]
26. Kwon, T.-W.; Cho, H.-S. Professional physical strength according to the level of training of university Taekwondo competition player and a comparative analysis of Trumk"s isokinetic myofunction. *Korean J. Sports Sci.* **2019**, *28*, 885–896. [CrossRef]
27. Lee, Y.-H.; Ham, W.-T. The effect of the short period high intensity winter training program on improvement of physical fitness in male university Taekwondo competition players. *Korean J. Sports Sci.* **2018**, *27*, 1127–1137. [CrossRef]
28. Monks, L. The Effects of 4 Weeks of High Intensity Interval Training on the Body Composition, Physical Fitness, Aerobic and Anaerobic Capacity and Isokinetic Muscle Strength of Collegiate Taekwondo Athletes. Graduate School of Kyunghee University. 2016. Available online: http://khu.dcollection.net/public_resource/pdf/200000056139_20210910092132.pdf (accessed on 10 September 2021).
29. Moon, H.-W.; Park, H.-Y.; Sunoo, S.; Nam, S.-S. The effect of short-term normobaric hypoxic training on maximal oxygen consumption, erythropoietin and blood lactate level in Taekwondo players. *Korean J. Sports Sci.* **2016**, *25*, 793–803.
30. Noh, J.-W. Analysis of Physical Characteristics of Elite Athletes in Martial Arts and Combat Sports for Orthopedic Manipulative Physical Therapy Research. Graduate School of Rehabilitation & Welfare Yongin University. 2015. Available online: http://yongin.dcollection.net/public_resource/pdf/000001952556_20210910092410.pdf (accessed on 10 September 2021).
31. Park, E.-H.; Yang, Y.-K. Effects of anaerobic exercise on physical strength according to Taekwondo weight class. *J. Converging Sport Exerc. Sci.* **2020**, *18*, 73–81.
32. Park, J.-H. The Effects of Caffeine Intake for 12 Weeks on Body Compositions, Physical Fitness, Stress, and Liver Functions of Elite Taekwondo Athletes. Graduate School of Physical Education Kyunghee University. 2016. Available online: http://khu.dcollection.net/public_resource/pdf/200000056132_20210910092541.pdf (accessed on 10 September 2021).
33. Song, J.-K.; Jung, H.-C.; Kang, H.-J.; Kim, H.-B. Gender-related Difference of Body Composition, Aerobic, Anaerobic Capacity and Isokinetic Muscle Strength in Collegiate Taekwondo Athletes. *J. Sport Leis. Stud.* **2010**, *40*, 699–708. [CrossRef]
34. Tak, H.-K.; Jang, J.-O.; Kim, J.-W.; Choi, H.-M. A Study on the Improvement of Competitiveness by Comparing Physical Fitness Factors among Demonstrators in Taekwondo Competition. *Taekwondo J. Kukkiwon* **2019**, *10*, 283–299. [CrossRef]
35. Yoo, D.-S.; Park, H.-Y.; Kim, H.-J.; Lee, M.-G. Effects of Types of Recovery Treatment and Glucose Supplementation on Physical Fitness in Male Collegiate Taekwondo Athletes. *J. Korean Alliance Martial Arts* **2015**, *17*, 33–44.
36. Yoo, D.-S.; Park, H.-Y.; Lee, M.-G. Effects of type of recovery treatment on fatigue-related blood variables and physical fitness in male collegiate taekwondo players. *Exerc. Sci.* **2011**, *20*, 261–272.

37. Han, D.-J. The Effects of 6 Week Conditioning Training on Body Composition, Physical Fitness, and Isokinetic Muscle Strength in Collegiate Female Taekwondo Athletes. Graduate School of Education Kyung Hee University. 2014. Available online: http://khu.dcollection.net/public_resource/pdf/200000055310_20210910092637.pdf (accessed on 10 September 2021).
38. Song, J.-K.; Han, D.-J.; Jung, H.-C.; Kang, H.-J.; Seo, M.-W.; Clarke, J.A.; Kim, H.-B. Does Pre-season Training Improve Body Composition, Physical Fitness, and Isokinetic Muscle Strength in Female Taekwondo Athletes? *Acta Taekwondo et Martialis Artium (JIATR)* **2015**, *2*, 6–15. Available online: https://preview.kstudy.com/kiss61/paperSearchPreview.asp?a_code=8091001073000v01&code=8639290019580013102&isDownLoad=0 (accessed on 10 September 2021).
39. Pieter, W. Performance characteristics of elite taekwondo athletes. *Korean J. Sport Sci.* **1991**, *3*, 94–117.
40. Bouhlel, E.; Jouini, A.; Gmada, N.; Nefzi, A.; Abdallah, K.B.; Tabka, Z. Heart rate and blood lactate responses during Taekwondo training and competition. *Sci. Sports* **2006**, *21*, 285–290. [CrossRef]
41. Cao, Z.-B.; Miyatake, N.; Higuchi, M.; Ishikawa-Takata, K.; Miyachi, M.; Tabata, I. Prediction of VO2max with daily step counts for Japanese adult women. *Graefe's Arch. Clin. Exp. Ophthalmol.* **2009**, *105*, 289–296. [CrossRef]
42. McArdle, W.D.; Katch, F.I.; Katch, V.L. Exercise physiology: Nutrition, Energy, and Human Performance. Lippincott Williams & Wilkins: Philadelphia, PA, USA, 2010.
43. Wier, L.T.; Jackson, A.S.; Ayers, G.W.; Arenare, B. Nonexercise models for estimating VO2max with waist girth, percent fat, or BMI. *Med. Sci. Sports Exerc.* **2006**, *38*, 555–561. [CrossRef]
44. Chun, S.-Y. Comparative of Angle of Calcaneus, Balance, Circumference of Calf and Isokinetic Strength of Ankle on Athletic Performances in Soccer Players. *Korean J. Sports Sci.* **2015**, *24*, 1101–1110.
45. Choi, D.-S.; Park, M.-H.; Kim, Y.-Y.; Kim, J.-G.; Chae, W.-S. Effects of 12-week core exercise program on isokinetic muscular function, balance and basic physical fitness of female high school volleyball players. *Korean J. Sports Sci.* **2019**, *28*, 1251–1263. [CrossRef]
46. Park, E. Overestimation and Underestimation: Adolescents' Weight Perception in Comparison to BMI-Based Weight Status and How It Varies Across Socio-Demographic Factors. *J. Sch. Health* **2011**, *81*, 57–64. [CrossRef]
47. Provencher, M.T.; Chahla, J.; Sanchez, G.; Cinque, M.E.; Kennedy, N.I.; Whalen, J.; Price, M.D.; Moatshe, G.; LaPrade, R.F. Body Mass Index Versus Body Fat Percentage in Prospective National Football League Athletes: Overestimation of Obesity Rate in Athletes at the National Football League Scouting Combine. *J. Strength Cond. Res.* **2018**, *32*, 1013–1019. [CrossRef]
48. Chiodo, S.; Tessitore, A.; Lupo, C.; Ammendolia, A.; Cortis, C.; Capranica, L. Effects of official youth taekwondo competitions on jump and strength performance. *Eur. J. Sport Sci.* **2012**, *12*, 113–120. [CrossRef]
49. Bridge, C.A.; Jones, M.A.; Hitchen, P.; Sanchez, X. Heart rate responses to Taekwondo training in experienced practitioners. *J. Strength Cond. Res.* **2007**, *21*, 718.
50. Ke-tien, Y. Training periodization in lower limb performance and neuromuscular controlling in taekwondo athletes. *Life Sci. J.* **2012**, *9*, 850–857.
51. Bridge, C.A.; Jones, M.A.; Drust, B. Physiological Responses and Perceived Exertion during International Taekwondo Competition. *Int. J. Sports Physiol. Perform.* **2009**, *4*, 485–493. [CrossRef]
52. Casolino, E.; Cortis, C.; Lupo, C.; Chiodo, S.; Minganti, C.; Capranica, L. Physiological Versus Psychological Evaluation in Taekwondo Elite Athletes. *Int. J. Sports Physiol. Perform.* **2012**, *7*, 322–331. [CrossRef] [PubMed]
53. Kim, H.-B.; Stebbins, C.L.; Chai, J.-H.; Song, J.-K. Taekwondo training and fitness in female adolescents. *J. Sports Sci.* **2011**, *29*, 133–138. [CrossRef]

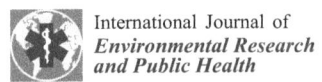

Article

Application of Real-Time Visual Feedback System in Balance Training of the Center of Pressure with Smart Wearable Devices

I-Lin Wang [1], Li-I Wang [2], Yang Liu [3], Yu Su [3], Shun Yao [3] and Chun-Sheng Ho [4,5,*]

[1] College of Physical Education, Hubei Normal University, Huangshi 435002, China; ilin@gms.ndhu.edu.tw
[2] Department of Physical Education and Kinesiology, National Dong Hwa University, Hualien 97046, Taiwan; tennis01@gms.ndhu.edu.tw
[3] Graduate Institute, Jilin Sport University, No. 2476, Freedom Road, Nanguan District, Changchun 130022, China; ly972226173@gmail.com (Y.L.); y.su825@gmail.com (Y.S.); yaoshun0330@gmail.com (S.Y.)
[4] Division of Physical Medicine and Rehabilitation, Lo-Hsu Medical Foundation, Inc., Lotung Poh-Ai Hospital, Yilan City 26546, Taiwan
[5] Department of Physical Therapy, College of Medical and Health Science, Asia University, Taichung 41354, Taiwan
* Correspondence: cochonho@gmail.com

Abstract: Balance control with an upright posture is affected by many factors. This study was undertaken to investigate the effects of real-time visual feedback training, provided by smart wearable devices for COP changes for healthy females, on static stance. Thirty healthy female college students were randomly divided into three groups (visual feedback balance training group, non-visual feedback balance training group, and control group). Enhanced visual feedback on the screen appeared in different directions, in the form of fluctuations; the visual feedback balance training group received real-time visual feedback from the Podoon APP for training, while the non-visual feedback balance training group only performed an open-eye balance, without receiving real-time visual feedback. The control group did not do any balance training. The balance training lasted 4 weeks, three times a week for 30 min each time with 1–2 day intervals. After four weeks of balance training, the results showed that the stability of human posture control improved for the one leg static stance for the visual feedback balance training group with smart wearable devices. The parameters of COP max displacement, COP velocity, COP radius, and COP area in the visual feedback balance training group were significantly decreased in the one leg stance ($p < 0.05$). The results showed that the COP real-time visual feedback training provided by smart wearable devices can better reduce postural sway and improve body balance ability than general training, when standing quietly.

Keywords: balance training; real-time visual feedback; smart wearable devices; center of pressure

1. Introduction

Balance ability refers to the human body's ability to adjust automatically to maintain postural stability when it moves or is subjected to external forces [1]. Balance control is usually affected by joint range of motion and muscle strength, which can be used to monitor the sensory information of the mechanism [2]. Therefore, good balance must be regulated by the sensory system and neuromuscular system. During upright posture control, people are clearly aware of their positional changes in space when they are given visual feedback (VF) based on the displacement of the center of pressure (COP) or body center of mass (COM) [3]. A visual system can provide the human body with information about the surrounding environment, location, direction, and speed during movement. When the visual information is removed or altered, the action system must rely on proprioceptive feedback and sensory information from the vestibular system in order to maintain

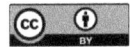

balance [4]. Therefore, VF can help increase the body's stability and balance ability, while controlling the posture of the human body.

In recent years, sensorimotor integration technology has been used to provide VF to improve the balance ability of people with disabilities and at high-risk of falls. Previous studies have indicated that internal feedback on one's own postural sway can be obtained through VF, so that the body can control its posture changes more autonomously [5]. In a study detailing the effect of VF from COP on the balance posture control of adolescents and the elderly, it was found that the use of VF for COP in the standing task is a common method for evaluating and training posture control [6]. Therefore, VF can improve upright posture control and change postural sway in the anterior–posterior and medial–lateral directions to maintain balance. In addition, further findings on ankle movement clarify the effect of different types of VF on body sway and ankle joint mechanisms that contribute to postural sway control [7]. A comparison between traditional body training and computer vision feedback training indicated that the computer vision feedback group had better effects on the balance posture control of the human body [8]. Therefore, providing VF in balance training can effectively improve the balancing ability of participants.

VF training to control body posture helps improve the body's ability to maintain balance and achieve stable standing. It can stabilize the body posture and significantly improve static and dynamic balance ability [9]. Previous studies have found that COP displacement and the mean velocity of patients with spinal cord injury decreased after VF standing balance training, indicating that the ability of static and dynamic stability improved significantly after training [9]. After applying wearable devices to balance training for the elderly, the COP area and COP parameters displayed a significant decrease, indicating that balance training is effective for improving postural control and functional performance in older adults [10]. These studies used visual feedback via a display of COP displacements as balance training to maintain stability. Therefore, appropriate external real-time VF information (the position of the real-time COP) should be provided during balance training to improve the control ability of postural balance and increase the benefit of training. In summary, effectively using real-time VF information of COP provided by smart wearable devices for balance control and training can benefit technology-assisted balance training at home, thereby aiding sports training and physical rehabilitation.

Our previous research explored the immediate effect of visual feedback provided by intelligent devices on the posture control of different genders [11]. It was found that visual feedback balance training with smart wearable devices can improve balance and there are differences in the visual feedback with smart wearable devices between males and females. After visual feedback balance training, females have better balance control ability than males. Therefore, this study aimed to explore the balance improvement of healthy females after visual feedback balance training in the one leg stance (OLS) or tandem stance (TS) postures.

2. Materials and Methods

2.1. Participants

Thirty healthy female college students were recruited and randomly assigned to the visual feedback balance training group (VFT), non-visual feedback balance training group (NVFT), or no balance training control group (CG), with 10 persons in each group. The basic characteristics of the participants, concerning age (21.30 ± 0.82, 21.44 ± 1.01, and 21.60 ± 1.71 years, respectively), height (168.10 ± 5.63, 164.67 ± 4.68, and 163.90 ± 3.75 cm, respectively), and weight (58.60 ± 6.60, 57.89 ± 7.17, and 56.00 ± 6.82 kg, respectively) in the VFT, NVFT, and CG groups were recorded. Meanwhile, there were no significant differences among the three groups. Exclusion criteria: any past history of injury or treatment of the lower limbs, any neurological or vascular deficit affecting balance, pain and swelling near the ankle and foot, or visual or vestibular impairment [12]. The participants were informed of the content, process, and precautions for the study group. The test instructions were read out to them and they understood and were willing to cooperate fully with the experimenter and signed the consent form. The study was approved by the Research Ethics Committee of Hualien Tzu Chi Hospital, Buddhist Tzu Chi Medical Foundation (IRB109-053-B) and was conducted in accordance with the Declaration of Helsinki.

2.2. Equipment

2.2.1. Evaluation Equipment

A force plate (BTS P6000, BTS Bioengineering, Italy) was used to calculate kinematic data: COP anteroposterior max displacement, COP mediolateral max dis-placement, COP anteroposterior velocity, COP mediolateral velocity, COP radius, and COP area. The force plate signals were collected at a sampling frequency of 300 Hz. In order to avoid the impact of different wear and tear during the test, all participants wore the same experimental tights and uniform sports shoes. The sports shoe incorporated a smart insole (Figure 1). The smart insole was linked to the Podoon APP in an iPad Pro (Apple, Cupertino, CA) to act as a smart wearable device to record COP changes. Podoon APP displays the dynamic points of COP, and participants tried to keep the dynamic points in the center circle [11].

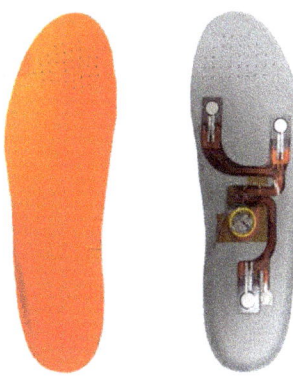

Figure 1. Smart insoles.

2.2.2. Training Equipment

The VF training group wore the experimental tights and uniform training shoes with smart insoles and used the Podoon APP on the iPad Pro during training. The NVF training group wore the same experimental tights and training shoes without smart wearable devices.

2.3. Experimental Protocol

2.3.1. Evaluation Protocol

Participants were recruited prior to the experiment, and their foot length was measured. Then, a smart foot pad matching their foot length was selected and cut. The participants had a five-minute warm-up run on a treadmill at 6 km/h to activate the lower extremity muscles for better balance control and one minute of rest. After the preparation, the thirty female college students were randomly divided into VFT, NVFT, or CG groups and completed tests before training as a pre-test. The pre-test consisted of 6 items, including one leg stance non-visual feedback (OLS-NF), one leg stance-visual feedback (OLS-VF), tandem stance (dominant leg in back)-non visual feedback (TSDL-NF), tandem stance (dominant leg in back)-visual feedback (TSDL-VF), tandem stance (non-dominant leg in back)-non visual feedback (TSNDL-NF), and tandem stance (non-dominant leg in back)-visual feedback (TSNDL-VF). Each item was measured three times, each time for 10 s. In order to ensure the consistency of the test, subjects in the study were all selected to have the right leg dominant. OLS is defined as the participant using the dominant leg to stand, while the non-supported leg was flexed at the knee with the plantar surface of the foot stabilized on the knee of the supporting leg [13]. TS is defined as the participant's feet (on a line, heel-toe position) placed on the center of the force plate [14]. The iPad Pro with Podoon APP was located at an eye-level height, 1 m apart from the participants during the pre-test. At the end of the four weeks balance training, all participants performed the balance test again as a post-test to measure the effect of visual feedback on improving balance. The post-test was the same as the pre-test.

2.3.2. Training Protocol

After the pre-test, the participants underwent four weeks balance training, three times a week for 30 min each time, with 1-2 day intervals. Training included the VFT using Podoon APP to perform OLS/TS-VF balance training. The NVFT was given an open-eye balance training without Podoon APP participation on OLS/TS-NF. The control group did not do any training. The iPad Pro with Podoon APP was located at an eye-level height, 1 m apart from the participants. Participants in the VFT were asked to keep the dynamic point in the central circle as much as possible.

2.4. Sample Size Estimation

A priori power analysis (G*Power version 3.1.9.4; Heinrich Heine University Düsseldorf, Düsseldorf, Germany) showed that a minimum of 10 participants was required on the basis of conventional α (0.05) and β (0.80) values, with an effect size of 3.05.

2.5. Statistical Analysis

In this study, the average values of three measurements for each item in each subject were calculated and used for statistical analysis. MATLAB (R2014a, The MathWorks Inc., Natick, MA, USA) was used for statistical analysis. The experiment used a mixed design two-way analysis of variance (ANOVA) (3 Group × 2 Times) to compare the differences between the pre-test and post-test of the three groups (VFT, NVFT, CG) in the six items: one leg stance non-visual feedback (OLS-NF), one leg stance-visual feedback (OLS-VF), tandem stance (dominant leg in back)-non visual feedback (TSDL-NF), tandem stance (dominant leg in back)-visual feedback (TSDL-VF), tandem stance (non-dominant leg in back)-non visual feedback (TSNDL-NF), and tandem stance (non-dominant leg in back)-visual feedback (TSNDL-VF). When the interaction was found to be significant, we used least significant difference comparisons between the three groups and t-test between the pre-test and post-test for post-hoc comparison. The level of significance was set at $\alpha < 0.05$.

3. Results

After four weeks of balance training with different interventions, balance postures were assessed immediately after the training was completed. The position balance of VFT was significantly improved in OLS when compared with pre ($p < 0.05$). In addition, COP max displacement, COP velocity, COP radius, and COP area after intervention were significantly lower than that before intervention, except for the CG group. The effect from these interventions for the above COP parameter varied from weak to moderate across the balance conditions.

3.1. Analysis of $COP_{ML/AP}$ Max Displacement

Figure 2 shows that significant interactions between Groups*Times were found in OLS-NF ($p < 0.05$). For the OLS-NF, post hoc analyses revealed that the $COP_{ML/AP}$ max displacement of the visual feedback balance training group decreased after visual feedback balance training and the COP_{ML} max displacement of the non-visual feedback balance training group also decreased after traditional balance training.

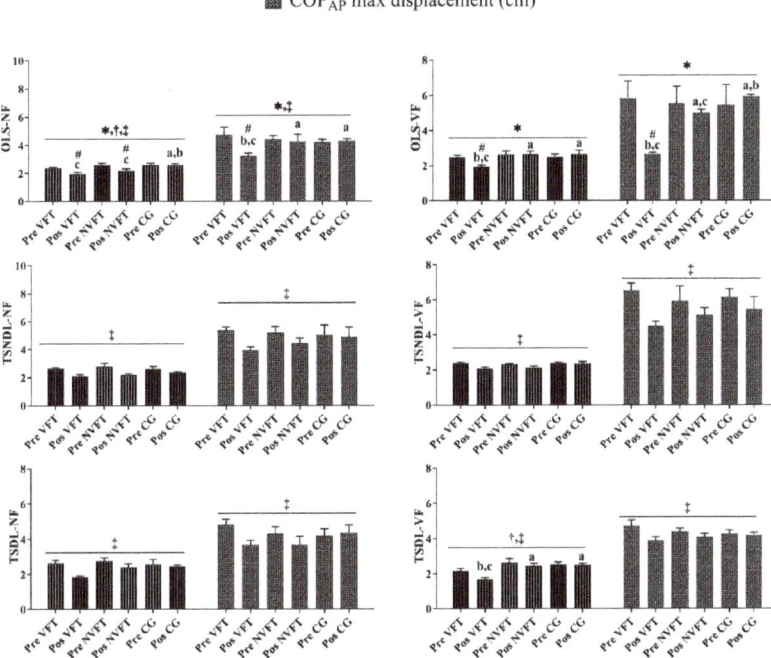

Figure 2. The training of group and time differences in the COP_{ML} and COP_{AP} maximum displacement parameters. Note: * Indicates a significant difference in interaction (Group*Times) ($p < 0.05$). † Indicates a significant difference in main effect (group) ($p < 0.05$). ‡ Indicates a significant difference in main effect (times) ($p < 0.05$). # Indicates a significant difference with pre-test. [a] Indicates a significant difference with VFT. [b] Indicates a significant difference with NVFT. [c] Indicates a significant difference with CG. VFT and NVFT before and after the test of various parameters of COP in OLS/TS. There was a significant difference in the interaction (Group*Times) of the COP_{ML} max displacement or COP_{AP} max displacement in OLS ($p < 0.05$). There was no significant difference in the interaction (Group*Times) of the COP_{ML} max displacement or COP_{AP} max displacement in TS ($p > 0.05$).

Figure 2 shows that significant interactions between Groups*Times were found in OLS-VF ($p < 0.05$). For the OLS-VF, post hoc analyses revealed that the $COP_{ML/AP}$ max displacement of the visual feedback balance training group decreased after visual feedback balance training.

Figure 2 shows that no significant interactions between Groups*Times were found for TSNDL-NF, TSNDL-VF, TSDL-NF, and TSDL-VF. There were time main effects for TSNDL-NF, TSNDL-VF, TSDL-NF, and TSDL-VF ($p < 0.05$). Post hoc analyses revealed that the COP_{ML}/COP_{AP} max displacement between the pre-test and the post-test decreased in TSNDL-NF, TSNDL-VF, TSDL-NF, and TSDL-VF.

3.2. Analysis of $COP_{ML/AP}$ Velocity

Figure 3 shows that significant interactions between Groups*Times were found in OLS-NF ($p < 0.05$). For the OLS-NF, post hoc analyses revealed that the $COP_{ML/AP}$ velocity of the visual feedback balance training group decreased after visual feedback balance training.

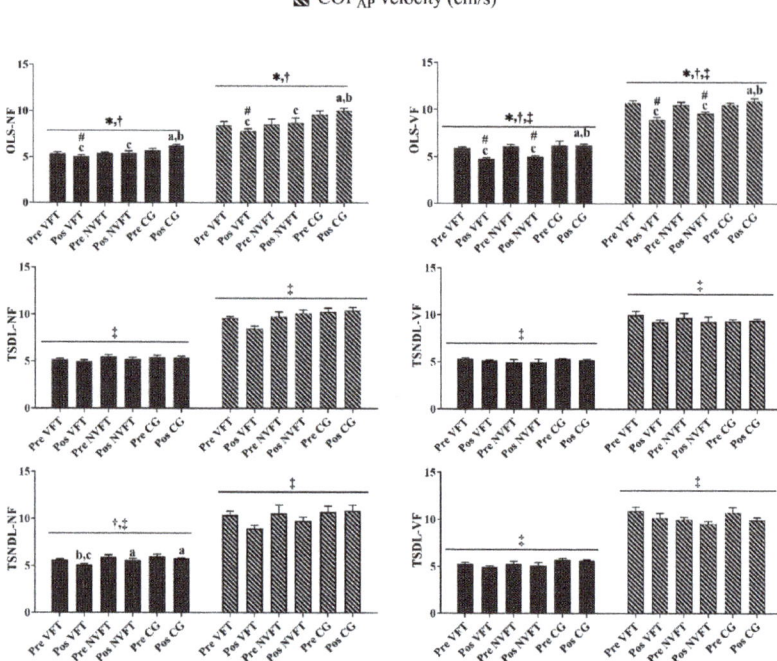

Figure 3. The training of group and time differences in the COP_{ML} and COP_{AP} velocity parameters. Note: * Indicates a significant difference in interaction (Group*Times) ($p < 0.05$). † Indicates a significant difference in main effect (group) ($p < 0.05$). ‡ Indicates a significant difference in main effect (times) ($p < 0.05$). # Indicates a significant difference with pre-test. a Indicates a significant difference with VFT. b Indicates a significant difference with NVFT. c Indicates a significant difference with CG. VFT and NVFT before and after the test of various parameters of COP in OLS/TS. There was a significant difference in the interaction (Group*Times) of the COP_{ML} velocity or COP_{AP} velocity in OLS ($p < 0.05$). There was no significant difference in the interaction (Group*Times) of the COP_{ML} velocity or COP_{AP} velocity in TS ($p > 0.05$).

Figure 3 shows that significant interactions between Groups*Times were found in OLS-VF ($p < 0.05$). For the OLS-VF, post hoc analyses revealed that the $COP_{ML/AP}$ velocity of the visual feedback balance training group decreased after visual feedback balance training; post hoc analyses revealed that the $COP_{ML/AP}$ velocity of NVFT decreased after traditional balance training.

Figure 3 shows that no Significant interactions between Groups*Times were found in TSNDL-NF, TSNDL-VF, TSDL-NF, and TSDL-VF. There were time main effects in TSNDL-NF, TSNDL-VF, TSDL-NF, and TSDL-VF ($p < 0.05$). Post hoc analyses revealed that the COP_{ML}/COP_{AP} velocity between the pre-test and the post-test decreased in TSNDL-NF, TSNDL-VF, TSDL-NF, and TSDL-VF.

3.3. Analysis of COP Radius and COP Area

Figure 4 shows that significant interactions between Groups*Times were found in OLS-NF ($p < 0.05$). For the OLS-NF, post hoc analyses revealed that the COP radius of the visual feedback balance training group and the COP area of the visual feedback balance training group decreased after visual feedback balance training.

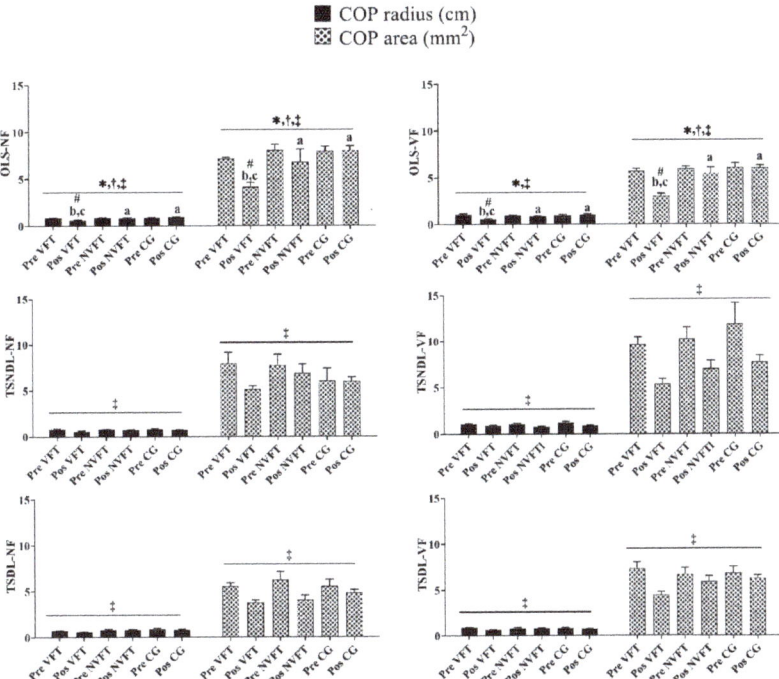

Figure 4. The training of group and times differences in the COP radius or COP area parameter. Note: * Indicates a significant difference in interaction (Group*Times) ($p < 0.05$). † Indicates a significant difference in main effect (group) ($p < 0.05$). ‡ Indicates a significant difference in main effect (times) ($p < 0.05$). # Indicates a significant difference with pre-test. a Indicates a significant difference with VFT. b Indicates a significant difference with NVFT. c Indicates a significant difference with CG. VFT and NVFT before and after the test of various parameters of COP in OLS/TS. There was a significant difference in the interaction (Group*Times) of the COP radius or COP area in OLS ($p < 0.05$). There was no significant difference in the interaction (Group*Times) of the COP radius or COP area in TS ($p > 0.05$).

Figure 4 shows that significant interactions between Groups*Times were found in OLS-VF ($p < 0.05$). For the OLS-VF, post hoc analyses revealed that the COP radius of the visual feedback balance training group and the COP area of the visual feedback balance training group decreased after visual feedback balance training.

Figure 4 shows that no significant interactions between Groups*Times were found in TSNDL-NF, TSNDL-VF, TSDL-NF, and TSDL-VF. There were time main effects in TSNDL-NF, TSNDL-VF, TSDL-NF, and TSDL-VF ($p < 0.05$). Post hoc analyses revealed that the COP radius and COP area between the pre-test and the post-test decreased in TSNDL-NF, TSNDL-VF, TSDL-NF, and TSDL-VF.

4. Discussion

The purpose of this study was to explore balance training effects for healthy females, with a real-time VF technique of COP changes provided by smart wearable devices, on static balance postural control. After four weeks of balance training, the results showed that visual feedback training can improve healthy female stability of postural control by OLS and TS static balance training with a VFT intelligent app.

In this study, the decrease in COP_{ML} and COP_{AP} displacement with VFT demonstrated that the participants could control body sway in a considerably more stable manner with the help of real-time VF information. A past study had shown that real-time visual feedback can provide sensory information to the central nervous system (CNS), helping to reduce motor output variability [15]. Visual feedback balance training can enhance sensorimotor integration by a recalibration of the sensory systems [16]. In addition, the maintenance of body balance requires the joint action of CNS, vision, and somatosensory [17]. Therefore, after VF training in this study, the decrease in COP_{ML} and COP_{AP} max displacement may have been due to the increased proprioceptive integration ability and the stability of motor output with VF training. In addition, visual feedback balance training can increase muscle activity around the ankle and isokinetic muscle strength to improve balance ability [18]. Therefore, in this study, VF training may have increased ankle stability, thereby reducing COP displacement and improving balance. In summary, the decrease in AP and ML displacement of COP indicates that technical assistance training may increase balance control ability for reducing body swing and displacement changes after VF participation.

Previous studies have found that the smaller the displacement velocity, the better the balance control ability when using VF training [19]. In this study, VF training using smart auxiliary equipment may have helped subjects maintain better physical stability. When the human body is performing visual feedback training, the central nervous system controls the body's goal-directed movements through relevant mechanisms [20]. The postural sway in the ML direction is controlled by adduction/abduction of the hip joint mechanism, while the posture sway in the AP direction is controlled by plantar flexion/dorsiflexion of the ankle joint mechanism [21]. Therefore, in this study, the decrease of the COP_{ML} velocity and the COP_{AP} velocity in the VFT may have been caused by the goal-directed movement of the ankle and hip joint mechanism, regulated by the CNS during VF training. In addition, past studies have found that balance training stimulates proprioception and increases sensory motor nerve signal transmission to improve balance control ability [18], while balance training also strengthens muscle activity and improves the stability of balance control [22]. Therefore, training without the assistance of smart devices will strengthen muscle activity. However, VFT gives visual feedback during the training process and the CNS controls the relevant muscle groups to perform goal-directed movements during training, so that the training effect of the visual feedback training group was higher than the general training group. In summary, the CNS mobilizes more motor neurons to increase the physical stability when performing VF training in OLS and TS.

Previous studies have shown that the COP radius and the COP area can reflect the static stability of the human body in the process of OLS; the larger the COP area and COP radius, the worse the stability [14]. Therefore, the results of this study show that balance training with visual feedback assisted by smart insoles can help subjects maintain better physical stability. The decrease in COP radius and COP area is mainly due to the conscious control by the human body, based on the visual information obtained from VF [23]. During the training process, the subjects could integrate VF information and motor sensory information to maintain physical stability under the control of the CNS [24]. Therefore, the decrease of COP area and COP radius after training with VF provided by smart insoles may have been due to the increase of visual information. In addition, past studies have pointed out that smart wearable devices give VF to the body's COM, and the COM VF will strengthen autonomous control and reduce postural sway, thereby achieving more efficient posture control or improving balance [9]. The training without smart auxiliary equipment only adjusts using the original sense organ system, and cannot judge the position effectively through VF [25]. Therefore, the balance ability of the NVFT cannot be significantly improved, and the use of VF assisted by smart insoles for training provides more VF information to strengthen the physical autonomous control ability and improve the physical balance ability.

A limitation of this study is that the experiment was conducted in a small sample of participants, and the small amount of training the participants received may not have been sufficient to measure the adaptation effect of the training. Therefore, although the value of COP of VFT after training was higher than CG/NVFT, the training effect needs more samples for further verification. In addition, the study only assessed the static standing of female subjects in stable postures, and no further discussion was made of postural balance with an unstable plane/external disturbance or the involvement of male subjects; our future research will address these issues.

5. Conclusions

Visual feedback training may increase the participants' visual information and promote the integration of the central nervous system, thereby assisting proprioception to reduce the center of pressure movement and enhance balance ability. In this study, the healthy females increased their balance ability after visual feedback training and found that the need for visual feedback in the balanced posture on one foot was significantly higher than that with two feet. It is particularly important to use smart wearable devices to improve the body's ability to maintain balance.

Author Contributions: Conceptualization, I.-L.W.; writing-original draft, L.-I.W.; data curation conceived, Y.L.; formal analysis, Y.S. and S.Y.; writing—review and editing, C.-S.H. All authors have read and agreed to the published version of the manuscript.

Funding: This research received a grant from the Lo-Hsu Medical Foundation, Inc., Lotung Poh-Ai Hospital (Number: E157).

Institutional Review Board Statement: The study was approved by the Research Ethics Committee of Hualien Tzu Chi Hospital, Buddhist Tzu Chi Medical Foundation (IRB109-053-B).

Informed Consent Statement: Participants were informed of the experimental procedures and risks and provided their written informed consent prior to attending several familiarization sessions.

Data Availability Statement: The datasets used and analyzed in the current study are included in this article.

Acknowledgments: The authors thank Shi-Jie Xue and Y.L. for conducting the biomechanical examinations.

Conflicts of Interest: The authors declare no potential conflicts of interest with respect to the research, authorship, and/or publication of this article. The funders had no role in the design of the study; in the collection, analyses, or interpretation of data; in the writing of the manuscript, or in the decision to publish the results.

Abbreviations

COP: center of pressure; VFT: visual feedback balance training group; NVFT: non-visual feedback balance training group; CG: control group; COPAP: COP anteroposterior; COPML: COP mediolateral; COM: center of mass; OLS: one leg stance; TS: tandem stance; OLS-NF: one leg stance non-visual feedback; OLS-VF: one leg stance-visual feedback; TSDL-NF: tandem stance (dominant leg in back)-non visual feedback; TSDL-VF: tandem stance (dominant leg in back)-visual feedback; TSNDL-NF: tandem stance (non-dominant leg in back)-non visual feedback; TSNDL-VF: tandem stance (non-dominant leg in back)-visual feedback; CNS: central nervous system.

References

1. Wang, J.; Xu, J.; An, R. Effectiveness of backward walking training on balance performance: A systematic review and meta-analysis. *Gait Posture* **2019**, *68*, 466–475. [CrossRef]
2. Horak, F.; Kuo, A. Postural adaptation for altered environments, tasks, and intentions. In *Biomechanics and Neural Control of Posture and Movement*; Springer: New York, NY, USA, 2000; pp. 267–281.
3. De Brito Silva, P.; Oliveira, A.S.; Mrachacz-Kersting, N.; Laessoe, U.; Kersting, U.G. Strategies for equilibrium maintenance during single leg standing on a wobble board. *Gait Posture* **2016**, *44*, 149–154. [CrossRef] [PubMed]

4. Shubert, T.E. Evidence-based exercise prescription for balance and falls prevention: A current review of the literature. *J. Geriatr. Phys. Ther.* **2011**, *34*, 100–108. [CrossRef]
5. Wulf, G. Attentional focus and motor learning: A review of 15 years. *J. Sport Exerc. Psychol.* **2013**, *6*, 77–104. [CrossRef]
6. Alfieri, F.M.; Riberto, M.; Gatz, L.S.; Ribeiro, C.P.C.; Lopes, J.A.F.; Battistella, L.R. Comparison of multisensory and strength training for postural control in the elderly. *Clin. Interv. Aging* **2012**, *7*, 119. [CrossRef] [PubMed]
7. Freitas, S.M.S.F.; Duarte, M. Joint coordination in young and older adults during quiet stance: Effect of visual feedback of the center of pressure. *Gait Posture* **2012**, *35*, 83–87. [CrossRef] [PubMed]
8. Sungkarat, S.; Fisher, B.E.; Kovindha, A. Efficacy of an insole shoe wedge and augmented pressure sensor for gait training in individuals with stroke: A randomized controlled trial. *Clin. Rehabil.* **2011**, *25*, 360–369. [CrossRef]
9. Sayenko, D.G.; Alekhina, M.I.; Masani, K.; Vette, A.; Obata, H.; Popovic, M.; Nakazawa, K. Positive effect of balance training with visual feedback on standing balance abilities in people with incomplete spinal cord injury. *Spinal Cord* **2010**, *48*, 886–893. [CrossRef]
10. Schwenk, M.; Grewal, G.S.; Honarvar, B.; Schwenk, S.; Mohler, J.; Khalsa, D.S.; Najafi, B. Interactive balance training integrating sensor-based visual feedback of movement performance: A pilot study in older adults. *J. Neuroeng. Rehabil.* **2014**, *11*, 164. [CrossRef]
11. Wang, I.-L.; Wang, L.-I.; Xue, S.-J.; Hu, R.; Jian, R.-J.; Ho, C.-S. Gender differences of the improvement in balance control based on the real-time visual feedback system with smart wearable devices. *Acta Bioeng. Biomech.* **2021**, *23*, 163–171.
12. Kulkarni, P.; Thosar, J. Effect of Arch Index of Foot on Dynamic Balance in Healthy Young Adults. *Indian J. Physiother. Occup. Ther.* **2020**, *14*, 134–140.
13. Alghadir, A.H.; Alotaibi, A.Z.; Iqbal, Z.A. Postural stability in people with visual impairment. *Brain Behav.* **2019**, *9*, e01436. [CrossRef]
14. Brown, C.N.; Ko, J.; Rosen, A.B.; Hsieh, K. Individuals with both perceived ankle instability and mechanical laxity demonstrate dynamic postural stability deficits. *Clin. Biomech. (Bristol Avon)* **2015**, *30*, 1170–1174. [CrossRef]
15. Vando, S.; Longo, S.; Cavaggioni, L.; Maurino, L.; Larion, A.; Invernizzi, P.; Padulo, J. The Effects of Short-Term Visual Feedback Training on the Stability of the Roundhouse Kicking Technique in Young Karatekas. *Int. J. Environ. Res. Public Health* **2021**, *18*, 1961. [CrossRef] [PubMed]
16. Li, Z.; Wang, X.-X.; Liang, Y.-Y.; Chen, S.-Y.; Sheng, J.; Ma, S.-J. Effects of the visual-feedback-based force platform training with functional electric stimulation on the balance and prevention of falls in older adults: A randomized controlled trial. *PeerJ* **2018**, *6*, e4244. [CrossRef] [PubMed]
17. Eils, E.; Behrens, S.; Mers, O.; Thorwesten, L.; Völker, K.; Rosenbaum, D.J.G. Reduced plantar sensation causes a cautious walking pattern. *Gait Posture* **2004**, *20*, 54–60. [CrossRef]
18. Nam, S.-M.; Kim, K.; Lee, D.Y. Effects of visual feedback balance training on the balance and ankle instability in adult men with functional ankle instability. *J. Phys. Ther. Sci.* **2018**, *30*, 113–115. [CrossRef] [PubMed]
19. Moraes, R.; Lopes, A.G.; Barela, J.A. Monocular vision and increased distance reducing the effects of visual manipulation on body sway. *Neurosci. Lett.* **2009**, *460*, 209–213. [CrossRef] [PubMed]
20. Kannape, O.A.; Barré, A.; Aminian, K.; Blanke, O. Cognitive loading affects motor awareness and movement kinematics but not locomotor trajectories during goal-directed walking in a virtual reality environment. *PLoS ONE* **2014**, *9*, e85560. [CrossRef] [PubMed]
21. Mochizuki, G.; Semmler, J.G.; Ivanova, T.D.; Garland, S.J. Low-frequency common modulation of soleus motor unit discharge is enhanced during postural control in humans. *Exp. Brain Res.* **2006**, *175*, 584–595. [CrossRef]
22. Nam, S.M.; Kim, K.; Lee, D.Y. Effects of balance training by knee joint motions on muscle activity in adult men with functional ankle instability. *J. Phys. Ther. Sci.* **2016**, *28*, 1629–1632. [CrossRef] [PubMed]
23. Rougier, P. Visual feedback induces opposite effects on elementary centre of gravity and centre of pressure minus centre of gravity motions in undisturbed upright stance. *Clin. Biomech. (Bristol Avon)* **2003**, *18*, 341–349. [CrossRef]
24. Brauer, S.G.; Woollacott, M.; Shumway-Cook, A. The interacting effects of cognitive demand and recovery of postural stability in balance-impaired elderly persons. *J. Gerontol. Ser. A Biol. Sci. Med Sci.* **2001**, *56*, M489–M496. [CrossRef] [PubMed]
25. Hsu, W.-L.; Scholz, J.P.; Schoner, G.; Jeka, J.J.; Kiemel, T. Control and estimation of posture during quiet stance depends on multijoint coordination. *J. Neurophysiol.* **2007**, *97*, 3024–3035. [CrossRef]

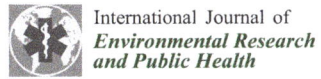

Article

Neuromuscular Fitness Is Associated with Success in Sport for Elite Female, but Not Male Tennis Players

Karoly Dobos [1,2], Dario Novak [3,4,*] and Petar Barbaros [3]

1. Pál Péter Domokos Elementary School, 1119 Budapest, Hungary; karoly.dobos93@gmail.com
2. Hungary and Department of Combat Sports, University of Physical Education, 1123 Budapest, Hungary
3. Faculty of Kinesiology, University of Zagreb, 10000 Zagreb, Croatia; petar.barbaros@kif.unizg.hr
4. Institute for Anthropological Research, 10000 Zagreb, Croatia
* Correspondence: dario.novak@kif.unizg.hr; Tel.: +385-99-4455699

Citation: Dobos, K.; Novak, D.; Barbaros, P. Neuromuscular Fitness Is Associated with Success in Sport for Elite Female, but Not Male Tennis Players. *Int. J. Environ. Res. Public Health* **2021**, *18*, 6512. https://doi.org/10.3390/ijerph18126512

Academic Editors: Mariusz Ozimek, Andrzej Ostrowski, Henryk Duda, Michał Spieszny and Tadeusz Ambrozy

Received: 22 April 2021
Accepted: 13 June 2021
Published: 17 June 2021

Publisher's Note: MDPI stays neutral with regard to jurisdictional claims in published maps and institutional affiliations.

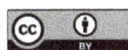

Copyright: © 2021 by the authors. Licensee MDPI, Basel, Switzerland. This article is an open access article distributed under the terms and conditions of the Creative Commons Attribution (CC BY) license (https://creativecommons.org/licenses/by/4.0/).

Abstract: Background: The purpose of the study was to examine whether neuromuscular fitness contributes significantly to the success of eAlite junior tennis players of differing ages and sexes. Methods: The 160 participants, who were elite Hungarian junior tennis players (aged 11–17), were separated into four groups within this study, and 10 different types of field tests were used. Results: A moderate significant correlation was found between the results of the 5 m run (r = −0.42; r = −0.45), standing long jump (r = 0.39; r = 0.56), overhand ball throw (r = 0.44; r = 0.53), serve (r = 0.39; r = 0.64), amount of push-ups in 30 seconds (r = 0.32; r = 0.48), 10 × 5 m run in a shuttle run (r = −0.34; r = −0.45), the spider run (r = −0.34; r = −0.52), and competitive tennis success among U14 and U18 girls. A significant correlation between the overhead medicine ball throw test value (r = 0.47) and the current competitive performance was found only among U18 elite female tennis players. In contrast, no correlation was found between the values of the U14 and U18 male tennis players and their current competitive performance. Conclusions: Additional studies are needed to identify interventions that can increase sport-specific neuromuscular fitness with the ultimate goal of achieving better performance.

Keywords: agility; explosive power; first quick quickness; flexibility; neuromuscular fitness

1. Introduction

Tennis has undergone dramatic changes in the past few decades. The technique, spin of the ball, speed of the game, anthropometric characteristics of the players, playing style, and strategy have developed significantly thanks to modern equipment, the modern court surface, and the precise selection and modern training methods. As a result, the physical fitness of tennis players has greatly increased in not only senior players, but junior players as well [1,2].

Tennis requires open skills and is an intermittent sport characterized by its repeated high-intensity efforts (i.e., first quick step, accelerations, decelerations, changes of direction and strokes, etc.) during a variable period of time (i.e., on average 90 min) [1–4]. Speed of the ball and movement of the players has an effect on both the upper and lower parts of the body. This is due to the players being required to execute movements and strokes of different directions and distances within a very short period of time. Furthermore, they are also required to adjust the movement and parameters of the ball trajectory. The average sprint distance performed in tennis is 5–7 m during an individual point, with an average of four to six changes of direction [2]. Movements in tennis can be characterized most frequently by the explosive power and the combination of medium to high aerobic and anaerobic capacity (endurance) [3,4]. This explosive power (that involves a stretching–shortening cycle) manifests itself during the rally through the number of repeated shots and tennis-specific footwork which occurs [5]. The average number of shots during a rally can be between five and six, with any given match lasting between 1–5 h depending on the type of competition [2,4]. Moreover, tennis requires the ability of a high level of coordination and proper dynamic flexibility due to the need to generate ball speed in extreme body positions [5]. Based on these facts, tennis players have to possess a high level of speed, agility, flexibility, and explosive power combined with well-developed aerobic and anaerobic endurance. However, the role of these physical variables in current competitive performance has to be examined especially in elite junior tennis players of differing ages and sexes, as they are at the beginning of their careers, and their physical characteristics, chronological age, and maturity differ from those of the adult professional players. It is well documented that the largest differences between juniors and professionals were in physical demands of play [3]. Professional players play longer matches, produce more shots, and cover more distance per match than junior players [3]. As far as measuring the physical variables, the current sport literature differs in both field and laboratory tests. Laboratory tests have high validity and authenticity and are very expensive, this being due to the quality and accuracy of the results that they can provide. However, field tests also model special movement patterns accurately, with physical variables and metabolic processes (compared to other tests) then being carried out in the laboratory, both of which characterize this sport. Furthermore, they are relatively simple and cost-effective and can be used for a high number of subjects [3].

In order to provide support in the development of young and talented athletes, it is essential to understand the factors that can have a positive influence on their sporting success. There is some evidence on the role of physical variables in the competitive performance of junior tennis players with the help of field tests [6–11]. In line with the above-mentioned, we hypothesized that neuromuscular fitness may be associated with sport success at the junior level. However, few studies have simultaneously examined the contribution of different neuromuscular factors to sport performance.

Accordingly, in the present study, we investigated the association of neuromuscular fitness with competitive tennis success among a sample of elite junior tennis players.

2. Materials and Methods

2.1. Participants

In total, 160 Hungarian junior tennis players (80 boys and 80 girls) aged between 11–17 took part in the study, with each participant having between 3 and 7 years' experience in international and national tennis competitions. Each participant had also played 40–60 matches per year and was ranked among the top 40 in Hungary in their respective age groups, this being the acceptance criteria for the participants to qualify to be a part of this study. The program G-power (version 3.1.9.2; Heinrich Heine University Dusseldorf, Dusseldorf, Germany) with the statistical power of 0.95 was used for estimating the appropriate number of participants. Subjects were selected through the stratified random sampling method.

The 4 age groups of the present study were formed in accordance with the United States Tennis Association guidelines [5]. Their chronological age was: mean $\pm$ SD = 12.44 + 1.35 years (boys U14, $n = 40$); mean $\pm$ SD = 12.50 + 1.37 years (girls U14, $n = 40$); mean $\pm$ SD = 16.16 + 1.57 years (boys U18, $n = 40$); and mean $\pm$ SD = 16.24 + 1.67 years (girls U18, $n = 40$).

2.2. Design and Procedures

Ten different types of field-tests (Table 1; for more details, please check Appendix A) were applied based on previous literary data and research [1,3,5,12–16].

Table 1. The sequence and variables of selected field test.

Code	Tests	Variables Measured
H	Hexagon (0.01 s)	Agility and coordination
R5	5 meter run (0.01 s)	Acceleration and speed of first-step
SLJ	Standing long jump (m)	Explosive power
OMBT	Overhead medicine ball throw (m)	Explosive power
OBT	Overhand ball throw (m)	Explosive power of the dominant side of the body
S	Serve (km/h)	Tennis-specific explosive power
PU30s	Push ups in 30 s (freq.)	Muscle endurance
SH10 × 5	10 × 5-m shuttle run (0.01 s)	Linear agility
SR	Spider run (0.01 s)	Multidirectional tennis-specific agility
STR	Sit and reach (cm)	Flexibility

The current competitive performance variable (elaborated and used by the Hungarian Tennis Federation for several years) was also used, which represented the average values of the points won in matches by each participant. A familiarization session was performed 1 week prior to the testing, where the participants were informed in both oral and written form about the aim, the testing process, and the testing protocol. No intense physical activity was performed by the players 48 h prior to the tests. The tests were then carried out on an indoor clay court, certified by the Hungarian Tennis Federation according to Hungarian and international rules and regulations, at a temperature of 15–25 °C. The players had to execute the tests in a given order (Table 1) after a 15-min standard warm-up, which consisted of 5 min of jogging; dynamic flexibility exercises; forward, backward, and sideways running; acceleration running; and the execution of fifteen flat serves. There was a period of 4-min between the warm-up and the tests, with there being a rest period of 2 min between the trials and a 25 s rest period between the serves; this was in order to limit the effects that fatigue may play on the results. The players had 3 trials in the 5 m run (R5), standing long jump (SLJ), overhead medicine ball throw (OMBT), overhand ball throw (OBT), 8 trials in the serve (S), 2 trials in the hexagon (H), sit and reach (STR), 10 × 5 m shuttle run (SH 10 × 5), spider run (SR), and the push-ups in 30 s (PU 30 s) in the testing process. Neither the measuring equipment nor the participants carrying out the work were modified in the repeated examinations. For the R5, SH10 × 5, and SR tests, the GUR-1 electric timer (within 0.01 seconds of accuracy) was used, and for the H and PU 30 s tests, the Casio stopwatch (within 0.01 s of accuracy) was used. During the measuring of the OMBT and OBT and SLJ tests, a 1 kg stuffed ball, a 103 g small ball (diameter 8 cm), and a calibrated tape measurer (marked at every cm) were used. For the S test, the "Stalker ATS II" serve speed measurer (within ±3 km/h of accuracy) and 53–56 g and 6.5 diameter "Slazenger Ultra Vis" balls as well as at the STR test 32 cm high, 45 cm wide, and 55 cm long box were used. The study met the guidelines of recommendations of the Declaration of Helsinki [17] and was approved by the Ethical Committee of Public Health Division of the Budapest Government Office (permission # 7878/2014). Furthermore, all the players had a medical screening and received declarations of consent from their parents prior to the study.

2.3. Statistical Analysis

The normality of the data was checked by the Shapiro–Wilk W test. In addition, the ICC was calculated to determine the reliability of the measurements (except S test) using the Spearman–Brown formula of calculation. The correlations between the physical variables and the current competitive performance were calculated with the Spearman's rank correlation methods. The correlations were considered as weak ($|r| < 0.3$), moderate ($0.3 < |r| < 0.7$), or strong ($|r| > 0.7$) [18] at a significance of $p < 0.05$. The statistical analysis of the data was carried out with the SPSS 21.0 software.

3. Results

Most of the data (H, R5, SLJ, SH10 × 5, SR, and PU 30s) did not fulfill the requirements of normal distribution, which was checked by the Shapiro–Wilk W test ($p < 0{,}05$); thus, at every variable, the basic statistical data were described as mean ± standard deviation and minimal and maximal result (Table 2). For all tests, an ICC of 80–94 was found and therefore all tests were considered to be reliable (Table 3). A moderate significant correlation was found between the R5, SLJ, OMBT, OBT, S, PU 30s, SH 10 × 5, and SR test values and the current competitive performance in girls, but not in boys (Table 4). A moderate significant correlation was found between the R5, SLJ, OBT, S, PU 30s, SH 10 × 5, and SR test values and the current competitive performance in the U14 and U18 female junior tennis players. Furthermore, in the U18 elite female junior tennis players, the OMBT test's value showed a moderate significance of correlation with the current competitive performance (Table 5.). The H, OMBT, and STR test values in the U14 females, H and STR test values in the U18 females, and all the test values of the U14 and U18 elite junior male tennis players did not show any correlation with the current competitive performance (Table 5).

Table 2. The descriptive statistics of the elite junior male and female tennis players ($n = 160$).

Tests	U14 Girls $n = 40$		U14 Boys $n = 40$		U18 Girls $n = 40$		U18 Boys $n = 40$	
	Mean ± SD	Min-Max	Mean ± SD	Min-Max	Mean ± SD	Min-Max	Mean ± SD	Min-Max
H (0.01 s) *	12.01 ± 1.12	1.34–14.52	12.18 ± 2.00	10.00–20.00	10.90 ± 0.84	9.14–2.40	10.76 ± 1.18	8.84–13.53
R5 (0.01 s) *	1.29 ± 0.07	1.15–1.44	1.27 ± 0.06	1.15–1.41	1.25 ± 0.04	1.16–1.38	1.14 ± 0.05	0.99–1.27
SLJ (m) *	1.69 ± 0.19	1.30–2.08	1.82 ± 0.16	1.30–2.21	1.85 ± 0.16	1.42–2.20	2.23 ± 0.23	1.72–2.88
OMBT (m)	8.84 ± 1.90	5.47–13.62	9.35–2.14	6.09–14.32	10.74 ± 1.61	7.88–14.48	14.50 ± 2.41	9.20–19.20
OBT (m)	27.03 ± 5.69	16.57–39.90	35.42 ± 6.20	25.75–50.30	30.65 ± 5.97	19.80–44.30	48.23 ± 7.54	32.36–66.8
S (km/h)	128.62 ± 18.42	87.00–176.00	140.52 ± 17.07	110.00–175.00	152.00 ± 10.31	133.00–169.00	174.60 ± 13.8	144.00–211
PU30s (freq.) *	8.66 ± 5.90	1–25.00	17.42 ± 4.51	9.00–28.00	10.89 ± 7.99	1.00–30.50	27.23 ± 8.05	11.00–44.00
SH10 × 5 (0.01 s) *	20.65 ± 1.47	18.48–26.40	19.95 ± 0.95	18.00–21.70	19.51 ± 0.83	18.04–21.40	18.52 ± 078	17.08–20.20
SR (0.01 s) *	21.80 ± 1.64	18.56–26.13	20.81–1.08	18.76–23.79	19.28 ± 0.94	17.10–21.90	18.05 ± 0.97	15.96–20.00
STR (cm)	20.18 ± 7.42	1.32–34.00	13.57–6.45	1.00–31.00	23.72 ± 7.04	9.00–37.00	17.56 ± 8.67	1.00–35.00

Legends: H—hexagon; R5—5 m run; SLJ—standing long jump; OMBT—overhead medicine; ball throw; OBT—overhead ball throw; S—serve; s; PU30—push ups in 30 s; SH10 × 5—10 × 5 m shuttle run; SR—spider run; STR—sit and reach; Shapiro-Wilk W test (* $p < 0{,}05$).

Table 3. Reliability values of selected field test for elite junior tennis players.

Tests	H	R5	SLJ	OMBT	OBT	S	PU 30 s	SH 1 × 5	SR	STR
ICC (95% CI)	0.91 (0.90–0.92)	0.93 (0.92–0.94)	0.82 (0.80–0.84)	0.89 (0.97–0.91)	0.86 (0.85–0.87)	0.87 (0.85–0.87)	0.85 (0.80–0.90)	0.87 (0.85–0.90)	0.90 (0.89–0.91)	0.92 (0.90–0.94)
CV%	3.1	2.3	3.5	3.9	3.8	2.3	3.8	2.9	2.1	1.5

Legends: H—hexagon; R5—5 m run; SLJ—standing long jump; OMBT—overhead medicine ball throw; OBT—overhead ball throw; S—serve; PU30s—push ups in 30 s; SH10 × −5—10 × 5 m shuttle run; SR—spider run; STR—sit and reach; ICC—intraclass correlation coefficient; CI—confidence interval; CV—coefficient of variation.

Table 4. Spearman correlation coefficients between physical variables of selected field tests and the current competitive performance of the same sex as a single group ($n = 160$).

Groups	H	R5	SLJ	OMBT	OBT	S	PU 30 s	SH 10 × 5	SR	STR
Girls	−0.16	−0.43 *	0.50 *	034 *	0.49 *	0.46 *	0.39 *	−0.41 *	−0.39 *	0.04
Boys	−0.19	−0.20	0.11	0.11	0.11	0.17	0.21	0.06	−0.21	−0.16	0.11

Legends: H—hexagon; R5—5 m run; SLJ—standing long jump; OMBT—overhead medicine ball throw; OBT—overhead ball throw; S—serve; PU30s—push ups in 30 s; SH10 × −5—10 × 5 m shuttle run; SR—spider run; STR—sit and reach (* denotes significant correlations at * $p < 0.05$).

Table 5. Spearman correlation coefficients between physical variable of selected field tests and the current competitive performance in elite junior tennis players (n = 160).

Groups	H	R5	SLJ	OMBT	OBT	S	PU 30 s	SH 10 × 5	SR	STR
U14 girls	−0.06	−0.42 *	0.39 *	0.29	0.44 *	0.39 *	0.32 *	−0.34 *	−0.34 *	0.08
U18 girls	−0.11	−0.45 *	0.56 *	0.47*	0.53 *	0.64 *	0.48 *	−0.45 *	−0.52 *	0.01
U14 boys	−0.15	−0.08	0.10	0.03	0.17	0.03	0.05	−0.22	−0.26	0.35
U18 boys	−0.11	−0.18	0.11	0.05	0.01	0.25	0.18	−0.16	−0.05	0.02

Legends: H—hexagon; R5—5 m run; SLJ—standing long jump; OMBT—overhead medicine ball throw; OBT—overhead ball throw; S—serve; PU30s—push ups in 30 s; SH10 × −5—10 × 5 m shuttle run; SR—spider run; STR—sit and reach (* denotes significant correlations at * $p < 0.05$).

4. Discussion

This study aimed to investigate the association of neuromuscular fitness in sporting success among a sample of elite junior tennis players. With regard to the study aim, we can conclude neuromuscular fitness is associated with sporting success in females but not male elite junior tennis players.

There is a positive role of physical fitness on the competitive performance of junior tennis players [6–11]. Comparing the present results with previous literature is difficult, as previous studies were conducted with a different sample size, participants of a differing sex, and different test protocols, although the results of the present study (a moderate correlation between the physical variables and the current competitive performance) of Hungarian junior female players reinforce the results of the previous research [6–11]; except for the H and the STR tests, this was not the case for the male Hungarian junior tennis players. Tennis is a tactical and technically dominant sport that can be characterized by the complex interaction of physical abilities and metabolism processes from a conditional point of view [3,6,7,10]. It is well documented that the sexual maturity of female adolescents is happening earlier compared to males of the same age, with females reaching their peak physical performance much earlier [19]. We can hypothesize that increases in mass and stature have a large influence on their physical fitness measures, whereas in junior males there are some qualitative differences in performance due to other factors (i.e., technical executions, tactical solutions, diversity of shorts). Elite junior male tennis players who possess better physical fitness than their peers cannot necessarily translate this advantage into a significantly higher chance of winning. In addition, it is possible that the examined junior male tennis players can play in a more versatile way than females. This meaning that during the game, due to slightly different playing style, the junior female tennis players prefer those simpler technical and tactical solutions in which their physical abilities (i.e., explosive power) can play a more significant and effective role.

However, it is surprising that the better H test value of the examined junior tennis players did not result in a better current competitive performance, which contrasts with previous studies [20]. The results observed may be due to several factors including a uniformly high level of fine motor co-ordination abilities, dynamic postural control, and balance of the examined players. Additionally, the movement patterns with the test are not related to the typical movements in tennis. The value of the STR test (which is often an official part of any assessments protocols) did not show a correlation with current competitive performance either in the examined junior tennis players, which might be explained by the fact that static flexibility performance could not be transferred to dynamic situations in tennis [21]. Nonetheless, static stretching was considered the safest and best method to improve a players' flexibility and decrease the risk of injury.

4.1. The First Step Quickness, Acceleration, and Agility

The R5 test value showed a moderate correlation with the current competitive performance in U14 and U18 females. This test measures the speed of the first step in running/sprinting forward. In tennis, the emphasis is on the speed of the first step in order for the player to reach an effective hitting position and how fast the player can get into motion, overcoming the inertia of his/her own body. The 5 m straight run models the launching of this motion effectively for observation [8]. Although the speed and frequency of the strokes executed by the junior female tennis players lag behind those of adult female players, especially in the U14 age group, the first step and the ability to speed up within a short distance are both essential requirements for handling the ball correctly to successfully solve the game situations [2]. Tennis is defined as a sport with continuous changing situations, as every ball hit or received has a different speed, position, and spin. It is important to point out that the functional mechanism for speed and agility is different. The way in which a player moves around the court determines the successfulness of the player [7,8], this being due to the fact that proper footwork makes for effective and successful execution of the strokes. The results show that the SH 10 × 5 and the SR test values in the U14 and U18 elite junior female tennis players show a moderate correlation with current competitive performance. The nature of tennis having fast exchanges requires a high level of linear and multi-directional agility, which is why explosive and controlled moves, direction changes, fast instances of slowing down, and proper support are also important requirements of competing successfully at this age, in addition to forming the basis of the technical execution of accurate and successful strokes.

4.2. Lower Body Explosive Power

The obtained data show that the explosive power of the lower limbs (SLJ test) in the U14 and U18 elite junior female categories show a moderate correlation with current competition performance. The contact of the legs with the ground creates a so-called starting force that provides the basis of all tennis strokes. Several studies have explored the correlation between the explosive power of the lower limbs as well as the sprinting of various distances [9], and the correlation between the lower body explosive power and running speed, modified by direction changes [22–24]. This is why the development of the lower body explosive power is of utmost importance in the preparation of elite junior players. A tennis player who is able to exert explosive power is also able to move quickly around the court and execute strokes with effective speed [22,23].

4.3. Upper Body Explosive Power

A moderate correlation was found between the values of OBT test of the U14 elite junior female players and the U18 elite junior tennis players and the OMBT test value of the U18 players and current competitive performance. The stretch and shortening cycle (the plyometric movements) is the most frequent contraction type in tennis, as the coordination pattern of most of the strokes is built up from this specific contraction. This is why the use of plyometric throwing exercises is indispensable in developing the most beneficial stroke power [1,3,13], with special consideration given to those athletic throwing forms (overhand ball throw, medicine ball throws from overhead and forehand and backhand side) that aid in the learning and perfecting process of the technical elements that occur in tennis.

4.4. Tennis-Specific Explosive Power

In professional tennis, the role of the serve being key is unquestionable. The serve is the only technical element that is executed by the player independent of the opponent's ball. This independent execution ensures the highest possible level of movement control by an individual player. However, the serve does not play such a dominant role in the game of junior female players, especially in the U14 age group. Nevertheless, the S test value of U14 and U18 elite junior female tennis players showed a moderate correlation with current competition performance, with the reason for that being the faster the serve hit, the shorter preparation time available for the receiving player. This is why the chance of the server to gain points increases, but that of the receiver decreases with high-speed serves, as the receiver has to match their movements to the trajectory parameters of the ball within a very short time, which is a great challenge in junior-level tennis due to the players having not yet perfected their skill set. At the same time, it must not be forgotten that the speed of stroke is only one factor determining the quality of the serve (reliability, assurance, accuracy, spinning, and speed). It is important to point out that the technical execution of the serve is an important factor affecting speed, and high-level competition performance cannot be completed without a reliable and accurate serve in the modern game [25].

4.5. Muscle Endurance

The obtained data show that the muscular endurance (PU 30s test) in U14 and U18 elite junior female players shows a moderate correlation with current competitive performance. The pectoralis and the muscles in the arm executing the stroke show great activity in the phases of speeding up the racket while executing different technical elements [26]. As well as this, there is also a high, repeated, and unbalanced load on the upper body of junior tennis players. The matches can last many hours, and during this time, a player may execute several hundred strokes; accordingly, if they want to maintain the level of their stroke quality whilst avoiding the risk of injury, they should develop the explosive power and muscle endurance required to do so.

This study has a number of limitations, which will be discussed below. Firstly, the subjects involved in this study were highly selected youth tennis players in a very sensitive and crucial developmental phase. Secondly, we did not evaluate the biological age of the participants, which is known to influence neuromuscular performance; thirdly, we did not have the possibility to look at the anthropometric variables and well as at the tennis-specific variables like technical execution of the serve or forehand/backhand medicine ball throw; and fourthly, we did not have the possibility to look at the mental and physical fatigue that may have occurred during the testing process; therefore, it could have potentially affected the most effective movement execution.

In summary, the present study suggests that neuromuscular fitness is associated with competitive tennis success in female junior tennis players, but not male elite junior tennis players. Our findings provide useful information for coaches to create a wide range of tennis-specific situations to develop a proper performance, especially for their player's neuromuscular fitness. Additional studies are needed to identify interventions that can increase sport-specific neuromuscular fitness with the ultimate goal of achieving better performance.

5. Conclusions

The result of the present study showed that the better performance in selected field tests (except for H, OMBT, and STR in the U14 girls, H and STR in U18 girls) showed a better current competitive performance in the U14 and U18 elite Hungarian female tennis players, but in contrast, U14 and U18 elite Hungarian male players did not show a better current competitive performance in selected fields. We can hypothesize that sexual maturation has a large influence on female physical fitness measures, and due to slightly different playing style, the importance of neuromuscular fitness is greater. In males, there are some qualitative differences in performance due to other factors. In addition, future research should focus on complex measuring of different performance variables that happen during a match or training (i.e., by taking the speed and accuracy of hitting on the serve, forehand, and backhand strokes as a criterion or indicator of competitive level). Furthermore, more research is required in order to develop a tennis-specific field test that can measure the key physical variables more precisely. Finally, future research should be extended to other age categories, taking into account biological age rather than chronological age.

Author Contributions: Conceptualization, K.D. and D.N.; methodology, K.D.; formal analysis, K.D. and D.N.; data collection, K.D.; resources, K.D. and P.B.; data curation, K.D.; writing—original draft preparation, K.D. and D.N.; writing—review and editing, K.D., D.N. and P.B.; visualization, K.D., D.N. and P.B.; supervision, D.N. and P.B. All authors have read and agreed to the published version of the manuscript.

Funding: This research received no external funding.

Institutional Review Board Statement: The study was conducted according to the guidelines of the Declaration of Helsinki and approved by the Ethical Committee of Public Health Division of the Budapest Government Office (Code: N° 7878/2014, Date: 23-08-2014).

Informed Consent Statement: Informed consent was obtained from all subjects involved in the study.

Data Availability Statement: The data presented in this study are available on request from the corresponding author.

Acknowledgments: The authors would like to thank the athletes for their willingness to participate in this investigation and the University of Physical Education for providing a framework for this study.

Conflicts of Interest: The authors declared no conflict of interest regarding the publication of this manuscript.

Appendix A

Description of Selected Field Tests

H: Participants started the test from a ready position and from the centre of the hexagon where they waited for a signal to begin. The player performed a jump motion in and out of the hexagon jumping across every line of the shape, using both legs and moving in a clockwise direction. The exercise finished after three completed circuits. During the execution, the player was not allowed to touch the lines of the hexagon, and the order of the jumps around the shape had to be maintained. A penalty of 0.5 s was given for each line that was touched or a 1 s penalty for failure to follow the proper sequence. The aim was to finish the test within the shortest amount of time. The time was measured in seconds, and the best recorded result was used for analysis [5,12]. The interclass correlation coefficient (ICC) for this test was 0.91 (0.90–0.92).

R5: The player stood in a ready position 50 cm behind the line, and the test started with a signal. The aim was to sprint the 5 m distance within the shortest time possible. The photocell gates were placed at the start and at the end point of the distance, as well as 1 m above the ground level. The time was measured in seconds and the best result recorded was used for analysis [1,3]. The ICC for this test was 0.93 (0.92–0.94).

SLJ: The player stood in a ready position behind starting line. Their toes were not allowed to touch the line. After gaining momentum (with knee-flexion and an arm-swing at the same time), the player executed a forward double leg jump with the aim to jump as far as possible. During the drive phase, the heels of the player had to be in full contact with the ground. The aim was to reach the highest possible height measured in meters. The best result recorded was used for analysis [1]. The ICC for this test was 0.82 (0.80–0.84).

OMBT: The player stood behind the line from which they were to from in a forward straddle with the ball held above the head with both hands. After gaining momentum, the medicine ball was tossed with a two-hand overhead throw. During the execution and after the release, the player was not allowed to touch or cross the line they threw from. The aim was to throw it as far as possible, with the distance being measured in meters. The best result recorded was used for analysis [1,3,5]. The ICC for this test was 0.89 (0.87–0.91).

OBT: The player stood in a forward straddle position behind the line from which they threw; the ball was held in the dominant arm and in front of their thigh. After gaining momentum, the ball was thrown in a one-handed overhand throw. During the execution of the throw and the release of the ball, the player was not allowed to touch or cross the line from which they threw. The aim was to throw the ball as far as possible, with the distance being measured in meters. The best result recorded was used for analysis [13]. The ICC for this test was 0.86 (0.85–0.87).

S: The player served from the deuce (right) side of the court and executed eight flatly hit serves into the 180 × 180 cm target zone, which was located in the corner nearest to the respective T-line of the tennis court. The radar instrument measuring the speed of the serve was located in the centre, 4 m behind the baseline, at a height covering the contact point of the serve. The player was instructed to execute the flat serve with maximal speed. Only the correctly executed serves that landed within the target area were measured in km/h, and the best result was used for later analysis. The intertrial reliability for serve velocity was 3.2% and the ICC for this test was 0.91–0.94, as found in previous research [1,3].

PU 30s: The player was in the push-up position, with only their toes and hands touching the floor. The player executed arm flexion and extension from a shoulder-width push-up position in such a way that a 12 cm high object located on the ground had to be touched by the chest. The aim was to do as many arm-flexions and extension (push-ups) as possible within the 30-s time frame. Only the correctly executed push ups were recorded and used for later analysis [14]. The ICC for this test was 0.85 (0.80–0.90).

SH 10 × 5: The player stood in the ready position behind the starting line. After the signal to begin, the participant ran to the line located 5 m away, crossed it with both legs, turned, and ran back; this had to be repeated four times during each test. During the task, the player was not allowed to use the sliding technique. The aim was to execute the exercise within the shortest possible time, measured in seconds, and the best result was used for later analysis. The photocell gate was placed at the starting point of the shuttle run and 1 m above ground level [15]. The ICC for this test was 0.87 (0.85–0.90).

SR: The player stood in a ready position in the middle of the court behind the baseline. Starting when signalled to, the participant had to collect the balls that were located on different parts of the court (cross point of the singles side-lines with the baseline and the service line and on the T-line), one after the other, in a pre-determined order, and put them onto a 30–45 cm quadrangle-shaped area drawn just behind the centre part of the baseline. The player was only allowed to run forward. The aim was to execute the test within the shortest possible time, measured in seconds, and the best result was used for later analysis. The photocell gate was placed at the starting point of the spider run and 1 m above ground level [5,16]. The ICC for this test was 0.90 (0.89–0.91).

STR: The player was seated in an L-shaped seated position with the soles of their feet firmly supported against the measuring box and their fingers positioned on the ruler located on the inner side of the upper surface of the box. Then, leaning forward, the participant had to push the ruler as far forward as they could and hold this position for 1 to 2 s. Their knees were not allowed to flex during the execution. The result was recorded in cm, and the best value was used for later analysis [5,15]. The ICC for this test was 0.92 (0.90–0.94).

Current competitive performance: The method of the Hungarian Tennis Federation was used as follows: (1) the total of the five best individual results over the past twelve months; (2) the bonus points gained; (3) one-fifth of the total of the five best results in pairs; (4) the division of the gained result by six; and (5) the corrections of the averaged points based on international results. Thus, the players were ranked on their averages (measured in two decimals) in a decreasing order, which meant that the player with the highest average had the highest ranking position.

References

1. Fernández-Fernández, J.; Saez De Villarreal, E.; Sanz-Rivas, D.; Moya, M. The Effects of 8-Week Plyometric Training on Physical Performance in Young Tennis Players. *Pediatr. Exerc. Sci.* **2016**, *28*, 77–86. [CrossRef]
2. Stephaine, A.K.; Reid, M. Comparing matchplay characteristics and physical demand of junior and professional tennis athletes in the era of big data. *J. Sci. Med. Sport* **2017**, *16*, 489–497.
3. Fernández-Fernández, J.; Ulbricht, A.; Ferrauti, A. Fitness testing of tennis players: How valuable is it? *Br. J. Sports Med.* **2014**, *48*, 22–31. [CrossRef]
4. Reid, M.; Duffield, R.; Minett, G.; Sibte, N.; Murphy, A.; Baker, J. Physiological, perceptual, and technical responses to on-court tennis training on hard and clay courts. J. Strength. *Cond. Res.* **2013**, *27*, 1487–1495. [CrossRef]
5. Roetert, E.P.; Ellenbecker, T. *Complete Conditioning for Tennis*; Human Kinetics: Champaign, IL, USA, 2007; pp. 17–41.
6. Baiget, E.; Fernández-Fernández, J.; Iglesias, X.; Vallejo, L.; Rodriguez, F.A. On-court endurance and performance testing in competitive male tennis players. *J. Strength Cond. Res.* **2014**, *28*, 256–264. [CrossRef] [PubMed]
7. Filipčič, A.; Pisk, L.; Filipčič, T. Relationship between the result of selected motor tests and competitive successfulness in tennis for different age categories. *Kinesiology* **2010**, *42*, 175–183.

8. Girard, O.; Millet, G. Physical Determinants of Tennis Performance in Competitive Teenage Players. *J. Strength Cond. Res.* **2009**, *23*, 1867–1872. [CrossRef] [PubMed]
9. Kramer, T.; Huijgen, B.; Elferink-Gemser, M.T.; Visscher, C. A longitudinal study of physical fitness in elite junior tennis players. *Pediatr. Exerc. Sci.* **2016**, *28*, 553–564. [CrossRef]
10. Kremer, T.; Huijgen, B.; Elferink-Gemser, M.T.; Visscher, C. Prediction of tennis performance in junior elite tennis players. *J. Sports Sci. Med.* **2017**, *16*, 14–21. [PubMed]
11. Ulbricht, A.; Fernandez-Fernandez, J.; Mendez-Villanueva, A.; Ferrauti, A. Impact of fitness characteristics on tennis performance in elite junior tennis players. *J. Strength Cond. Res.* **2016**, *30*, 989–998. [CrossRef]
12. Beekhuizen, K.S.; Davis, M.D.; Kolber, M.J.; Cheng, M.S.S. Test retest reliability and minimal detectable change of the hexagon agility test. *J. Strength Cond. Res.* **2009**, *23*, 2167–2171. [CrossRef]
13. Dobos, K.; Nagykaldi, C. The relationship between distance of overhand ball throw and maximal ball speed of serve in elite junior tennis players. *ITF CSSR* **2017**, *73*, 22–23.
14. Augustsson, S.R.; Bersås, E.; Thomas, E.M.; Sahlberg, M.; Augustsson, J.; Svantesson, U. Gender differences and reliability of selected physical performance tests in young women and men. *Adv. Physiother.* **2009**, *11*, 64–70. [CrossRef]
15. Tsigilis, N.; Douda, H.; Tokmakidis, S.P. Test-Retest Reliability of the Eurofit Test Battery Administered to University Students. *Percept. Mot. Skills* **2002**, *95*, 1295–1300. [CrossRef]
16. Huggins, J.; Jarvis, P.; Brazier, J.; Kyriacou, Y.; Bishop, C. Within—and between—Session Reliability of the Spider Drill Test to Assess Change of Direction Speed in Youth Tennis Athletes. *Int. J. Sports Exerc. Med.* **2017**. [CrossRef]
17. Harriss, J.; MacSween, A.; Atkinson, G. Ethical Standard in Sport and Exercise Science Research. *Int. J. Sports Med.* **2019**, *40*, 813–817. [CrossRef] [PubMed]
18. Dancey, C.; Reidy, J.; Rowe, R. *Statistics for the Health Sciences: A Non-Mathematical Introduction*; SAGE: London, UK, 2012; pp. 288–289.
19. Ochi, S.; Campbell, M.J. The progressive physical development of a high-performance tennis player. *Strength Cond. J.* **2009**, *31*, 59–68. [CrossRef]
20. Roetert, E.P.; Garrett, G.E.; Brown, S.W.; Camaione, D.N. Performance profiles of nationally ranked junior tennis players. *J. Appl. Sport Sci. Res.* **1992**, *6*, 225–231. [CrossRef]
21. Kovacs, M. Strength and Conditioning for Tennis. *ITF. CSSR.* **2010**, *50*, 13–14.
22. Asadi, A. Effects of six weeks depth jump and countermovement jump training on agility performance. *Sports Sci.* **2012**, *5*, 67–70.
23. Thomas, K.; French, D.; Hayes, P.R. The effect of two plyometric training techniques on muscular power and agility in youth soccer players. *J. Strength Cond. Res.* **2009**, *23*, 332–335. [CrossRef]
24. Váczi, M.; Tollár, J.; Meszler, B.; Juhász, I.; Karsai, I. Short-term high intensity plyometric training program improves strength, power and agility in male soccer players. *J. Hum. Kinet.* **2013**, *36*, 17–26. [CrossRef] [PubMed]
25. Fernandez-Fernandez, J.; Ellenbecker, T.; Sanz-Rivas, D.; Ulbricht, A.; Ferrauti, A. Effects of a 6-week junior tennis conditioning program on service velocity. *J. Sports Sci. Med.* **2013**, *12*, 232–239. [PubMed]
26. Ulbricht, A.; Fernandez-Fernandez, J.; Ferrauti, A. Conception for fitness testing and individualized training program in the German Tennis Federation. *Sport Orthop. Traumatol.* **2013**, *29*, 180–192. [CrossRef]

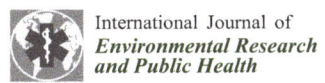

Article

Sex Disparity in Bilateral Asymmetry of Impact Forces during Height-Adjusted Drop Jumps

Chin-Yi Gu [1], Xiang-Rui Li [2], Chien-Ting Lai [2], Jin-Jiang Gao [2], I-Lin Wang [3,*] and Li-I Wang [2,*]

[1] Department of Education and Human Potentials Development, National Dong Hwa University, No. 1, Sec. 2, Da Hsueh Rd., Shoufeng, Hualien 97401, Taiwan; stronggu@gmail.com
[2] Department of Physical Education and Kinesiology, National Dong Hwa University, No. 1, Sec. 2, Da Hsueh Rd., Shoufeng, Hualien 97401, Taiwan; s86919177@gmail.com (X.-R.L.); 610789004@gms.ndhu.edu.tw (C.-T.L.); kao974129@gmail.com (J.-J.G.)
[3] College of Physical Education, Hubei Normal University, Huangshi 435002, China
* Correspondence: ilin@gms.ndhu.edu.tw (I.-L.W.); tennis01@gms.ndhu.edu.tw (L.-I.W.)

Abstract: Side-to-side asymmetry of lower extremities may influence the risk of injury associated with drop jump. Moreover, drop heights using relative height across individuals based on respective jumping abilities could better explain lower-extremity loading impact for different genders. The purpose of the current study was to evaluate the sex differences of impact forces and asymmetry during the landing phase of drop-jump tasks using drop heights, set according to participants' maximum jumping height. Ten male and ten female athletes performed drop-jump tasks on two force plates, and ground reaction force data were collected. Both feet needed to land entirely on the dedicated force plates as simultaneously as possible. Ground reaction forces and asymmetry between legs were calculated for jumps from 100%, 130%, and 160% of each participant's maximum jumping height. Females landed with greater asymmetry at time of contact initiation and time of peak impact force and had more asymmetrical peak impact force than males. Greater values and shorter time after ground contact of peak impact force were found when the drop height increased to 160% of maximum jumping ability as compared to 100% and 130%. Females exhibited greater asymmetry than males during drop jumps from relative heights, which may relate to the higher risk of anterior cruciate ligament injury among females. Greater sex disparity was evident in impact force asymmetry than in the magnitude of peak impact force; therefore, it may be a more appropriate field-screening test for risk of anterior cruciate ligament injury.

Keywords: anterior cruciate ligament; ground reaction force; knee injuries; leg dominance

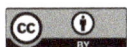

1. Introduction

Compared to males, females have a high rate of noncontact anterior cruciate ligament (ACL) injuries during athletic competition [1]. Many studies have reported that females showed greater impact in vertical ground reaction forces (I-vGRF) and have a strong trend toward one-leg dominance with greater bilateral asymmetry during landing tasks compared to males [2–4]. Previous research has revealed that females have larger I-vGRF in the nondominant limb compared to that in the dominant limb during the landing phase of the drop-jump (DJ) task [5]. Greater I-vGRF can create knee instability and increase loading both on the knee joint and ACL [6]. Leg dominance theories may explain reports that side-to-side imbalances predict future ACL injury risk during bilateral tasks [2], and side-to-side asymmetries of I-vGRFs during bilateral landing tasks may be an important predictor for ACL injury risk [7]. Despite the many studies that have focused on asymmetry of the lower extremity during landing in females, little research has looked specifically at I-vGRF parameters to measure asymmetry during bilateral landing tasks between sexes.

Drop jumps (DJs), a popular plyometric exercise method for improving the neuromuscular strength and power of lower extremities, are widely used in biomechanical studies to investigate lower-extremity injury risk [8–10]. The DJ involves stepping off a fixed drop height, briefly landing, and immediately taking off from the ground to achieve maximum jump height. Previous studies have investigated DJ performance under various height and loading parameters and indicated that the choice of appropriate drop height is important [9,11]. Some studies suggested that during double-legged DJ training, the drop height should not exceed 40 cm [8,10]. Some studies indicated that bilateral DJs from lower heights, such as 20 cm, caused greater asymmetry in leg power required, which may cause an asymmetrical bilateral training stimulus. [12].

Previous studies often investigated the sex disparities in injury risk in controlled laboratory experiments using the same drop heights (absolute height) in males and females [13,14]. However, Komi and Bosco have suggested that the appropriate DJ height differs between males and females [15], and that the capacity to endure the impact forces is weaker for females, both of which jointly contributed to the sex disparity in the stiffness alterations when the drop height increased to 60 cm [14]. Therefore, the most appropriate drop heights for plyometric training may vary across individuals according to jumping ability [16]. To our knowledge, this study is among the first to investigate sex disparity in bilateral asymmetry using drop jumps from heights set relative to individuals' jump ability.

The few studies comparing the I-vGRF of males and females dropping from relative height (RH) have found that there are no sex differences during unilateral landings [17,18]. However, these studies were only focused on one RH (100% jump height of the countermovement jump). Increased drop height during bilateral DJ would generate greater perturbation of landing and likely affect the landing impact and bilateral asymmetry [7,10]. The purpose of the current study was to examine the differences in bilateral landings between male and female athletes performing two-legged DJs from RHs. We hypothesized that: (a) there would be no sex differences in landing impact; (b) females would exhibit greater bilateral asymmetry compared to males when performing DJs from RHs. We also aimed to explore the impact force of incremental drop height changes on the DJ for determining an appropriate RH.

2. Materials and Methods

2.1. Participants

Ten male (1.75 ± 0.07 m and 69.9 ± 8.9 kg) and ten female (1.61 ± 0.04 m and 52.4 ± 4.2 kg) college athletes from the physical education department participated, and their written informed consent was collected. Males included 7 basketball, 2 track and field, and 1 field hockey athletes. Females included 5 basketball, 4 track and field, and 1 field hockey stick athletes. All participants had plyometric training experience and were familiar with double-legged drop jumps. Participants had been free of any lower-extremity injury in the past 6 months prior to the experiment. The study met the principles outlined in the Declaration of Helsinki [19].

2.2. Countermovement Jump Testing Procedures

For all testing, the participants warmed up by running 10 min at a comfortable self-selected pace on a motorized treadmill and dynamically stretching the lower extremity prior to the testing protocol. At least one week before DJ experimentation, the participants' jumping ability was measured using the countermovement jump task. After the warm-up, there was a 3 min rest. Participants were then instructed to stand erect on a force plate (BP600900, AMTI Inc., Watertown, MA, USA) and with their hands placed on their waist. Three maximum-effort vertical countermovement jumps were performed with a 1 min rest between trials, and ground reaction forces (GRFs) were recorded at 2000 Hz with KwonGRF software (VISOL Inc., Seoul, Korea). Jump height (JH) was calculated using the formula: $JH = gT^2/8$ ($g = 9.81$ m/s^2; T = flight time) [9]. The greatest JH was used to determine each participant's RHs for the subsequent DJ experimental session.

2.3. Drop-Jump Testing Procedures

Three minutes after the warm-up, the participants completed 3–4 practice jumps to become familiar with the appropriate DJ technique under the guidance of the Strength and Conditioning Coach. The drop-jump tasks consisted of three RHs (JH × 100% (males: 46.70 ± 3.90 cm; females: 31.30 ± 2.24 cm), JH × 130% (males: 60.71 ± 5.34 cm; females: 40.69 ± 3.07 cm), and JH × 160% (males: 74.72 ± 6.58 cm; females: 50.08 ± 3.78 cm) ($RH_{100\%}$, $RH_{130\%}$, and $RH_{160\%}$, respectively)), and the trial height order was randomized for each participant. The double-legged DJ tasks comprised dropping with both feet off a raised platform onto two force plates and then jumping off the ground as fast and high as possible. Participants were instructed to keep their hands on their waist. During the DJ task instructions, the participants were asked to control their legs in the same way. Each entire foot needed to land on a separate force plate at the same time as possible. Each participant was asked to complete three successful DJs (as described previously) for each RH with a 30 s rest between trials. Data were averaged across the three trials for each DJ.

2.4. Data Collection and Analysis

The GRF data were collected and analyzed with the Qualisys Track Manager motion capture and analog data acquisition system (Qualisys, Gothenburg, Sweden). Two force plates (BP600900; AMTI, Inc., Watertown, MA, USA) at a 2000 Hz sampling rate were used. The force plates were synchronized using a Qualisys 64-channel A/D board. The ground contact phase was defined as the time interval from foot contact to the foot leaving the ground. Parameters were calculated for the participants' dominant and nondominant limbs. The dominant limb was determined using a ball-kicking test. The leg they chose to kick with was deemed the dominant leg, whereas the plant leg was deemed the nondominant leg [20]. The instant of ground contact commencement (t1) was determined by assessing the 10 N vGRF threshold of the force plate. I-vGRFpeak was defined as the maximum vGRF during the landing phase of the DJ. Time to I-vGRFpeak after ground contact was considered as the time interval from t1 to the time of I-vGRFpeak (t2): t2-t1. Absolute difference in t1, t2, and I-vGRFpeak per leg during the landing phase was used to calculate side-to-side asymmetry [7,12,21]. The I-vGRFs were normalized using two methods: (a) normalized to body weight (BW) [7], and (b) normalized to body weight × $RH^{-\frac{1}{2}}$ ($BW \times RH^{-\frac{1}{2}}$) to minimize the variation due to individual differences in body weight and drop height [17].

2.5. Statistical Analysis

Data were analyzed using the Statistical Program for the Social Sciences 14.0 for Windows (SPSS, Inc., Chicago, IL, USA). Variables were analyzed with a two-way mixed-model ANOVA for sex and three RHs. If statistically significant interactions existed, a post-hoc using independent *t*-test for sex difference and one-way ANOVA for each RH were performed. If no statistically significant interaction existed, main effects between sexes or among RHs were analyzed. If a difference of main effects among RHs existed, the post-hoc test was assessed using the least significant difference (LSD) method of variances. Sphericity was analyzed using Mauchly's test, followed by a Greenhouse–Geisser correction when the results were nonspherical. The significance level was set at $\alpha = 0.05$. A priori power analysis (G × Power version 3.1.9.4; Heinrich Heine University Düsseldorf, Düsseldorf, Germany), with a power level of 80% and an α level of 0.05 [22], was performed. The expected effect size was calculated using the means (2.16 and 2.98) and standard deviation (0.46 and 0.78) of the peak impact force under DJH30 and DJH40 conditions [23]. It revealed that the sample size of 14 participants would be sufficient for the analysis.

3. Results

The time to peak I-vGRFpeak variables are shown in Table 1. No interaction between height and sex was observed in time to I-vGRFpeak after ground contact (dominant limb: $p = 0.238$; nondominant limb: $p = 0.203$). A significant main effect of height was observed (dominant limb: ES 0.8, $p = 0.024$; nondominant limb: ES 0.1, $p = 0.009$). Times to I-vGRFpeak after ground contact in $RH_{160\%}$ were significantly shorter than in $RH_{100\%}$ (dominant limb: $p = 0.021$; nondominant limb: $p = 0.013$) and $RH_{130\%}$ (dominant limb: $p < 0.001$; nondominant limb: $p = 0.012$). No difference was found between $RH_{100\%}$ and $RH_{130\%}$ (dominant limb: $p = 0.925$; nondominant limb: $p = 0.467$). No significant main effect of sex was found (dominant limb: $p = 0.124$; nondominant limb: $p = 0.154$).

Table 1. Time to I-vGRFpeak after ground contact for both limbs.

	$RH_{100\%}$	$RH_{130\%}$	$RH_{160\%}$	RH × sex	RH	Sex
Dominant limb (ms) [†]						
Females	47.60 (10.43)	50.60 (7.60)	43.60 (4.40)	$p = 0.238$	$p = 0.024$	$p = 0.124$
Males	45.70 (7.32)	43.10 (6.85)	40.50 (5.42)			
Post Hoc					$RH_{100\%}, RH_{130\%} > RH_{160\%}$	
Nondominant limb (ms) [†]						
Females	47.10 (10.14)	48.80 (7.64)	44.10 (5.17)	$p = 0.203$	$p = 0.009$	$p = 0.154$
Males	47.10 (6.40)	42.90 (6.42)	39.50 (3.31)			
Post Hoc					$RH_{100\%}, RH_{130\%} > RH_{160\%}$	

Values are presented with mean and standard error of the mean. I-vGRFpeak = peak impact force during the landing phase; RH = relative height. [†] Significant RH main effect ($p < 0.05$).

The I-vGRFpeak variables are shown in Table 2. When the I-vGRFpeak was normalized by BW, no interaction between height and sex was observed (dominant limb: $p = 0.541$; nondominant limb: $p = 0.144$). A significant main effect of height was observed (dominant limb: ES 0.25, $p < 0.001$; nondominant limb: ES 0.30, $p < 0.001$). The I-vGRFpeak significantly increased with each drop height increment in the dominant limb ($RH_{100\%}$ and $RH_{130\%}$: $p < 0.001$; $RH_{100\%}$ and $RH_{160\%}$: $p < 0.001$; $RH_{130\%}$ and $RH_{160\%}$: $p < 0.001$) and in the nondominant limb ($RH_{100\%}$ and $RH_{130\%}$: $p < 0.001$; $RH_{100\%}$ and $RH_{160\%}$: $p < 0.001$; $RH_{130\%}$ and $RH_{160\%}$: $p < 0.001$). The I-vGRFpeak of males was significantly greater than females (dominant limb: $p = 0.007$; nondominant limb: $p = 0.013$). When the I-vGRFpeak was normalized by $BW \times RH^{-\frac{1}{2}}$, no interaction between height and sex was observed (dominant limb: $p = 0.853$; nondominant limb: $p = 0.513$), but a significant main effect of height was observed (dominant limb: ES 0.08, $p = 0.001$; nondominant limb: ES 0.05, $p = 0.003$). The I-vGRFpeak of $RH_{160\%}$ was significantly greater than of $RH_{100\%}$ in both limbs (dominant limb: $p = 0.006$; nondominant limb: $p = 0.003$) and $RH_{130\%}$ in dominant limb ($p = 0.017$). No difference was found between $RH_{100\%}$ and $RH_{130\%}$ in both limbs dominant limb: $p = 0.083$; nondominant limb: $p = 0.086$) and between $RH_{130\%}$ and $RH_{160\%}$ in the nondominant limb ($p = 0.061$). No significant main effect was found between sexes (dominant limb: $p = 0.493$; nondominant limb: $p = 0.524$).

The absolute differentials in time of I-vGRFpeak between the dominant and nondominant limbs are shown in Figure 1. No interaction between height and sex was observed in the absolute time differentials of the I-vGRFpeak ($p = 0.184$). No significant main effect of height variables was observed ($p = 0.084$). The absolute time differentials in the I-vGRFpeak of females were significantly greater than males (ES 0.20, $p = 0.010$).

Table 2. I-vGRFpeak for both limbs.

	$RH_{100\%}$	$RH_{130\%}$	$RH_{160\%}$	RH × sex	RH	Sex
I-vGRFpeak (BW)						
Dominant limb [†, ‡]						
Females	1.63 (0.53)	1.98 (0.49)	2.44 (0.40)	$p = 0.541$	$p < 0.001$	$p = 0.007$
Males	2.11 (0.36)	2.64 (0.52)	3.10 (0.68)			
Post Hoc				$RH_{100\%} < RH_{130\%} < RH_{160\%}$; Females < Males		
Nondominant limb [†, ‡]						
Females	1.62 (0.29)	1.91 (0.52)	2.27 (0.58)	$p = 0.144$	$p < 0.001$	$p = 0.013$
Males	2.01 (0.45)	2.55 (0.59)	3.02 (0.69)			
Post Hoc				$RH_{100\%} < RH_{130\%} < RH_{160\%}$; Females < Males		
I-vGRFpeak ($BW \times RH^{-\frac{1}{2}}$)						
Dominant limb [†]						
Females	2.92 (0.96)	3.11 (0.78)	3.45 (0.61)	$p = 0.853$	$p = 0.001$	$p = 0.493$
Males	3.10 (0.57)	3.40 (0.69)	3.60 (0.81)			
Post Hoc				$RH_{100\%} = RH_{130\%} < RH_{160\%}$		
Nondominant limb [†]						
Females	2.91 (0.61)	3.00 (0.82)	3.21 (0.85)	$p = 0.513$	$p = 0.003$	$p = 0.524$
Males	2.96 (0.68)	3.28 (0.81)	3.50 (0.81)			
Post Hoc				$RH_{100\%} < RH_{160\%}$		

Values are presented with mean and standard error of the mean. I-vGRFpeak = peak impact force during the landing phase; BW = body weight; RH = relative height. [†] Significant RH main effect ($p < 0.05$), [‡] significant sex main effect ($p < 0.05$).

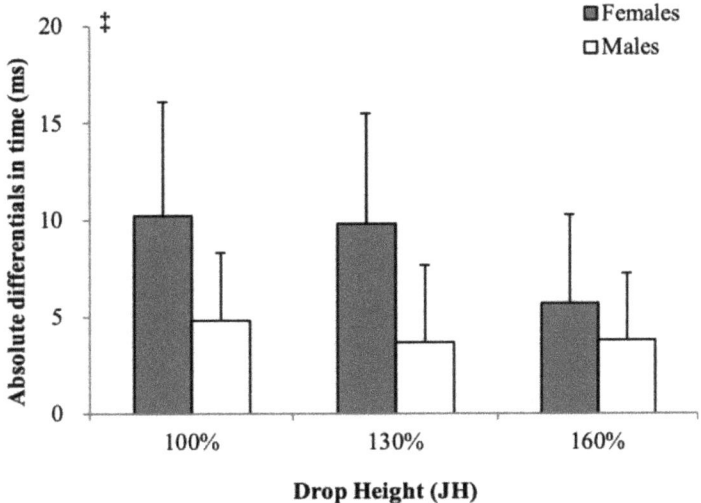

Figure 1. The side-to-side differentials in time of I-vGRFpeak between the dominant and nondominant limbs. I-vGRFpeak = peak impact force during the landing phase; JH = jump height of the countermovement jump. ‡ Significant sex main effect ($p < 0.05$).

The absolute differentials in starting contacts between the dominant and nondominant limbs are shown in Figure 2. Significant effects were not found for the interaction of height and sex on the absolute differentials in time of starting dominant limb and nondominant limb contacts ($p = 0.333$). No significant main effect of height variables was observed ($p = 0.918$). The absolute time differentials of starting contacts of females were significantly greater than males (ES 0.25, $p = 0.007$).

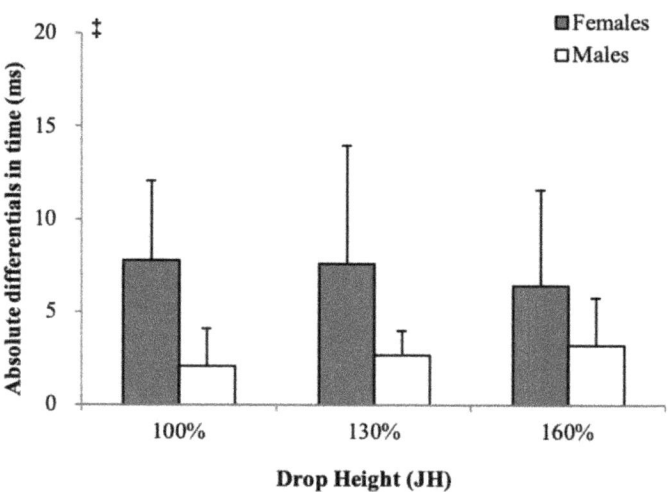

Figure 2. The side-to-side differentials in starting contacts between the dominant and nondominant limbs. JH = jump height of the countermovement jump. ‡ Significant sex main effect ($p < 0.05$).

The absolute differences in I-vGRFpeak between the dominant and nondominant limbs are shown in Table 3. No interaction between height and sex was observed when normalized by BW ($p = 0.926$) or by BW $\times$ RH$^{-\frac{1}{2}}$ ($p = 0.773$). No significant main effect of height was observed (BW: $p = 0.110$; BW $\times$ RH$^{-\frac{1}{2}}$: $p = 0.472$). The absolute differentials of females were significantly greater compared to those of males (BW: $p = 0.014$; BW $\times$ RH$^{-\frac{1}{2}}$: $p = 0.002$).

Table 3. Side-to-side differences of the I-vGRFpeak.

	RH$_{100\%}$	RH$_{130\%}$	RH$_{160\%}$	RH × sex	RH	Sex
I-vGRFpeak (BW)‡						
Females	0.46 (0.28)	0.58 (0.26)	0.54 (0.31)	$p = 0.926$	$p = 0.110$	$p = 0.014$
Males	0.25 (0.08)	0.37 (0.20)	0.37 (0.12)			
Post Hoc						Males < Females
I-vGRFpeak (BW $\times$ RH$^{-\frac{1}{2}}$)‡						
Females	0.82 (0.49)	0.90 (0.39)	0.76 (0.43)	$p = 0.773$	$p = 0.472$	$p = 0.002$
Males	0.37 (0.12)	0.48 (0.27)	0.43 (0.14)			
Post Hoc						Males < Females

Values are presented with mean and standard error of the mean. I-vGRFpeak = peak impact force during the landing phase; BW = body weight; RH = relative height. ‡ Significant sex main effect ($p < 0.05$).

4. Discussion

The aim of this study was to compare the I-vGRFs of bilateral legs between males and females to assess the symmetry of impact induced by DJ from different RHs according to an individuals' jump ability. Females and males were found to have a similar I-vGRFpeak overall. However, females had greater asymmetry in starting contact times, time of I-vGRFpeak, and I-vGRFpeak than males. A greater I-vGRFpeak and shorter time to I-vGRFpeak after ground contact was found at $RH_{160\%}$ than $RH_{100\%}$ and $RH_{130\%}$ overall.

Previous studies have indicated that the risk of lower-extremity injuries may be associated with the magnitude of peak impact and time between peak impact and ground contact [9,10]. Our study showed that the time to I-vGRFpeak during DJ was earlier at $RH_{160\%}$ than $RH_{100\%}$ and $RH_{130\%}$, and I-vGRFpeak was increased with incremental RH, which could increase the risk of injury [6,24]. This study followed the normalized suggestion by [17] to minimize the variation due to individual differences in body weight and drop height. However, the impact force was still significantly greater in $RH_{160\%}$ than $RH_{100\%}$ and $RH_{130\%}$ after normalization, which suggests that the increase in impact force at $RH_{160\%}$ is not only affected by the increase in drop height. These data suggest that a relatively high impact load of the lower extremity may be linked to practices of the double-legged DJ from a height above 160% height of the countermovement jump.

It is important to note that the height of the countermovement jump for males is nearly 15 cm higher than that for females; this disparity implies that males have greater muscle performance in the lower extremity [25]. Therefore, it is necessary to consider that DJs of absolute height may create an inequitable task demand and unrealistic impact on the lower extremities of female participants [17]. The present study found that peak I-vGRFs were greater in males than females during DJs from RHs. As previously described, greater drop heights prior to landing incrementally increase peak I-vGRFs on the lower extremity. The higher drop height in males in our study was set relative to the higher jump height of the countermovement jump, which may have caused the contrary finding with previous research on the experimental design of absolute drop height [4] but may justify the greater peak I-vGRFs recorded in males. Interestingly, while these peak I-vGRFs were normalized by the square root of drop height, the sex disparities disappeared. Wang et al. reported that the capacity to dissipate or endure the impact forces experienced by the lower extremity might be stronger in males compared with that of their female counterparts [14]. Therefore, it remains to be clarified whether males will have a greater injury risk when the DJ is adjusted for RH. Regardless of which normalization method is selected, females do not experience greater impact than males when the drop height of the DJ task is set relative to jumping ability.

A previous study found females to have greater side-to-side asymmetries than males during landing tasks, but the measurement was limited to kinematic and kinetic parameters from the absolute drop height [3]. To the best of our knowledge, ours is the first study to demonstrate that side-to-side asymmetries in the I-vGRFpeak parameters during bilateral RH DJ tasks differ between males and females. The present study found that females exhibit more asymmetrical magnitude and timing in the I-vGRFpeak than males during RH DJ. The greater imbalance of the I-vGRFpeak supports the idea that females may adopt a leg-laterality strategy during landing, relying on laterality of the limb to resist and absorb GRFs and possibly increasing the risk of knee injury [5,17]. A greater asymmetrical I-vGRFpeak between sides may generate greater knee instability and a high risk of second ACL injury [11,26,27]. Variation within side-to-side asymmetry in the I-vGRFpeak may provide clinicians and scientists with a method to identify athletes predisposed to potential future knee injury [7], especially females, whose greater asymmetry of impact may explain their greater risk of ACL injury. In the current study, male and female subjects used the same instructions of the DJ task and had similar sports experiences. Among them, athletes of the ipsilateral sports, such as badminton, table tennis, and tennis, were not included.

Therefore, we infer that female had larger bilateral asymmetry, which may be due to an individual's undesirable neuromuscular control.

The current study found a significantly greater time difference between starting dominant and nondominant limb contacts in females relative to males. The bilateral differentials in the timing of contact initiation could cause an asymmetrical bilateral stimulus and will affect the neuromuscular load between legs [21,28,29]. Ball et al. attributed the asymmetry in contact initiation to an insufficient drop time from lower heights [12]. Because of their lower average jump heights, females had lower drop heights in our study, but there was no difference found in the side-to-side asymmetry of starting contact times at different heights. The difference in the findings of the two studies may be explained by the different methodology, particularly the different platform-leaving movement: we asked participants to leave the raised platform symmetrically, while the previous participants were asked to leap off the platform with the right foot leading and needed to bring their trailing foot into position to become bilaterally coordinated before landing [12]. This indicates that the females DJs from lower heights with shorter drop times should not be the cause of greater asymmetry of starting contact times. This result showed that females might be more prone to preferential use of one leg over the other in DJ tasks [30].

This study had several limitations. First, joint movement and internal kinetics of the lower extremity were not measured. Therefore, future studies should use kinematical analysis and the inverse dynamic method to confirm the method by which I-vGRF side-to-side imbalances may cause ACL injury. Second, the sample of this study was also healthy and without pathology, and the cross-sectional design cannot assess injury risk. Otherwise, we assume, based on previous studies, that a greater jumping height is relative to high strength levels of the lower extremity. Therefore, the RHs used in this study were according to individual jumping ability instead of controlling for strength levels. We must also be aware of the inconsistency of statistical results found between different normalization methods of I-vGRFpeak; the question of whether males will exhibit greater impact load during DJs from RHs is still unanswered.

5. Conclusions

According to the results of this study, the use of relative height may be a better choice rather than absolute height, and it is not recommended that athletes practice double-legged drop jumps from heights above 160% of maximum jump height. In addition, athletes must pay attention to the bilateral asymmetries in the risk of lower limb injury during the drop-jump task, especially female athletes. Impact force asymmetry may be a better screening tool for lower-extremity injury risk than magnitude. The impact force of asymmetry may serve as useful monitoring information for practitioners.

Author Contributions: Conceptualization, L.-I.W.; methodology, C.-Y.G. and X.-R.L.; software, X.-R.L., C.-T.L., and J.-J.G.; formal analysis, I.-L.W. and L.-I.W.; writing—original draft preparation, C.-Y.G.; writing—review and editing, I.-L.W. and C.-Y.G. All authors have read and agreed to the published version of the manuscript.

Funding: This research received no external funding.

Institutional Review Board Statement: The study was approved by the Antai Medical Care Corporation Memorial Hospital (No. 18-149-B).

Informed Consent Statement: Informed consent was obtained from all subjects involved in the study.

Data Availability Statement: The data used to support the findings of this study are available from the corresponding author upon request.

Acknowledgments: The authors are grateful for the financial support from the Ministry of Science and Technology, ROC (MOST-105-2815-C-259-015-H).

Conflicts of Interest: The authors declare no conflict of interest.

References

1. Arendt, E.; Dick, R. Knee injury patterns among men and women in collegiate basketball and soccer: NCAA data and review of literature. *Am. J. Sports Med.* **1995**, *23*, 694–701. [CrossRef] [PubMed]
2. Hewett, T.E.; Ford, K.R.; Myer, G.D.; Wanstrath, K.; Scheper, M. Gender differences in hip adduction motion and torque during a single-leg agility maneuver. *J. Orthop. Res.* **2006**, *24*, 416–421. [CrossRef] [PubMed]
3. Pappas, E.; Carpes, F.P. Lower extremity kinematic asymmetry in male and female athletes performing jump-landing tasks. *J. Sci. Med. Sport* **2012**, *15*, 87–92. [CrossRef]
4. Salci, Y.; Kentel, B.B.; Heycan, C.; Akin, S.; Korkusuz, F. Comparison of landing maneuvers between male and female college volleyball players. *Clin. Biomech.* **2004**, *19*, 622–628. [CrossRef]
5. Cowley, H.R.; Ford, K.R.; Myer, G.D.; Kernozek, T.W.; Hewett, T.E. Differences in neuromuscular strategies between landing and cutting tasks in female basketball and soccer athletes. *J. Athl. Train.* **2006**, *41*, 67.
6. Hewett, T.E.; Myer, G.D.; Ford, K.R.; Heidt, R.S., Jr.; Colosimo, A.J.; McLean, S.G.; Van den Bogert, A.J.; Paterno, M.V.; Succop, P. Biomechanical measures of neuromuscular control and valgus loading of the knee predict anterior cruciate ligament injury risk in female athletes: A prospective study. *Am. J. Sports Med.* **2005**, *33*, 492–501. [CrossRef]
7. Bates, N.A.; Ford, K.R.; Myer, G.D.; Hewett, T.E. Impact differences in ground reaction force and center of mass between the first and second landing phases of a drop vertical jump and their implications for injury risk assessment. *J. Biomech.* **2013**, *46*, 1237–1241. [CrossRef]
8. Bobbert, M.F.; Huijing, P.A.; Van Ingen Schenau, G.J. Drop jumping. II. The influence of dropping height on the biomechanics of drop jumping. *Med. Sci. Sports Exerc.* **1987**, *19*, 339–346. [CrossRef]
9. Wang, L.-I.; Peng, H.-T. Biomechanical comparisons of single-and double-legged drop jumps with changes in drop height. *Int. J. Sports Med.* **2014**, *35*, 522–527. [CrossRef] [PubMed]
10. Peng, H.-T. Changes in biomechanical properties during drop jumps of incremental height. *J. Strength Cond. Res.* **2011**, *25*, 2510–2518. [CrossRef]
11. Paterno, M.V.; Schmitt, L.C.; Ford, K.R.; Rauh, M.J.; Myer, G.D.; Hewett, T.E. Effects of sex on compensatory landing strategies upon return to sport after anterior cruciate ligament reconstruction. *J. Orthop. Sports Phys. Ther.* **2011**, *41*, 553–559. [CrossRef]
12. Ball, N.B.; Stock, C.G.; Scurr, J.C. Bilateral contact ground reaction forces and contact times during plyometric drop jumping. *J. Strength Cond. Res.* **2010**, *24*, 2762–2769. [CrossRef]
13. Herrington, L.; Munro, A. Drop jump landing knee valgus angle; normative data in a physically active population. *Phys. Ther. Sport* **2010**, *11*, 56–59. [CrossRef] [PubMed]
14. Wang, I.-L.; Wang, S.-Y.; Wang, L.-I. Sex differences in lower extremity stiffness and kinematics alterations during double-legged drop landings with changes in drop height. *Sports Biomech.* **2015**, *14*, 404–412. [CrossRef] [PubMed]
15. Komi, P.V.; Bosco, C. Utilization of stored elastic energy in leg extensor muscles by men and women. *Med. Sci. Sports* **1978**, *10*, 261–265.
16. Weinhandl, J.T.; Irmischer, B.S.; Sievert, Z.A. Sex differences in unilateral landing mechanics from absolute and relative heights. *Knee* **2015**, *22*, 298–303. [CrossRef] [PubMed]
17. Weinhandl, J.T.; Irmischer, B.S.; Sievert, Z.A.; Fontenot, K.C. Influence of sex and limb dominance on lower extremity joint mechanics during unilateral land-and-cut manoeuvres. *J. Sports Sci.* **2017**, *35*, 166–174. [CrossRef]
18. Weinhandl, J.T.; Joshi, M.; O'Connor, K.M. Gender comparisons between unilateral and bilateral landings. *J. Appl. Biomech.* **2010**, *26*, 444–453. [CrossRef] [PubMed]
19. Association, W.M. World Medical Association Declaration of Helsinki: Ethical principles for medical research involving human subjects. *JAMA* **2013**, *310*, 2191–2194.
20. Wang, J.; Fu, W. Asymmetry between the dominant and non-dominant legs in the lower limb biomechanics during single-leg landings in females. *Adv. Mech. Eng.* **2019**, *11*, 1687814019849794. [CrossRef]
21. Ball, N.B.; Scurr, J.C. Bilateral neuromuscular and force differences during a plyometric task. *J. Strength Cond. Res.* **2009**, *23*, 1433–1441. [CrossRef]
22. Huang, Y.-P.; Peng, H.-T.; Wang, X.; Chen, Z.-R.; Song, C.-Y. The arch support insoles show benefits to people with flatfoot on stance time, cadence, plantar pressure and contact area. *PLoS ONE* **2020**, *15*, e0237382. [CrossRef] [PubMed]
23. Chen, Z.-R.; Peng, H.-T.; Siao, S.-W.; Hou, Y.-T.; Wang, L.-I. Whole body vibration immediately decreases lower extremity loading during the drop jump. *J. Strength Cond. Res.* **2016**, *30*, 2476–2481. [CrossRef] [PubMed]
24. Yu, B.; Garrett, W.E. Mechanisms of non-contact ACL injuries. *Br. J. Sports Med.* **2007**, *41*, i47–i51. [CrossRef] [PubMed]
25. Michailidis, Y. Effect of plyometric training on athletic performance in preadolescent soccer players. *J. Hum. Sport Exerc.* **2015**, *10*, 15–23. [CrossRef]
26. Hewett, T.E.; Stroupe, A.L.; Nance, T.A.; Noyes, F.R. Plyometric training in female athletes: Decreased impact forces and increased hamstring torques. *Am. J. Sports Med.* **1996**, *24*, 765–773. [CrossRef] [PubMed]
27. Paterno, M.V.; Ford, K.R.; Myer, G.D.; Heyl, R.; Hewett, T.E. Limb asymmetries in landing and jumping 2 years following anterior cruciate ligament reconstruction. *Clin. J. Sport Med.* **2007**, *17*, 258–262. [CrossRef]
28. Hay, D.; De Souza, V.A.; Fukashiro, S. Human bilateral deficit during a dynamic multi-joint leg press movement. *Hum. Mov. Sci.* **2006**, *25*, 181–191. [CrossRef] [PubMed]

29. Santello, M.; McDonagh, M. The control of timing and amplitude of EMG activity in landing movements in humans. *Exp. Physiol. Transl. Integr.* **1998**, *83*, 857–874. [CrossRef]
30. McLean, B.; Tumilty, D. Left-right asymmetry in two types of soccer kick. *Br. J. Sports Med.* **1993**, *27*, 260–262. [CrossRef] [PubMed]

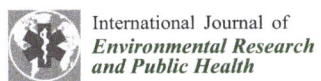

Article

Characteristics of Technical and Tactical Preparation of Elite Judokas during the World Championships and Olympic Games

Wiesław Błach [1], Łukasz Rydzik [2,*], Łukasz Błach [1], Wojciech J. Cynarski [3], Maciej Kostrzewa [4] and Tadeusz Ambroży [2,*]

1. Faculty of Physical Education & Sport, University School of Physical Education, 51-612 Wroclaw, Poland; wieslaw.judo@wp.pl (W.B.); blachlukas@gmail.com (Ł.B.)
2. Institute of Sports Sciences, University of Physical Education, 31-571 Krakow, Poland
3. Institute of Physical Culture Studies, College of Medical Sciences, University of Rzeszow, 35-959 Rzeszów, Poland; ela_cyn@wp.pl
4. Department of Sports Training, Jerzy Kukuczka Academy of Physical Education in Katowice, 40-065 Katowice, Poland; m.kostrzewa@awf.katowice.pl
* Correspondence: lukasz.gne@op.pl (Ł.R.); tadek@ambrozy.pl (T.A.); Tel.: +48-730-696-377 (Ł.R.); +48-126-831-068 (T.A.)

Abstract: The basis for achieving success in sport is technical preparation supported by adequate level of physical fitness. During judo competitions, athletes use technique to meet tactical objectives aimed to achieve victory. The modification of the rules of combat in judo that has been carried out in recent years has changed the course of competition. It seems to be interesting if there are relations between technical and tactical preparation expressed by means of indices and modification of the course of the fight caused by changes in the rules. The purpose of the paper was to determine the values of technical and tactical preparation of judokas during competition at the elite level. A hundred and twenty bouts during the Olympic Games in London in 2012 as well as 136 bouts fought during the World Championships in Rio de Janeiro in 2013 were analyzed. Verification was performed by calculating indicators of technical and tactical preparation. The results show a significant correlation between the indicators of technical and tactical preparation and the ranking in the general classification of the analyzed competitions. There were no statistically significant correlations between the change of fighting rules and the level of the examined indices of technical and tactical preparation. The results of the study verified the appropriate method of preparation for the competitions analyzed.

Keywords: judo; martial arts; technical and tactical preparation; fighting rules

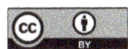

1. Introduction

Judo is a combat sport that includes many techniques of the fight and requires proper motor and physiological preparation [1]. This sport features open sensory and motor abilities with a dynamic sequence of events, and success is a result of the efficiency of the athlete's actions and the number of the rival's errors [2]. The analysis of the different techniques of performing, as well as many more details related to somatic and anthropometric changes during the athlete's development, makes sports training more and more sophisticated, while the coaching staff are supported by specialists from various fields of science, and the athlete becomes a source of valuable feedback [3–5]. Moreover, judo bouts force versatile technical and tactical preparation on competitors, which is the core of sports and decides sports championships [6,7].

According to the experts in the field, it is not possible to achieve excellent results in combat sports without earlier technical preparation [8–10]. To rationally plan the training process, it is necessary to recognize which techniques and tactical activities are effective in modern sport judo fights [11]. The most significant factors contributing to success in sports include proper technical and tactical preparation as well as the ability to apply them efficiently [12].

Currently, there are many up-to-date developments that analyze judo bouts in terms of technical and tactical actions [10,13–16]. Gutiérrez-Santiago et al. [7] analyzed the fights during the World Championships in judo in 2017 in the 66–73 kg weight division. The indicators of technical and tactical training in terms of activity, efficiency, and effectiveness of attack operations of judokas of national teams of Japan and Russia fighting during the World Championships in 2013–2015 were also analyzed [9]. Maduro et al. [17] estimated the technical profile of judokas and their coaches. The relationship between the short-term changes of results and the results achieved in World Championships was also subject to study [18]. The analysis of bouts fought during the Olympic Games found a relationship between the increase in the values of technical–tactical indicators and success in elite judo [19]. Calmet et al. [20] also showed the evolution of judo caused by the impact of new competition rules. As the result of the study, the variables of technical and tactical training of the participants (the weight divisions all together) were determined.

In the examination of the variables affecting the efficiency of the fighting technique, and consequently the level of sporting achievements, attempts have been made to verify the athlete's technical parameters in terms of activeness during competitions [21,22]. The course of the fight is determined by the rules affecting the quantitative and qualitative structure. When describing the sports fight in judo, one should mention such elements as the actual time of the fight, the time of work and rest, the number of technical and tactical activities and their types, activity, efficiency, and effectiveness [23–25]. The analysis of judo fighting conducted to date indicates the necessity to divide it into offensive and defensive fighting systems [26,27]. Both actions in attack and effective defense affect the final result of the fight, providing the athlete with points [28,29]. In planning a rational training program to ensure the achievement of the sports champion level, one should use the information obtained during the fight monitoring [30]. The most common form of determining the sports skill level of an athlete is the values of indices of technical and tactical preparation, which are used for training correction and determining the current skill level. The research on technical and tactical indicators has been the subject of many studies on combat analysis in Judo [31–33]. Monitoring of the changes within the sports fight in judo following the modification of the sports' rules seems to be an important part of the research [24].

The research was inspired by the change of the rules introduced before the World Championships in Rio. The main changes included:

(a) techniques using catching a competitor's lower limbs below the belt were banned (in 2012, they were allowed if they were used after a different allowed technique);
(b) the time limit of a golden score (overtime) was cancelled;
(c) durations of holds were shortened;
(d) many limitations in fighting for a hold were introduced.

They were supposed to make the fight more spectacular, attract media, and bring it closer to the original traditional version. Calculation and compilation of the values of indicators of technical and tactical preparation of judokas during competition at the elite level allows for the determination of the current level of competition in terms of the preparation of competitors and changes in the course of judo fights following the introduction of new regulations, and also for linking it with technical and tactical skill level [34].

The purpose of this paper was to determine the indicators of the technical and tactical skill level of judokas during competition at the elite level in two competitions of the highest rank, in between which a modification of the rules was made.

Answers for the following study questions were sought:

(1) What are the values of the indicators of technical and tactical preparations of judokas competing in the World Championships in Rio de Janeiro in 2013?

(2) What are the values of the indicators of technical and tactical preparations of judokas competing in the Olympic Games in London in 2012?
(3) What are the differences in the indicators between the members of both study groups?

The research hypothesis assumes that modifications in judo fighting rules may have led to changes in the level of technical and tactical training indicators of elite judo athletes.

2. Materials and Methods

The study was based on the analyses of bouts fought during the Olympic Games in London in 2012 and the World Championships in Rio de Janeiro in 2013. The participants of the study were medalists in seven weight divisions. Technical and tactical actions taken by 56 judokas included 28 athletes participating in the Olympic Games and 28 judokas that took part in the World Championships. Altogether, 256 men's fights were registered, including 120 bouts fought during the Olympics and 136 bouts fought during the World Championships. To determine the scores and places in the general classification, in addition to video analysis, we reviewed referee documentation and tournament reports made available by the International Judo Federation.

Age and height of the participants are shown in Table 1. Body height and age were determined based on anthropometric data from competition entry forms obtained from the International Judo Federation (IJF).

Table 1. Descriptive characteristics of the study participants.

Stats Features	Mean	± SD	Q1	ME	Q2	Min–Max
Age (years)	26.32	3.59	24	26	29	20–34
Height (cm)	178.42	11.48	170.00	176	188	160–204

SD—standard deviation, Q1—first quartile, ME—median, Q2—second quartile, Min–Max—minimum–maximum.

The analysis included judokas of different weight divisions who had various numbers of bouts fought during the competition (Table 2).

Table 2. Number and duration of bouts fought during the Olympic Games in London in 2012 and the World Championships in Rio de Janeiro in 2013, including weight divisions.

Weight Division	Olympic Games London	World Championships Rio
	Number of Bouts	Number of Bouts
60 kg	16	20
66 kg	16	21
73 kg	18	22
81 kg	18	21
90 kg	18	18
100 kg	17	18
+100 kg	17	16
Σ	120	136

Sports fight analysis was performed by three champion-level judo coaches, based on the digital recording of selected tournament fights of the athletes studied. The recording was made with three cameras (Sony HDR-CX115, Manufacturer, Tokyo, Japan). Movavi Video Editor 14 software (Movavi, Wildwood, MO, USA) was used to merge the images. The setting of cameras allowed continuous observation of the athletes, referees, and the scoreboard. A single sheet was developed as the essential research tool. The sheet consisted of a time line of the fight, on which all the performed techniques were marked with symbols [35] at the appropriate time points, along with the number of points scored for a given technique. Data from the worksheets were entered into Excel (Microsoft, Redmond, WA, USA). Then, the values of technical and tactical preparation indices were calculated.

Variables of the technical and tactical training were determined based on videos of the bouts, and the computations were made of the following, Equations (1)–(6) [10]:

1. The efficiency of the attack

$$Sa = \frac{(M \times 5) + (M \times 7) + (M \times 10)}{N} \quad (1)$$

M—number of attacks awarded according to the attack performed (yuko—5, wazari—7, ippon—10)
Sa—the efficiency of the attack
N—number of observed bouts

2. The efficiency of the defense

So is equal to the value of the indicator of the efficiency of the attack of the opponent of a given fighter.

3. Total efficiency

$$Sk = Sa - So \quad (2)$$

where Sa is the indicator of the efficiency of the attack and So is the indicator of the efficiency of the defense.
Sk—total efficiency

4. The effectiveness of the attack

$$Ea = \frac{\text{number of effective attacks}}{\text{number of all attacks}} \times 100 \quad (3)$$

Ea—Effective attack is an offensive activity that scored points. An attack is any offensive action.
Number of all attacks is the sum of all athlete's actions that are offensive in nature

5. The effectiveness of the defense

$$Eo = \left(1 - \frac{As}{Ap}\right) \times 100 \quad (4)$$

Eo—the effectiveness of the defense
Where As is a number of effective attacks performed by the opponent and Ap is the number of all attacks by the opponent.

6. The activeness of the attack

$$Aa = \frac{\text{number of recorded attacks of the competitor}}{\text{number of bouts}} \quad (5)$$

7. The activeness of the defense

Ao is equal to the value of the indicator Aa of the activeness of the attack of the opponent.

8. Total activeness

$$A = Aa - Ao \quad (6)$$

A—total activeness
Aa—the activeness of the attack
Ao—the activeness of the defense

Methods of Statistical Analysis

The statistical analysis of the data was made using R ver. 3.6.3. The chosen variables were the arithmetic mean with standard deviation ($\pm$ SD).

The differences between paired data (London and Rio comparison) were analyzed with the paired Students t-test or Wilcoxon test. Before the appropriate method was selected, the assumption about normality of distribution was verified for the difference between both features with the Shapiro–Francia test. When the test confirmed the normality of the distribution, the Students t-test was selected for analyzing the difference. Otherwise, the Wilcoxon test was used.

Firstly, it was verified whether both variables were normally distributed. If non-normality was detected, the Spearman correlation test was applied. Otherwise, Pearson's test was used. For all tests, we assumed the significance of $p < 0.05$.

In this paper, a single judoka is a statistical unit in both paired (comparison between London and Rio) and non-paired tests. Each competitor's statistics are computed based on all his bouts.

3. Results

Most of the indicators turned out to be higher during the World Championships (Rio de Janeiro 2013, Brazil). The only lower value compared to the Olympic Games (London 2012, UK) was recorded for the efficiency. There were no statistically significant differences in all indicators measured ($p > 0.05$) (Table 3).

Table 3. The efficiency, activeness, and effectiveness of the attack and defense in London and Rio.

	Indicator	Mean	SD	Q1	ME	Q2	Min–Max	p
The efficiency of the attack (Sa)	Sa London	5.92	2.49	4.00	5.20	8.10	2.00–10.02	0.083
	Sa Rio	7.79	2.47	5.90	7.91	9.75	3.50–13.83	
The efficiency of the defense (So)	So London	1.24	1.04	0.00	1.08	2.00	0.00–3.40	0.715
	So Rio	1.44	1.29	0.00	1.53	2.07	0.00–4.50	
Total efficiency (Sk)	Sk London	4.68	2.57	2.96	4.45	6.50	−0.60–10.00	0.233
	Sk Rio	6.35	2.77	4.41	6.36	7.83	1.50–13.83	
The activeness of the attack (Aa)	Aa London	1.52	0.61	1.01	1.61	1.93	0.47–3.00	0.063
	Aa Rio	1.81	0.54	1.50	1.80	2.10	0.77–3.23	
The activeness of the defense (Ao)	Ao London	1.23	0.51	0.93	1.21	1.59	0.30–2.30	0.162
	Ao Rio	1.60	1.52	1.29	1.52	1.70	1.07–2.89	
Total activeness (A)	A London	0.29	0.59	0.01	0.23	0.65	−0.74–1.61	0.73
	A Rio	0.21	0.77	−0.45	0.11	0.71	−1.21–1.73	
The effectiveness of the attack (Ea)	Ea London	12.96	6.51	7.78	13.33	17.26	3.33–26.31	0.269
	Rio	17.25	7.81	11.58	16.32	24.16	5.76–33.33	
The effectiveness of the defense (Eo)	Eo London	76.78	2.70	95.11	96.87	100.00	90.90–100.00	0.927
	Rio	96.40	3.47	94.42	96.42	100.00	85.00–100.00	

SD—standard deviation, Q1—first quartile, ME—median, Q2—second quartile, Min-Max—minimum–maximum.

There are several significant relations between the described variables. Total activeness is moderately positively related to the activeness of the attack and negatively related to the activeness of the defense (0.69 and −0.54, respectively). Total activeness and the activeness of the attack are negatively correlated to the effectiveness of the attack (−0.36 and −0.37, respectively). Activeness of the attack is also positively correlated to the efficiency of the attack (0.33). The efficiency of the defense is negatively correlated to both effectiveness of the defense and total efficiency (−0.82 and −0.33, respectively) (Table 4).

Table 4. Correlation coefficient for indicators of technical and tactical preparations.

Variable	Correlation Coefficient, No Weight Divisions,							
	Sa	So	Sk	Ea	Eo	Aa	Ao	A
Sa	-	0.09	**0.91**	**0.61**	−0.05	**0.33**	**0.31**	0.06
So	0.09	-	−**0.33**	−0.18	−**0.82**	0.21	**0.44**	−0.14
Sk	**0.91**	−**0.33**	-	**0.65**	0.28	0.23	0.11	0.12
Ea	**0.61**	−0.18	**0.65**	-	0.09	−**0.37**	**0.04**	−**0.36**
Eo	−0.05	−**0.82**	0.28	0.09	-	−0.04	−**0.03**	−0.05
Aa	**0.33**	0.21	0.23	−**0.37**	−0.04	-	0.23	**0.69**
Ao	**0.31**	**0.44**	0.11	**0.04**	−**0.03**	0.23	-	−**0.54**
A	0.06	−0.14	0.12	−**0.36**	−**0.05**	**0.69**	−**0.54**	-

Sa—the efficiency of the attack, So—the efficiency of the defense, Sk—total efficiency, Ea—the effectiveness of the attack, Eo—the effectiveness of the defense, Aa—the activeness of the attack, Ao—the activeness of the defense, A—the activeness; Statistically significant values are in bold ($p < 0.05$).

There is a positive relationship between the rank of a competitor and the values of the efficiency of the defense (So) for London (0.45) and Rio (0.5) competitions as well as for the competitions altogether (0.47). There is a moderate negative correlation between total efficiency (S) and the rank in Rio (−0.54) and both competitions together (−0.41). There is a similar relationship between the effectiveness of the defense (Eo) and the rank in Rio (−0.42) and both contests (−0.31) (Table 5).

Table 5. Relationship between the indicators of technical and tactical preparations and the rank in the general classification of the analyzed competitions.

Spearman's Rank Correlation Coefficient	Sa	So	S	Ea	Eo	Aa	Ao	A
OG 2012 London	−0.23	**0.45**	−0.33	−0.11	−0.20	−0.06	0.24	−0.30
WC 2013 Rio	−0.29	**0.50**	−**0.54**	−0.33	−**0.42**	0.08	0.20	−0.10
Altogether	−0.23	**0.47**	−**0.41**	−0.20	−**0.31**	0.00	0.22	−0.18

Sa—the efficiency of the attack, So—the efficiency of the defense, S—total efficiency, Ea—the effectiveness of the attack, Eo—the effectiveness of the defense, Aa—the activeness of the attack, Ao—the activeness of the defense, A—the activeness; Statistically significant values are in bold, Coefficients in bold are significant $p < 0.05$, OG—Olimpic Game, WC—World Championship.

4. Discussion

This paper aimed to evaluate the indicators of the level of technical and tactical skills in elite judokas in competitive settings, i.e., the World Championship and Olympic Games, with the fighting rule change occurring between the two events.

The indicator of the efficiency of the attack in both groups was different, but the differences were not statistically significant. Therefore, it should be concluded that the modification of the rules did not affect the efficiency of the athlete's attack. Such results also indicate that changes in regulations do not significantly influence the evolution of fighting techniques in Judo. Other findings are presented in the analysis of rule change and performance evolution in judo based on the analysis of Olympic Games in 2012 and 2016 and World Championships in 2015 and 2017 at which there were statistically significant differences in terms of technical and tactical preparation indicators [20]. Similarly, Adam et al. analyzed the efficiency of offensive technical actions of athletes in the context of changes in the sports fighting rules. These authors analyzed championship tournaments from 2008–2012. Based on the observations in 2008, 2009, and 2012, they presented the technical evolution of judo in terms of the most efficient technical actions. Both the development of the sport and the changes in the fighting rules resulted in shifting the burden of combat towards hand techniques (throws from the te-waza group). The values of efficiency indicators during this period were almost twice smaller than those presented in this paper and were 2.88, 3.46, and 2.35, respectively [10]. Such a difference indicates an increase in the technical and tactical skill levels of judo players. The efficiency of the defense during the Olympic Games was 1.24, while during the World Championships, it reached a higher value (1.44). There is a noticeable difference, but it is not statistically significant. Therefore, it can be considered that the elimination of lower limb catching does not significantly affect the course of the fight. No statistically significant differences were also observed in the remaining indicators of technical and tactical preparation (activeness, effectiveness of the attack, and defence). The course of the fight does not depend on the changes in the rules, and it can be assumed that it is determined by the level of technical skills and the method of implementation of the training process.

A statistically significant positive correlation was found between the medal positions and the efficiency of defense during the world championships, Olympic Games, and without the division into groups. This demonstrates the crucial role of defense, which appears to be a necessary factor for success [23]. Defensive actions are a fundamental factor in athletic competition in grappling sports [36]. The efficiency of the defense is understood to mean defending the opponent's attack even with his or her high efficiency of the attack. Not allowing the opponent to perform offensive actions is the basis for winning in combat sports. In judo, a large part of the preparatory period during the pre-competition mesocycle is devoted to the technical and tactical training of defensive actions [37].

In the present study, there was a negative relationship between total efficiency and the efficiency of the defense and medal position in the Rio Championships and without division into groups. This demonstrates that a higher index of technical and tactical preparation corresponds to a lower medal position, i.e., to a better final result. Therefore, the accumulation of the efficiency of the attack, efficiency of the defense, and the effectiveness of the defense is an essential factor in the success of an athlete. According to Sterkowicz [38], top-class judokas should have a wide range of tactical actions, and in particular, be able to force penalties on the opponent. Franchini's research [39] indicated that top-class judokas use significantly more technical actions in different directions that lead to a scoring advantage. Such results confirm the conclusions of our research. They show that the number of different technical actions and the variety of sides on which they were performed depended on the number of fights won and ippon scored. Therefore, the greater number of technical actions used and the variation in the directions of attack seem to be important factors causing unpredictability during judo fights.

In the analysis of the relationships between indicators of technical and tactical preparation of judo competitors in elite championships (World Championships and Olympic Games), the influence of changes in the rule change in terms of technique and the limitation of the number of allowed actions was mainly analyzed, without finding any relations between these variables. Smaruj et al. [40] analyzed 1643 fights of female judo players that took place between 2001 and 2004 during national classification tournaments. These authors emphasized that the effective duration of a women's judo bout has changed in 2002 from 5 min to 4 min [40]. This change could have affected the values of the indicators of technical and tactical preparation achieved by the athletes. It can be presumed that changes in technique were compensated for by the players with a high level of physical fitness and by replacing forbidden techniques with others. Therefore, preparation indicators did not change, whereas shortening of the fight time caused the necessity of changing the physiological profile of the female players. The necessity to modify the method of endurance training caused by this fact could have influenced the profile of technical and tactical preparation [15].

The high positive correlation between the effectiveness and efficiency of the attack and the negative correlation with activeness may indicate a trend caused by the evolution of judo's way of fighting. New combat sport rules force fighters to strive for high point advantage [41]. This can result in forcing athletes' activity using penalties and limiting defensive options as a result of the ban on blocking by catching the opponent judogi's leg or lower limbs with upper limbs below the waist [42]. It should be added that the effectiveness of the attack (Ea) and the effectiveness of the defense (Eo) are characterized by a high universality, consisting in an objective characterization of the technical actions of competitors, regardless of the number of analyzed fights and the duration and the way the fight is resolved [10].

Therefore, to optimize the coaching process in combat sports, the emphasis should be on the development of natural aptitudes and methods of fighting, depending on functional potential. During the bout, motor abilities are most often manifested in a complex manner. Therefore, the development of technical and tactical skills in individual athletes should take into consideration their profile of motor abilities.

Limitation of the Study

Nonetheless, the findings of this study have to be seen in light of some limitations. The indicators determining the level of technical and tactical preparation of judokas were analyzed only during two competitions of different ranks. Thus, it may be speculated that if competitions of the same rank were compared (Olympic Games vs. Olympic Games), different results would be obtained. Additionally, there was about a year of differences between the compared occupations; it is possible that a comparison of competition with a longer time interval would show the impact of training or tactical preparation to a greater extent. Moreover, only elite male judokas were analyzed, and it cannot be excluded that these results may differ among females or sub-elite judokas.

5. Conclusions

Between the 2012 Olympic Games in London and the 2013 World Championships, there were no statistically significant differences in the level of technical and tactical preparation despite the change of fighting rules that took place between the competitions.

The level of technical and tactical preparation is closely related to the medal place achieved by the athletes at the elite level.

For achieving high medal positions in championships, more attention should be paid to the level of defensive actions in the process of sports training of judokas.

Application

Because the changes in the rules of judo fights in terms of technique do not significantly differentiate the level of technical and tactical preparation of the competitors, modifications to the training process should go in the direction of the most comprehensive training of the player in terms of technique and physical fitness.

Author Contributions: Conceptualization, T.A., Ł.R., and W.J.C.; methodology, Ł.B., W.J.C., T.A., W.B., and Ł.R.; software, M.K., Ł.B., Ł.R., and T.A; validation, W.B., Ł.R., Ł.B., and T.A.; formal analysis, W.B., Ł.R., Ł.B., W.J.C., and T.A.; investigation, W.B., Ł.B., Ł.R., T.A; resources, W.B., Ł.R., Ł.B., and T.A.; data curation, W.J.C., Ł.R., T.A., and M.K.; writing—original draft preparation, W.B., Ł.B., Ł.R., W.J.C., and T.A.; writing—review and editing, Ł.R. and T.A.; visualization, W.B. and Ł.B.; supervision, T.A., Ł.R and W.J.C.; project administration, Ł.R., W.B., and T.A.; funding acquisition, W.B. and T.A All authors have read and agreed to the published version of the manuscript. Please turn to the CRediT taxonomy for the term explanation. Authorship must be limited to those who have contributed substantially to the work reported.

Funding: This research received no external funding.

Institutional Review Board Statement: The study was conducted according to the guidelines of the Declaration of Helsinki, and approved by the Bioethics Committee at the Regional Medical Chamber (No. 287/KBL/OIL/2020).

Informed Consent Statement: Informed consent was obtained from all subjects involved in the study.

Data Availability Statement: The data presented in this study are available on request from the corresponding author.

Conflicts of Interest: The authors declare no conflict of interest.

References

1. Agostinho, M.F.; Olivio Junior, J.A.; Stankovic, N.; Escobar-Molina, R.; Franchini, E. Comparison of special judo fitness test and dynamic and isometric judo chin-up tests' performance and classificatory tables' development for cadet and junior athletes. *J. Exerc. Rehabil.* **2018**, *14*, 244–252. [CrossRef] [PubMed]
2. Osipov, A.Y.; Kudryavtsev, M.D.; Iermakov, S.; Jagiełło, W. Topics of doctoral and postdoctoral dissertations devoted to judo in period 2000-2016-the overall analysis of works of Russian experts. *Arch. Budo* **2017**, *13*, 1–10.
3. Bompa, T.; Haff, G. *Periodization: Theory and Methodology of Training*; Human Kinetics: Champaign, IL, USA, 2009.
4. Smaruj, M.; Orkwiszewska, A.; Adam, M.; Jeżyk, D.; Kostrzewa, M.; Laskowski, R. Changes in Anthropometric Traits and Body Composition Over a Four-Year Period in Elite Female Judoka Athletes. *J. Hum. Kinet.* **2019**, *70*, 145–155. [CrossRef]
5. Gepfert, M.; Filip, A.; Kostrzewa, M.; Królikowska, P.; Hajduk, G.; Trybulski, R.; Krzysztofik, M. Analysis of power output and bar velocity during various techniques of the bench press among women. *J. Hum. Sport Exerc.* **2020**, *16*. [CrossRef]
6. Burns, A.; Rosenblatt, B.; Macdonald, A. Physical preparation for judo. *Sci. Judo* **2018**, 120–129.
7. Gutiérrez-Santiago, A.; Gentico-Merino, L.A.; Prieto-Lage, I. Detection of the technical-tactical pattern of the scoring actions in judo in the men's category of −73 kg. *Int. J. Perform. Anal. Sport* **2019**, *19*, 778–793. [CrossRef]
8. Adam, M.; Tabakov, S.; Klimowicz, P.; Paczoska, B.; Laskowski, R.; Smaruj, M. The efficiency of judo techniques In the light of amendments to the rules of a sports contest. *J. Combat Sport Martial Arts* **2012**, *3*, 115–120. [CrossRef]
9. Adam, M.; Sterkowicz-Przybycień, K. The efficiency of tactical and technical actions of the national teams of Japan and Russia at the World Championships in Judo (2013, 2014 and 2015). *Biomed. Hum. Kinet.* **2018**, *10*, 45–52. [CrossRef]
10. Adam, M.; Smaruj, M.; Pujszo, R. Charakterystyka indywidualnego przygotowania techniczno-taktycznego zawodników judo, zwycięzców Mistrzostw Świata z Paryża w 2011 oraz z Tokio w 2010 roku. *IDO Mov. Cult. J. Martial Arts Anthr. Poland* **2012**, *12*, 60–69.
11. Mihalache, G. Psychological Preparedness in judo and its role in the multilateral preparedness of the future officers. *J. Def. Resour. Manag.* **2018**, *9*, 172–179.
12. Soto, D.A.S.; Aedo-Muñoz, E.; Brito, C.J.; Camey, S.; Miarka, B. Making Decisions and Motor Actions with Technical Biomechanical Classifications in Male Judo Weight Categories. *J. Hum. Kinet.* **2020**, *72*, 241–252. [CrossRef]
13. Soriano, D.; Irutia, A.; Tarragó, R.; Tayot, P.; Millá-Villaroel, R.; Iglesiss, X. Time-motion analysis during elite judo combats (defragmenting the gripping time). *Arch. Budo* **2019**, *15*, 33.
14. Segedi, I.; Sertić, H.; Franjić, D.; Kuštro, N.; Rožac, D. Analysis of judo match for seniors. *J. Combat Sport Martial Arts* **2014**, *5*, 57–61. [CrossRef]
15. Miarka, B.; Pérez, D.I.V.; Aedo-Muñoz, E.; da Costa, L.O.F.; Brito, C.J. Technical-Tactical Behaviors Analysis of Male and Female Judo Cadets' Combats. *Front. Psychol.* **2020**, *11*, 1389. [CrossRef]
16. Kłys, A.; Sterkowicz-Przybycień, K.; Adam, M.; Casals, C. Performance analysis considering the technical-tactical variables in female judo athletes at different sport skill levels: Optimization of predictors. *J. Phys. Educ. Sport* **2020**, *20*, 1775–1782. [CrossRef]
17. Maduro, L.A.R.; Guedes, A.B.; Guedes, A.; Vieira, D. O perfil dos técnicos de judô formadores dos atletas das seleções brasileiras de base e suas condições estruturais de trabalho. *Conexões* **2018**, *16*, 539–552. [CrossRef]
18. Velloso Breviglieri, P.; Soares Possa, M.E.; Moura Campos, V.; Humberstone, C.; Franchini, E. Judo world ranking lists and performance during cadet, junior and senior World Championships. *Ido Mov. Cult. J. Martial Arts Anthropol.* **2018**, *18*, 48–53.
19. Brustio, P.R.; Boccia, G.; Moisè, P.; Laurenzano, L.; Lupo, C. Relationship between stature level and success in elite judo: An analysis on four consecutive Olympic Games. *Sport Sci. Health* **2018**, *14*, 115–119. [CrossRef]
20. Calmet, M.; Pierantozzi, E.; Sterkowicz, S.; Takito, M.Y.; Franchini, E. Changes rules and evolution of results in judo, an analysis: Of the 2012 and 2016 Olympic Games and 2015 and 2017 World Championships. *HAL* **2018**, hal-017914, 1–6.
21. Adam, M. Ocena przygotowania techniczno taktycznego zawodników. *Judo Sport Wyczyn Poland* **2008**, 1–3, 40–47.
22. Rydzik, Ł.; Ambroży, T. Physical fitness and the level of technical and tactical training of kickboxers. *Int. J. Environ. Res. Public Health* **2021**, *18*, 3088. [CrossRef]
23. Adam, M.; Tyszkowski, S.; Smaruj, M. The Contest Effectiveness of the Men's National Judo Team of Japan, and Character of Their Technical-Tactical Preparation during the World Judo Championships 2010. *Balt. J. Heal. Phys. Act.* **2011**, *3*, 65. [CrossRef]
24. Suzuki, K.; Saito, H.; Tanaka, C.; Maekawa, N.; Kameyama, A.; Kanemochi, T.; Tamura, M. Research about the influence of changes on player's defense action according to revision of IJF rules. *Res. J. Budo* **2014**, *46*, 78.
25. Błach, W.; Migasiewicz, J. *Wpływ Zmian Przepisów Sędziowskich Na Obraz Walki w Judo*; AWF: Warszawa, Poland, 2006.
26. Nakamura, I.; Tanabe, Y.; Nanjo, M.; Narazaki, N. *Analysis of winning points in World Senior Championships from 1995*; Bulletin of the Association for the Scientific Studies on Judo; Kodokan Report: Tokyo, Japan, 2002; Volume 9, pp. 147–156.
27. Ito, K.; Hirose, N.; Nakamura, M.; Maekawa, N.; Tamura, M. Judo kumit-te pattern and technique effectiveness shifts after the 2013 International Judo Federation rule revisions. *Arch. Budo* **2014**, *10*, 1–9.

28. Laskowski, R. *Skuteczność Techniczna i Taktyczna Zawodniczek Reprezentacji Polski w Judo w Wieloletnim Procesie Treningowym*; Wydawnictwo Uczelniane AWFiS: Gdańsk, Poland, 2006.
29. Sertić, H.; Segedi, I. Structure of importance of techniques of throws in different age groups in men judo. *J. Combat Sport. Martial Arts* **2012**, *3*, 59–62. [CrossRef]
30. Kuźmicki, S. *Historia i metodyka nauczania, wybrane aspekty*; Akademii Wychowania Fizycznego: Warszawa, Poland, 2011.
31. Miarka, B.; Del Vecchio, F.B.; Franchini, E. Acute Effects and Postactivation Potentiation in the Special Judo Fitness Test. *J. Strength Cond. Res.* **2011**, *25*, 427–431. [CrossRef]
32. Miarka, B.; Fukuda, H.D.; Heinisch, H.-D.; Battazza, R.; Del Vecchio, F.B.; Camey, S.; Franchini, E. Time-motion analysis and Decision Making in Female Judo Athletes during Victory or Defeat at Olympic and Non-Olympic Events: Are Combat Actions Really Unpredictable? *Int. J. Perform. Anal. Sport* **2016**, *16*, 442–463. [CrossRef]
33. Calmet, M.; Ahmaidi, S. Survey of Advantages Obtained by Judoka in Competition by Level of Practice. *Percept. Mot. Skills* **2004**, *99*, 284–290. [CrossRef] [PubMed]
34. Segedi, I.; Sertić, H. Classification of judo throwing techniques according to their importance in judo match. *Kinesiol. Int. J. Fundam. Appl. Kinesiol.* **2014**, *46*, 107–112.
35. Adam, M.; Laskowski, R.; Smaruj, M. Ocena indywidualnego przygotowania techniczno-taktycznego zawodników judo. In *Proces Doskonalenia Treningu i Walki Sportowej*; AZS AWFiS Gdańsk: Warszawa, Poland, 2005; p. 192.
36. Otaki, T.; Draeger, D.F. *Judo Formal Techniques: A Complete Guide to KodokanRandori No Kata*; Tuttle Publishing: Clarendon, VT, USA, 2019.
37. Jagiełło Władysław *Wieloletni Treningu Judoków*; Centralny Ośrodek Sportu Biblioteka Trenera: Warszawa, Poland, 2000; ISBN 83-866504-69-2.
38. Sterkowicz, S.; Lech, G.; Rukasz, W. Charakterystyka rywalizacji w kolejnych fazach Mistrzostw Świata w Judo 2003 r. In *Proces Doskonalenia Treningu i Walki Sportowej. Tom 3*; Kuder, A., Perkowski, K., Śledziewski, D., Eds.; AWF: Warszawa, Poland, 2006; pp. 89–93.
39. Franchini, E.; Sterkowicz, S.; Meira, C.M.; Gomes, F.R.F.; Tani, G. Technical Variation in a Sample of High Level Judo Players. *Percept. Mot. Skills* **2008**, *106*, 859–869. [CrossRef]
40. Smaruj, M.; Laskowski, R.; Adam, M. Częstotliwość i efektywność ataków zawodniczek judo na podstawie walk w czteroletnim okresie treningowym. In *Proces doskonalenia Treningu i Walki Sportowej, Tom 5*; Sozański, H., Perkowski, K., Śledziewski, D., Eds.; AWF: Warszawa, Poland, 2008; pp. 102–106.
41. Chirazi, M. Consequences of the new specifications of the judo regulations. *Sport Soc. siSocietate* **2013**, *13*, 225–231.
42. Brito, C.J.; Miarka, B.; de Durana, A.L.D.; Fukuda, D.H. Home Advantage in Judo: Analysis by the Combat Phase, Penalties and the Type of Attack. *J. Hum. Kinet.* **2017**, *57*, 213–220. [CrossRef]

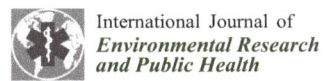

Article

Indicators of Targeted Physical Fitness in Judo and Jujutsu—Preliminary Results of Research

Wojciech J. Cynarski [1], Jan Słopecki [2], Bartosz Dziadek [1], Peter Böschen [3] and Paweł Piepiora [4],*

1. Institute of Physical Culture Studies, University of Rzeszów, 35-959 Rzeszów, Poland; ela_cyn@wp.pl (W.J.C.); bdziadek@ur.edu.pl (B.D.)
2. Idokan Poland Association, 35-959 Rzeszów, Poland; slopecki_jan@onet.eu
3. World Alliance of Martial Arts, 28197 Bremen, Germany; peter.boschen@gmail.com
4. Faculty of Physical Education and Sport, University School of Physical Education in Wrocław, 51-612 Wrocław, Poland
* Correspondence: pawel.piepiora@awf.wroc.pl

Abstract: (1) Study aim: This is a comparative study for judo and jujutsu practitioners. It has an intrinsic value. The aim of this study was to showcase a comparison of practitioners of judo and a similar martial art jujutsu with regard to manual abilities. The study applied the measurement of simple reaction time in response to a visual stimulus and handgrip measurement. (2) Materials and Methods: The group comprising $N = 69$ black belts from Poland and Germany (including 30 from judo and 39 from jujutsu) applied two trials: "grasping of Ditrich rod" and dynamometric handgrip measurement. The analysis of the results involved the calculations of arithmetic means, standard deviations, and Pearson correlations. Analysis of the differences (Mann–Whitney U test) and Student's t-test were also applied to establish statistical differences. (3) Results: In the test involving handgrip measurement, the subjects from Poland (both those practicing judo and jujutsu) gained better results compared to their German counterparts. In the test involving grasping of Ditrich rod, a positive correlation was demonstrated in the group of German judokas between the age and reaction time of the subjects ($r_{xy} = 0.66$, $p < 0.05$), as well as in the group of jujutsu subjects between body weight and the reaction time ($r_{xy} = 0.49$, $p < 0.05$). A significant and strong correlation between handgrip and weight was also established for the group of German judokas ($r_{xy} = 0.75$, $p < 0.05$). In Polish competitors, the correlations were only established between the age and handgrip measurements ($r_{xy} = 0.49$, $p < 0.05$). (4) Conclusions: Simple reaction times in response to visual stimulation were shorter in the subjects practicing the martial art jujutsu. However, the statement regarding the advantage of the judokas in terms of handgrip force was not confirmed by the results.

Keywords: martial arts; combat sports; physical fitness; dexterity; handgrip

Citation: Cynarski, W.J.; Słopecki, J.; Dziadek, B.; Böschen, P.; Piepiora, P. Indicators of Targeted Physical Fitness in Judo and Jujutsu—Preliminary Results of Research. *Int. J. Environ. Res. Public Health* **2021**, *18*, 4347. https://doi.org/10.3390/ijerph18084347

Academic Editor: Paul B. Tchounwou

Received: 16 February 2021
Accepted: 17 April 2021
Published: 20 April 2021

Publisher's Note: MDPI stays neutral with regard to jurisdictional claims in published maps and institutional affiliations.

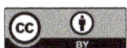

Copyright: © 2021 by the authors. Licensee MDPI, Basel, Switzerland. This article is an open access article distributed under the terms and conditions of the Creative Commons Attribution (CC BY) license (https://creativecommons.org/licenses/by/4.0/).

1. Introduction

Combat sports involving wrestling have their special characteristics, which include both performance training, specialist training, and teaching of technical–tactical skills. This applies to both training of judo as well as jujutsu as a sport discipline [1]. Both these disciplines have their sources in the old Japanese martial art jujutsu. However, due to the different objective sought in these disciplines, the results of the training involving the practitioners of sport jujutsu and traditional jujutsu assumes different directions [2]. The practitioners of the traditional martial arts jujutsu should be capable of combat in actual conditions of self-defense in the situation of a direct attack of several opponents on one and in various non-standard circumstances. In turn, judo forms a sport in which an emphasis is placed on the athletic preparation. In both cases (both in combat sports and martial arts), it is necessary to develop a high level of motor coordination skills [3–5]. The comprehensive array of these issues is best explained by the General Theory of Fighting Arts [6,7]. The *modern* jujutsu analyzed here is practiced as a traditional martial art and does not involve sport competition. However, both judo and jujutsu are open skill sports [8].

The authors of this paper adopted certain initial assumptions imposed by the needs of the study into motor skills in humans. The motor skills are therefore understood broadly. The authors assumed that the specific motor skills and the ability to perform specific motor activities are determined by the structure and functions of the organism. These motor abilities can be identified and developed as part of the structure and functions of the living organisms [6,9–16]. Among the various motor skills, we can distinguish skills that are especially important for particular sports.

The "targeted physical fitness" is the targeted physical fitness for judo and jujutsu. It involves the development of "manual skills" or "manual abilities" that determine the effectiveness of technical-tactical activities. Most of the fighting techniques in both fighting arts are so-called hand techniques (grips, throws, etc.).

The aim of the research was to compare two groups of subjects training in fighting arts, judo, and related jujutsu, with regard to manual capabilities. On the basis of long-term participant observation in the environment of the practitioners of sport judo and martial arts jujutsu, the authors collected data by performing observations and taking notes. The applicability of selected tests for research results from the experience gained by these authors. The focus in the study was placed on the phenomena (abilities) characteristic for the subjects practicing the martial arts jujutsu and the sport judo. On the basis of their experiences, the authors decided to apply a passive participant observation so as to be able to select the adequate abilities applied in the testing and analysis. The perception of these dependencies is not incidental but was performed in a continuous and systematic manner. Judo and jujutsu are both grappling sports. Most (in judo, almost all) techniques are performed in the grip. Therefore, the grip strength is a very important parameter here. On the basis of the above assumptions, we developed the main hypothesis and two detailed hypotheses. The main hypothesis was assumed in the form: there are differences in the motor abilities of practitioners of the martial art of jujutsu and judo. The detailed hypotheses assume that

1. Simple reaction time in response to a visual stimulus is shorter in the subjects practicing martial arts jujutsu.
2. Handgrip in practitioners of judo is greater than in the ones practicing martial art jujutsu.

The research results are useful for trainers and researchers, presenting a tool that is easy to apply in the conditions of a training room and a short training unit time. The ease of testing strength and dexterity and their connection with "grappling" sports constitute a valuable resource for the practice of sports training.

2. Material and Methods

The study purposefully selected subjects with a similar training experience in judo and jujutsu in the range from 10 to 30 years, with a note that all those involved in the study have master ranks in their disciplines (a minimum of 1 dan); the age range of the subjects was 18 to 45 years. For the purpose of reliability of the results, the group selected for the present study had to be carefully selected. In the case of jujutsu, they were people more active in the study of this martial art—participants of international training seminars. In judo, only activity and sports results enable the achievement of higher technical degrees. Therefore, the selection concerned people with higher grades (black belts). The purposeful selection carried out in this way can be considered representative here. As a result, the group comprising Polish and German practitioners was selected, $N = 69$ in total, including 40 subjects from Poland (20 judoka and 20 jujutsuka) and 29 from Germany (10 judoka and 19 jujutsuka).

The group of Polish jujutsu was represented by 20 *jujutsuka*, all members of the "Budokan Poland" team. The subjects practicing martial arts jujutsu often practice it for several dozen years, which has a big impact on the level of physical coordination in these people, and therefore we decided to perform a comparison using a similar group of study subjects (on the basis of training experience, age, and dan level) practicing judo in two clubs located in Warsaw—University of Warsaw and Warsaw University of Technology, comprising 20 judokas in total.

The group originating from Germany was made up of participants of the following training seminars: "Allen Sally Seminar" in Delmenhorst (19 November 2017), "ACS meets Friends Seminar" in Bremen (10 March 2018), and "Ronnin Ju-Jitsu" in Wolfenbüttel (11 March 2018). The black belts in judo comprised the subjects who attended seminars in Bremen and Wolfenbüttel—10 people in total. The remaining 19 people were representatives of jujutsu and related martial arts. They train 3 times a week in each group.

2.1. Methods and Technique Applied in Study

Coordination ability and reaction time seem to be dominant and characteristic of jujutsu practitioners. In turn, among judokas, the handgrip may be of particular importance, which is used, for example, in the *keikogi* grip.

Selected motor and psychomotor abilities, which are characteristic and dominant among subjects practicing the martial art such as judo and jujutsu, were chosen to measure and compare. The study applied testing of the reaction force performed by grasping of Ditrich rod and a dynamometric handgrip measurement. The selected scope of the testing is characteristic for each of these disciplines, and their selection is closely related to the type of data that are recorded and focused on in the anticipated results. The knowledge about the characteristics of the subjects (such as age, weight, training experience, attained master rank) and the respective measurements that are carried out have a direct effect on the course of the statistical analysis. The study applied the measurements of grip strength and reaction time, capabilities and behaviors of the individuals, combined with in-depth knowledge of the various complex motor skills resulting from variable ontogenetic and environmental circumstances, and related to the specific characteristics of the practiced discipline.

The grasping of Ditrich rod is often applied and recommended for analytical testing in combat sports. It involves a test in which the reaction speed is measured, that is, an extremely important aspect of movement coordination in the art of jujutsu combat. The description of the testing procedure is as follows: The subject sits astride a chair, facing the rest, on which he places his forearm (resting it halfway down); four fingers are straightened and tightened, and the thumb is abducted. The tester holds a stick with a diameter and length of 50 cm, on which a centimeter scale is marked along its entire length. The lower end of the cane (0 cm) is at the level of the lower edge of the patient's hand, approximately 1 cm from his hand. The tester lets go of the cane at any time. The subject's task is to grasp the cane by clenching the hand. The distance from point 0 to the grip point (bottom edge) is measured. The present experiment followed the procedure developed by Ditrich [17]. The study subjects performed the procedure 5 times, and 2 extreme results were rejected. The arithmetic mean was calculated from the remaining trials.

The test involving the dynamometric measurement of hand force was carried out as follows: Dynamometer model: KERN MAP 130K1 palm hand dynamometer was used. The subject squeezes the hand dynamometer with their stronger hand. The wrist should lie in the extension line of the forearm. During the test, the test hand must not touch any part of the body. The strength of the hand is measured in kilograms. The better measurement of the 2 tests was selected for further analysis. The dynamometer should be adjusted to the size of the hand of the subjects so that the more distal finger joints fit in its handle. Hand swings during measurement are not allowed, because they can alter the results. Subjects need to focus mentally on the task, since the goal was to perform the measurement of the maximum handgrip force of the subjects.

2.2. Statistical Methods

In order to carry out analyses, taking into account the country of origin and the fighters' style, for hand grip strength and Ditrich rod reaction time, we examined the normality of distribution in groups (Shapiro–Wilk test). Therefore, to test the significance of differences between the groups for the analyzed variables (handgrip, Ditrich's measures), we used appropriate tests (t-test, UMW test—Mann–Whitney U test), and their effect size was given. The dominant hand was always examined.

All analyses were performed using the Statistica 13.3 software [18]. The R programming language with additional packages [19] was used to present the results in the form of graphs.

3. Results

The characteristics of the research group are presented in Table 1. The results of the tests performed showed that only reaction time (Ditrich's measures) had a distribution close to normal.

Table 1. Basic characteristics of sample.

Variables	p	Judo		Jujutsu		p
		Poland	Germany	Poland	Germany	
N		20	10	20	19	
Age (years) [1]	0.3434	33.3 ± 8.03	30.1 ± 4.46	33.25 ± 7.29	45.42 ± 7.17	0.0001 *
Weight (kg) [1]	0.7747	83.45 ± 14.22	86.4 ± 12.66	85.6 ± 11.78	95.68 ± 13.94	0.0151 *
Years of training (years) [1]	0.7738	16.25 ± 6.87	15.7 ± 2.91	15.7 ± 3.96	28.84 ± 6.83	0.0001 *
Dominant hand, n (%)						
Left	—	—	—	—	—	—
Right		20 (100)	10 (100)	20 (100)	19 (100)	
Training experience (dan), n (%)						
1		18 (90.00)	8 (80.00)	19 (95.00)	7 (36.84)	
2	0.3540	1 (5.00)	2 (20.00)	1 (5.00)	4 (21.05)	0.0179 *
3		1 (5.00)	—	—	3 (15.79)	
4–10		—	—	—	5 (26.31)	

[1]—mean ± SD, p—probability obtained in the UMW test (χ^2—for training experience variable); * statistical significance at the 0.05 level.

The mean values obtained by the subjects from each group in the tests are presented in Figures 1 and 2. Analyzing the average results characterizing hand strength (Figure 1), we found that the Polish competitors practicing judo (91.5 ± 9.05 kg) had the greatest hand strength, and the Germans practicing jujutsu had the weakest (average hand strength was 74.11 ± 12.00 kg). Hand grip strength among judokas and jujutsu practitioners significantly differed by country of origin (Figure 1).

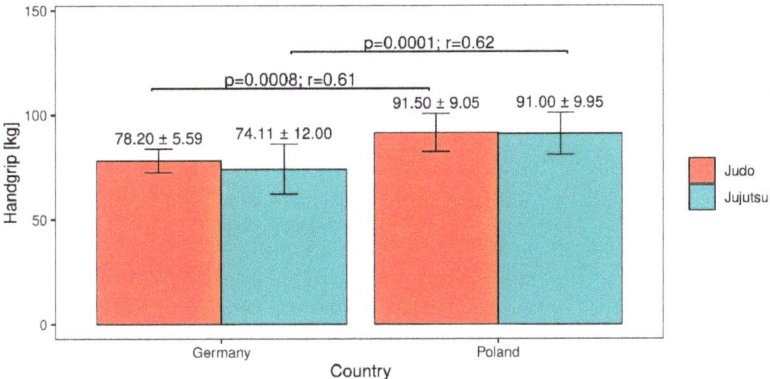

Figure 1. Mean values (±SD) obtained in the hand strength dynamometric test.

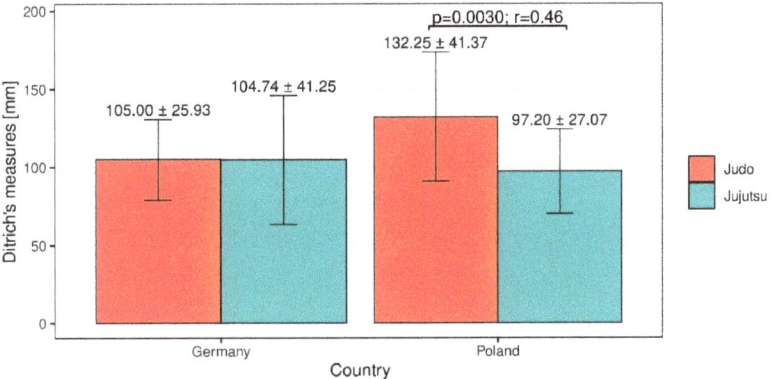

Figure 2. Mean values (±SD) obtained in the reaction speed test (Ditrich rod).

On the basis of the average results obtained in the reaction speed test (Figure 2), we observed the best results among Polish jujutsu participants (average 97.2 mm), and the weakest among judo participants (Poland). Additionally, the average results of Polish players training in different fighting styles differed statistically significantly at the level of $\alpha = 0.05$ (Figure 2).

For the variable characterizing the reaction speed of the subjects, we also performed a two-factor analysis of variance in the 2 × 2 scheme. Its aim was to investigate the influence of factors related to the origin of fighters (country) and the martial arts training style on the variability of reaction speed. The analysis of variance (Table 2) showed statistical significance for the main effect of country ($p = 0.0499$, $\eta^2 = 0.06$) and the interaction of independent variables (country * martial arts—$p = 0.0400$, $\eta^2 = 0.06$). The main effect related to the origin of the players indicated statistically significant differences in the average reaction speeds between Polish and German players.

Table 2. The result of the two-way analysis of variance for the variable reaction speed.

Effect	F	p	η²
Country	3.9896	0.0499 *	0.06
Martial arts	0.7075	0.4033	0.01
Country * martial arts	4.3881	0.0400 *	0.06

* Statistical significance at the 0.05 level.

Subsequently, the individual simple effects were analyzed, as shown in Figure 3. On the basis of the interaction graph, we found that there was a simple country effect in the judo group, where the respondents from Poland obtained weaker results than the respondents in the German group. Additionally, a simple effect of the origin of the respondents in the group of jujutsu practitioners was observed. Here, in turn, the Polish players were characterized by a better reaction speed than the players from Germany. The graph also showed a simple effect of the fighting style in the Polish group, where the jujutsu practitioners obtained better average reaction speed results than the judo practitioners. When analyzing the simple effect of martial arts in the German competitors' group, we found comparable average levels of reaction speed of competitors practicing judo and jujutsu.

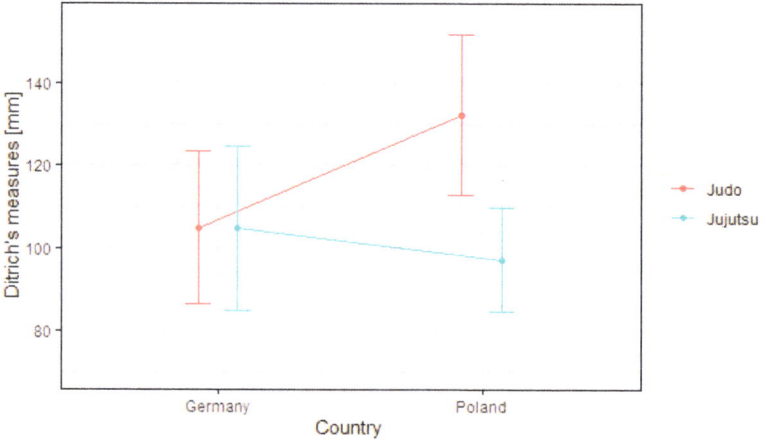

Figure 3. Simple effects interaction chart for country * martial arts effect.

For the collected statistical material, the influence of the variables age, body weight, and competitor training experience on the results obtained in the tests of hand strength and reaction speed was also examined. On the basis of the results obtained (Table 3), we found that there were statistically significant correlations between the analyzed variables. Moreover, the positive direction of the relationship between the analyzed variables and the results of the Ditrich stick test indicated the higher the value of the tested feature, the slower the player's reaction speed. In the case of measuring hand strength, the positive value of the coefficient indicated a directly proportional influence of the variable on the test result. The strongest relationships were established among German judo players. In this group, the hand strength obtained in the test was significantly influenced by the weight of the respondents ($r_{xy} = 0.75$), while the variable age had a significant influence on the reaction speed ($r_{xy} = 0.66$). In another group of players (Germany, jujutsu), the relationship between the weight of the subject and the speed of reaction also turned out to be significant. A statistically significant relationship between age and hand strength among Polish judo players was observed ($r_{xy} = 0.49$—Poland, judo).

Table 3. The results of the Pearson linear correlation analysis for the studied variables.

	Variables	Poland		Germany	
		Handgrip	Ditrich's Measures	Handgrip	Ditrich's Measures
Overall	Age (years)	0.31 *	0.04	−0.14	0.26
	Weight (kg)	0.39 *	−0.10	0.13	0.35
	Years of training	0.17	0.12	−0.14	0.07
Judo	Age (years)	0.49 *	−0.19	0.48	0.66 *
	Weight (kg)	0.42	−0.26	0.75 *	−0.02
	Years of training	0.17	0.15	0.39	0.49
Jujutsu	Age (years)	0.14	0.43	−0.07	0.36
	Weight (kg)	0.36	0.28	0.09	0.49 *
	Years of training	0.17	0.02	−0.04	0.06

* Statistical significance at the 0.05 level.

4. Discussion

The issue related to the handgrip force and manual abilities concerns almost the entire range of the related combat sports, including judo, sambo, and wrestling. The central consideration seems to lie in the handgrip, which forms an important parameter to determine the abilities in wrestling sports [16,20]. In contrast, the techniques and tactics adopted in the combat of the traditional jujutsu are similar to *aikido*, and dissimilar from judo, with a note that the range of the available techniques also includes the category named *atemi kogeki waza*, which includes strikes and kicks (performed in various positions and distances) [1]. As was stated in similar research, "Contribution of grip strength in system permits to consider them important for successfulness in wrestling, judo etc. At the same time in kicking martial arts these indicators are not very important and their absolute contribution in system formation is much lower" [16]. The strong grip is particularly important in such combat sports, such as judo, sambo, wrestling, and MMA [21,22].

In the case of judo and sports jujutsu, special fitness tests are often used, on the basis of acceptable throws in sports combat [23]. Intermediate performance tests (reaction speed and manual efficiency), such as the Batak Lite test [15,24] or the balance test, as an element of the motor coordination ability, have an indirect effect on the combat effectiveness [25–28]. The test involving gripping of Ditrich rod deserved its role in the sports that require fast reaction, such as in fencing [29,30]. The level of manual abilities is often examined as well. This tool can be applied in sports and movement rehabilitation—namely, in the tests involving speed of reaction and hand–eye coordination [12,31,32]. However, we are familiar with the dependencies that occur between the type of the training and the level of various motor abilities. To provide an insight from literature, "the training period with intensive judo-specific drills that engage cognitive functions and require hand's maximal static efforts improve psycho-motor ability but may impair hand grip strength" [6]. On the example of judo, it was also stated that "the use of standardized, specific tests seems to be a diagnostic tool for the rating of psycho-motor abilities in judo contestants" [20], where the handgrip force is one of indicators.

The level of motor abilities forms an important component of the positive health-related potential and is known to affect the level of the subjectively understood well-being. Hence, its role in sports cannot be underestimated. In particular jujutsu is commonly taken up for the reasons associated with the ability of self-defense as well as for recreation [4]. In addition, it can provide individuals with a feeling of personal security.

The way to gain the master rank in martial arts is not related to the results of sport competition; however, it is known to depend primarily on the involvement of the individuals and on various environmental and institutional determinants [5,7]. Therefore, it seems less important to analyze whether the study subjects come from Poland or Germany, and instead to assess their level of overall activity. Thus, the participants of seminars in martial arts (subjects from Germany) could form a group with a more active lifestyle. In addition, judokas from Germany participated in seminars concerned mainly with the practice of jujutsu. Therefore, their very good results in the "Ditrich rod" test (manual efficiency and speed of reaction) could be slightly better than judokas from Poland. Would it be a recommendable complementary sport for judokas? Perhaps it would be useful for coaches.

5. Conclusions

The results of the analysis allowed the authors to formulate the following conclusions:

- Simple reaction time in response to a visual stimulus is shorter in jujutsu practitioners ($p = 0.003$).
- There were no statistically significant differences between jujutsu and judo players in the dynamometric handgrip measurement.
- The two-factor analysis of variance showed a statistically significant effect of the interaction of country and martial arts variables on the results obtained by the respondents in the reaction speed test. Moreover, regardless of the type of martial arts, the average results obtained in the test with the Ditrich rod was significantly different between the country of origin of the participants.
- The Pearson's linear correlation values determined for the studied groups indicate a negative impact of ageing players on their reaction speed. The weight of the players also had a negative influence on the reaction speed.
- The weight and age of the competitors (especially in judo) had a significant ($p < 0.05$) influence on the results obtained in the dynamometer measurement of hand strength.

With the help of these two tools, we were able to establish the difference in the result in favor of people practicing jujutsu (which is a more comprehensive martial art according to the technical repertoire). The simple research tools of the Ditrich rod and hand grip dynamometer can still be very useful in the practice of sport, particularly in the fighting arts analyzed here. Ease of use is an advantage here.

Author Contributions: Conceptualization, J.S. and W.J.C.; methodology, B.D.; software, B.D.; validation, W.J.C. and B.D.; formal analysis, W.J.C., B.D. and J.S.; investigation, P.B. and J.S.; resources, P.B. and J.S.; data curation, J.S.; writing—original draft preparation, W.J.C. and J.S.; writing—review and editing, P.P. and B.D.; visualization, B.D.; supervision, P.P.; project administration, W.J.C.; funding acquisition, W.J.C. All authors have read and agreed to the published version of the manuscript.

Funding: This research received no external funding.

Institutional Review Board Statement: The study was conducted according to the guidelines of the Declaration of Helsinki, and approved by the Bioethical Committee at the University of Rzeszów, approval no. 3/11/2017.

Informed Consent Statement: Informed consent was obtained from all subjects involved in the study.

Data Availability Statement: The authors confirm that the data supporting the findings of this study are available within the article.

Conflicts of Interest: The authors declare no conflict of interest.

References

1. Kuboyama, K. The Mind-Set of jujutsuka in the Edo period in Japan as described in five historical documents (scrolls) from the Yoshin-ryu jujutsu school. *Ido Mov. Culture. J. Martial Arts Anthropol.* **2015**, *15*, 26–32.
2. Kons, R.L.; Ache-Dias, J.; Detanico, D. Can physical tests predict the technical-tactical performance during official judo competitions? *Arch. Budo Sci. Martial Arts Extrem. Sports* **2017**, *13*, 143–151.
3. Castelli, D.M.; Hillman, C.H.; Buck, S.M.; Erwin, H.E. Physical fitness and academic achievement in third- and fifth-grade students. *J. Sport Exerc. Psychol.* **2007**, *29*, 239–252. [CrossRef]
4. Cynarski, W.J.; Yu, J.H.; Pawelec, P. Changes in the level of physical fitness on the way to mastery in martial arts according to activity. *Ido Mov. Culture. J. Martial Arts Anthropol.* **2017**, *17*, 38–44.
5. Witkowski, K.; Piepiora, P.; Grochola, M. The knee joint extensor and flexor strength indicators in judo female athletes. *Arch. Budo Sci. Martial Arts Extrem. Sports* **2018**, *14*, 215–225.

6. Cynarski, W.J. Polish achievements in the theory of physical education and new directions. *Ido Mov. Culture. J. Martial Arts Anthropol.* **2014**, *14*, 1–14.
7. Cynarski, W.J.; Sieber, L.; Kudłacz, M.; Telesz, P. A Way Mastery. Mastery Martial Arts. *Ido Mov. Culture. J. Martial Arts Anthropol.* **2015**, *15*, 16–22.
8. Fontani, G.; Lodi, L.; Felici, A.; Migliorini, S.; Corradeschi, F. Attention in athletes of high and low experience enganged in different open skill sports. *Percept. Mot. Ski.* **2006**, *102*, 791–816. [CrossRef]
9. Cohen, J. *Statystyczna Analiza Mocy dla Nauk Behawioralnych*; Erlbaum Associates: New York, NY, USA, 1988.
10. Collardeau, M.; Brisswalter, J.; Audiffren, M. Effects of a prolonged run on simple reaction time of well-trained runners. *Percept. Mot. Ski.* **2001**, *93*, 679. [CrossRef]
11. Belej, M.; Junger, J. *Motor Tests of Coordination Abilities*; Presov University: Presov, Slovakia, 2006.
12. Borysiuk, Z.; Sadowski, J. Time and spatial aspects of movement anticipation. *Biol. Sport* **2007**, *24*, 63–82.
13. Chih, C.H.; Chen, J.F. The relationship between physical education performance, fitness tests, and academic achievement in elementary school. *Int. J. Sport Soc.* **2011**, *2*, 65–73.
14. Hassmann, M.; Buchegger, M.; Stollberg, K.-P. Judo Performance Tests Using a Pulling Force Device Simulating a Seoi-Nage Throw. *Ido Mov. Culture. J. Martial Arts Anthropol.* **2011**, *11*, 47–51.
15. Gierczuk, D.; Bujak, Z. Reliability and accuracy of Batak Lite tests used for assessing coordination motor abilities in wrestlers. *Pol. J. Sport Tour.* **2014**, *21*, 72–76. [CrossRef]
16. Iermakov, S.S.; Podrigalo, L.V.; Jagiełło, W. Hand-grip strength as an indicator for predicting the success in martial arts athletes. *Arch. Budo* **2016**, *12*, 179–186.
17. Raczek, J.; Juras, G.; Waśkiewicz, Z. The diagnosis of motor coordination. *J. Hum. Kinet.* **2001**, *6*, 113–125.
18. *TIBCO Statistica 13.3*; TIBCO Software, Inc.: Palo Alto, CA, USA, 2017. Available online: http://statistica.io (accessed on 8 October 2020).
19. R Core Team R. *A Language and Environment for Statistical Computing 3.6.2*; R Foundation for Statistical Computing: Vienna, Austria, 2019. Available online: https://www.R-project.org/ (accessed on 20 December 2019).
20. Obminski, Z.; Litwiniuk, A.; Staniak, Z.; Zdanowicz, R.; Zhu, W. Intensive specific maximal judo drills improve psycho-motor ability but may impair hand grip isometric strength. *Ido Mov. Culture. J. Martial Arts Anthropol.* **2015**, *15*, 52–58.
21. Chernozub, A.; Korobeynikov, G.; Mytskan, B.; Korobeinikova, L.; Cynarski, W.J. Modelling Mixed Martial Arts Power Training Needs Depending on the Predominance of the Strike or Wrestling Fighting Style. *Ido Mov. Culture. J. Martial Arts Anthropol.* **2018**, *18*, 28–36. [CrossRef]
22. Podrihalo, O.; Podrigalo, L.; Bezkorovainyi, D.; Halashko, O.; Nikulin, I.; Kadutskaya, L.; Jagiello, M. The analysis of handgrip strength and somatotype features in arm wrestling athletes with different skill levels. *Phys. Educ. Stud.* **2020**, *24*, 120–126. [CrossRef]
23. Arazi, H.; Noori, M.; Izadi, M. Correlation of anthropometric and bio-motor attributes with Special Judo Fitness Test in senior male judokas. *Ido Mov. Culture. J. Martial Arts Anthropol.* **2017**, *17*, 19–24.
24. Etnyre, B.; Kinugasa, T. Postcontraction influences on reaction time (motor control and learning). *Res. Quaterly Exerc. Sport* **2002**, *73*, 271–282. [CrossRef]
25. Maśliński, J.; Witkowski, K.; Jatowtt, A.; Cieśliński, W.B.; Piepiora, P. Physical fitness 11-12 years boys who train judo and those who do not practise sport. *Arch. Budo Sci. Martial Arts Extrem. Sports* **2015**, *11*, 41–46.
26. Ceylan, B.; Serdar Balci, S. The Comparison of Judo-Specific Tests. *Ido Mov. Culture. J. Martial Arts Anthropol.* **2018**, *18*, 54–62. [CrossRef]
27. Kristulovic, S.; Kuvacic, G.; Erceg, M.; Franchini, E. Reliability and Validity of the New Judo Physical Fitness Test. *Ido Mov. Culture. J. Martial Arts Anthropol.* **2019**, *19*, 41–55.
28. Kons, R.L.; Franchini, E.; Detanico, D. Neuromuscular and judo-specific tests: Can they predict judo athletes' ranking performance? *Ido Mov. Culture. J. Martial Arts Anthropol.* **2020**, *20*, 15–23. [CrossRef]
29. Peters, M.; Ivanoff, J. Performance asymmetries in computer mouse control of right-handers and left handers with left- and right-handed mouse experience. *J. Mot. Behav.* **1999**, *31*, 86–94. [CrossRef]
30. Avdeeva, M.S.; Tulyakova, O.V. Indicated factors of physical development, physical readiness, functional condition and efficiency of fimale students in the process of adaptation to training. *Phys. Educ. Stud.* **2018**, *22*, 4–11. [CrossRef]
31. Collins, M.W.; Field, M.; Lovell, M.R.; Iverson, G.; Johnston, K.M.; Maroon, J.; Fu, F.H. Relationship between postconcussion headache and neuropsychological test performance in high school athletes. *Am. J. Sports Med.* **2003**, *31*, 168–174. [CrossRef]
32. Perruchet, P.; Cleeremans, A.; Destrebecqz, A. Dissociating the effects of automatic activation and explicit expectancy on reaction times in a simple associative learning task. *J. Exp. Psychol. Learn. Mem. Cogn.* **2006**, *32*, 955–966. [CrossRef]

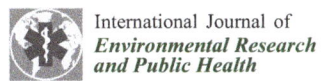

Brief Report

Effects of 4 Weeks of a Technique-Specific Protocol with High-Intensity Intervals on General and Specific Physical Fitness in Taekwondo Athletes: An Inter-Individual Analysis

Alex Ojeda-Aravena [1,2,*], Tomás Herrera-Valenzuela [3,4], Pablo Valdés-Badilla [5], Jorge Cancino-López [6], José Zapata-Bastias [7] and José Manuel García-García [2]

1. Department of Physical Activity Sciences, Universidad de los Lagos (ULA), 5290000 Osorno, Chile
2. Faculty of Sports Sciences, Universidad de Castilla-La Mancha (UCLM), 45071 Toledo, Spain; JoseManuel.Garcia@uclm.es
3. School of Sport Sciences, Universidad Santo Tomás (UST), 8370003 Santiago, Chile; tomas.herrera@usach.cl
4. School of Physical Activity, Sport and Health Sciences, Universidad de Santiago de Chile (USACH), 8370003 Santiago, Chile
5. Department of Physical Activity Sciences, Faculty of Education Sciences, Universidad Católica del Maule, 3530000 Talca, Chile; pvaldes@ucm.cl
6. Exercise Science Laboratory, School of Kinesiology, Faculty of Medicine, Universidad Finis Terrae, 8370003 Santiago, Chile; jcancino@uft.cl
7. Sports Coach Career, School of Education, Universidad Viña del Mar, 2520000 Viña del Mar, Chile; jzapata@uvm.cl
* Correspondence: alex.ojeda@ulagos.cl

Abstract: The aim of this research was to compare the effects of a technique-specific high-intensity interval training (HIIT) protocol vs. traditional taekwondo training on physical fitness and body composition in taekwondo athletes, as well as to analyse the inter-individual response. Utilising a parallel controlled design, sixteen male and female athletes (five females and 11 males) were randomly divided into an experimental group (EG) that participated in the technique-specific HIIT and a control group (CG) that participated in traditional taekwondo training. Both groups trained three days/week for four weeks. Squat jump (SJ), countermovement jump (CMJ), 5-metre sprint (5M), 20-metre shuttle run (20MSR), taekwondo specific agility test (TSAT), multiple frequency speed of kick test ($FSKT_{MULT}$), total kicks, and kick decrement index (KDI), as well as body composition were evaluated. Results indicate that there are no significant differences ($p > 0.05$) in the factors group and time factor and group by time interaction ($p > 0.05$). Although percentage and effect size increases were documented for post-intervention fitness components in TSAT, total kicks, KDI, and 20MSR, responders and non-responders were also documented. In conclusion, a HIIT protocol based on taekwondo-specific technical movements does not report significant differences in fitness and body composition compared to traditional taekwondo training, nor inter-individual differences between athletes.

Keywords: martial arts; athletes; physical fitness; body composition

1. Introduction

Olympic taekwondo is described as a modern and constantly evolving combat sport whose performance requires athletes to develop and maintain a high level of physical fitness as part of their preparation [1]. Therefore, it is important to understand the characteristics of the components involved in physical performance in this sport in order to apply appropriate training stimuli in the preparation of athletes. In this sense, taekwondo, specifically the combat modality, is classified as an activity of an intermittent nature (effort: pause ratio: 1:7 to 1:2) [2] of high physiological intensity (>90% HRmax: lactate 5.0 to 14 Mmol L^{-1}) with motor actions executed at high speed, mainly of the lower limbs [2,3].

In turn, in metabolic terms, it is described as a mixed sport, in which athletes use different proportions of energy substrates during combat (aerobic component: 58–66%, ATP-PCr: 26–30%, and glycolytic 4–5%) [4]. In addition to the above, competition categories are divided by body weight, which means that body composition has an important role [4,5].

Accordingly, considering the specific characteristics of this sport, the application of the high-intensity interval training (HIIT) model in the field of athletic performance in team and individual sports has grown exponentially in recent years [6]. Evidence in combat sports includes systematic reviews with [7] and without [8] meta-analyses, showing significant increases ($p < 0.05$) in cardiorespiratory capacity, physiological parameters, and physical skills, without reporting conclusive data on body composition. Specifically, in taekwondo, HIIT studies include the application of protocols based on repeated sprints [9,10] and recently HIIT protocols with specific technical characteristics [11,12]. However, these reports use interventions that add sessions to the usual training, which could influence the results of the studies analysed. On the other hand, only a few authors [11,12]. have documented increases in general and specific physical fitness using the temporal structure of combat as a work interval in the application of HIIT protocols [13]; however, the results are still controversial. Another element to consider is that usually the results of sport science interventions are interpreted in group terms, without considering the inter-individual variability of the athletes' response [14]. To address this limitation, some authors have dealt with this situation by classifying athletes into two types: responders (Rs) and non-responders (NRs) [14,15]. For example, Bonafiglia et al. [16] analysed the inter-individual response comparing sprint interval training with endurance training for three weeks using a crossover design on physiological parameters in recreationally physically active adults, reporting individual increases in both training protocols. In addition, Ramirez-Campillo, R et al. [14] analysed the inter-individual response after seven weeks of plyometric training on components of athletic performance in football players, documenting greater individual increases in physical fitness parameters with respect to habitual training. In contrast, to the best of our knowledge, studies in combat sports are unknown.

From the perspective of optimising training processes, HIIT shock microcycles show a positive impact on athletic development [17]. In this context, incorporating technique-specific HIIT protocols into regular training sessions could be effective in optimising physical preparation time, bearing in mind the multiple annual competitions taekwondo athletes face. Moreover, it represents a training modality similar to the intermittent and physiological characteristics of this sport, which may be useful for training dosage and control.

Consequently, the main purpose of the present study was to compare the effects of a technique-specific HIIT protocol vs. traditional taekwondo training on general and specific physical fitness and body composition in taekwondo athletes and specifically, to analyse the inter-individual response of the athletes. The hypothesis of this study is that the technique-specific HIIT protocol would be significantly superior to traditional training for general and specific physical fitness components and modify body composition in taekwondo athletes. In addition, a higher rate of responders would be expected in the technique-specific HIIT group than in the traditional training group.

2. Material and Methods

2.1. Experimental Approach to the Problem

The present study used a parallel controlled, randomised, single-blind, non-probabilistic convenience sample design. Together with the coach, a HIIT protocol was designed and planned that adhered to the usual training session, with specific technical characteristics based on repeated kicks, using the taekwondo temporal structure (effort: pause 4 s: 28 s; 1:7) of the HIIT work interval and a workload similar to the total duration of the combat (10 min). The athletes were distributed in experimental group (EG; $n = 8$) and control group (CG; $n = 8$) (for details see Figure 1). The effect of this training on components of the general and specific physical fitness and body composition in taekwondo athletes of both sexes was compared with the effect of a traditional taekwondo training. Athletes were invited to participate in the study before the end of the pre-season general physical preparation period (March 2019). The increase in the external training load during the application of the HIIT programme was based on the decrease in the pause times without modifying the work time. In turn, the internal training load considered the intensity, which was controlled by means of the rate perceived exertion or RPE (RPE 0–10) in both study groups. The HIIT group used the all-out format for the application of the training protocol [18].

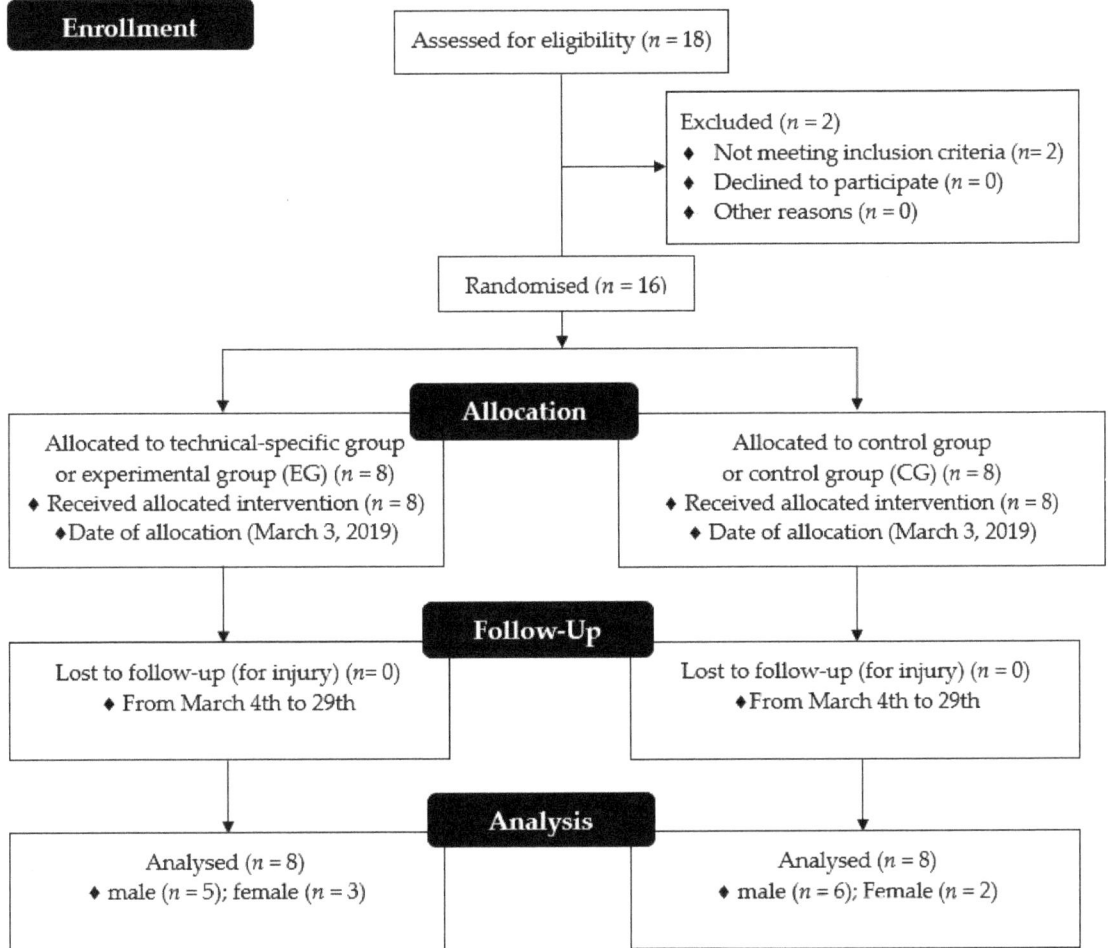

Figure 1. Participants flow.

2.2. Participants

Sixteen taekwondo athletes of both sexes voluntarily completed this study: five females with a mean age of 17.4 ± 2.9 years, height of 158.6 ± 6.9 cm, body mass of 58.6 ± 9.0 kg, and experience of 5.8 ± 1.7 years; and 11 males with a mean age of 20.5 ± 5.0 years, height of 169.5 ± 11.4 cm, body mass of 61.6 ± 12.7 kg, and experience of 7 ± 2 years, who compete annually in national-level tournaments. All athletes had to meet the following inclusion criteria to participate in the study: (i) four or more years of experience competing in taekwondo; (ii) training three or more times per week; (iii) preparing for competitions or tournaments organised by the Federación Nacional de Taekwondo Deportivo (FEDENAT, Chile), an organisation recognised by World Taekwondo; (iv) being enrolled in a club affiliated to FEDENAT; (v) all taekwondo athletes had to be free of injuries and neuromuscular problems in the last ten weeks; (vi) not being in a period of body mass reduction. All athletes and/or family members of athletes under 18 years of age were informed in advance of the study objectives, associated benefits, experimental procedures, and potential risks and provide informed consent or informed assent prior to the assessments and training sessions. The study was conducted in accordance with the Declaration of Helsinki on work with humans [19] and implemented after approval by the institutional ethics committee.

2.3. Assessments

2.3.1. Jump Ability

Jump ability was assessed by the squat jump (SJ) and countermovement jump (CMJ) tests through the maximum height reached (cm) using an electronic contact platform (Ergojump; Globus, Codogne, Italy; accuracy: 0.01 m). The SJ test was used to evaluate dynamic muscle-shortening actions [20]. For this, each athlete was previously instructed to place their hands on their hips, feet, and shoulders wide apart, and adopt a bent-knee position (approximately 90°) for 3 s, and then perform a maximal effort vertical jump. Meanwhile, the CMJ test was used to assess dynamic muscle actions, specifically the slow stretch-shortening cycle [20]. Prior to this, each athlete was instructed to rest hands on hips, feet and shoulders wide apart, and perform a downward movement (no restriction was placed on the knee angle achieved) followed by a maximal effort vertical jump [21]. Two trials were completed, with a one-min pause between attempts [22], and the highest performing trial was used for subsequent statistical analysis (intra-class correlation; ICC SJ pre = 0.90 [CI95% 0.76 to 0.96]; ICC SJ post = 0.92 [CI95% 0.80 to 0.97]), (ICC CMJ pre = 0.95 [CI95% 0.90 to 0.98]; ICC CMJ post = 0.95 [CI95% 0.90 to 0.98]).

2.3.2. Linear Sprint in 5 Metre (5M)

The speed to complete a linear sprint from 0 to 5 m was recorded using electrical photocells (Brower Timing System, Salt Lake City, UT, USA; accuracy: 0.001 s). Photocells were positioned 0.5 m after the starting line and 0.7 m above the floor (i.e., at hip level) to capture trunk movement rather than a false trigger of a limb [22]. Each participant placed the front foot 0.5 m before the first timing gate and began running when ready, thus eliminating reaction time [22]. Athletes performed two practice trials run at submaximal intensity after a thorough warm-up to familiarise them with the test. Three min after the warm-up, they completed two trials with two min of passive pause between trials, using the highest performing trial of 5M for subsequent statistical analysis (ICC pre = 0.85 [CI95% 0.58 to 0.93], ICC post = 0.87 [CI95% 0.62 to 0.94]).

2.3.3. Taekwondo Specific Agility Test (TSAT)

Specific agility was assessed through the taekwondo-specific agility test (TSAT) following previous recommendations [23]. From a guard position with both feet behind the start/finish line, the performer had to (a) move forward in guard position, without crossing feet, as quick as possible to the centre point; (b) turn toward partner 1 by adopting a lateral shift and perform a roundhouse kick with the left leg (i.e., leading-roundhouse kick; *dollyo tchagui*); (c) move toward partner 2 and perform a roundhouse kick with the right leg (i.e., leading-roundhouse kick; *dollyo-chagi*); (d) return to the centre; (e) move forward in guard position and perform a double-roundhouse kick (i.e., *narae-chagi*) toward partner 3; and (f) move backward to the start/finish line in a guard position. Sparring partners 1 and 2 hold a kick-target, whereas partner 3 holds two kick-targets. Sparring partners were instructed to maintain the kick-target at the torso height of the tested athlete. If a participant failed to follow these instructions (e.g., crossed one foot in front of the other during the various displacements, or failed to touch the kick-target powerfully when kicking), the trial was terminated and restarted after a three-minute recovery period. The time needed to complete the test was used as performance outcome, and it was assessed with an electronic timing system (Brower Timing Systems, Salt Lake City, UT, USA). Two trials were accorded to each athlete, with the best one maintained for later analysis (ICC pre = 0.90 [CI95% 0.87 a 0.92], ICC post = 0.86 [CI95% 0.78 a 0.87]).

2.3.4. Multiple Frequency Speed of Kick Test (FSKT$_{MULT}$)

The ability to repeat specific high-intensity efforts was assessed using the FSKT$_{MULT}$ test designed for taekwondo following previously described protocols [24]. Each of the five FSKT$_{MULT}$ sets had a duration of 10 s, with a pause interval of 10 s between sets. To perform the FSKT$_{MULT}$, each athlete faced a partner using a trunk protector (breastplate). After the sound signal, the athlete performed the maximum number of kicks possible, alternating right and left legs. Performance was determined by the number of kicks in each series, the total number of kicks (total kicks), and the kick decrement index (KDI) during the test. The KDI indicates that the performance decreases during the test. To calculate the KDI, the number of kicks applied during the FSKT$_{MULT}$ was taken into account. The calculation was performed using an equation that considers the results of all frequency speed of kick test (FSKT) series (Equation (1)).

$$KDI\ (\%) = \left[1 - \frac{FSKT1 + FSKT2 + FSKT3 + FSKT4 + FSKT5}{Best\ FSKT\ \times\ Number\ of\ Sets}\right] \times 100 \quad (1)$$

2.3.5. 20-Metre Shuttle Run Test (20MSR)

Aerobic fitness was assessed indirectly through the 20-metre shuttle run (20MSR) test according to the procedures of Leger and Lambert [25] and previous studies in taekwondo [12]. For its execution, athletes had to run back and forth between two lines separated by 20 m, at a pace set by an audio signal from an electronic recording. Each run was successful upon completion of the 20 m distance. The signal sounded at an increasing pace with each minute of the test, at which point the athletes had to increase their speed. They were warned once when they failed to reach the finish line within a certain period of time. The test was terminated when the examinee (i) could not follow the set pace of the signal for two successive runs; or (ii) when he/she voluntarily stopped. Scores were expressed as the last minute that athletes managed to complete during the test. One trial was completed, which was used for subsequent statistical analysis.

2.3.6. Anthropometric and Body Composition Assessments

Height (cm) was assessed with a stadiometer (Bodymeter 206, SECA, Germany, accuracy 1 mm) following standard protocols [26]. Each athlete stood without shoes, with heels together, back and buttocks touching the vertical surface of the stadiometer and head positioned in the Frankfort plane. Body composition, including body mass (BM), percentage fat mass (FM%), fat mass (FM), and muscle mass (MM), was assessed using an electrical bioimpedance scale (InBody120, 20 100 kHz tetrapolar tactile electrode sys-tem, model BPM040S12F07, Biospace, Inc, Seoul, Korea with an accuracy of 0.1 kg, with a measurement range of 5 to 250 kg and suitable for individuals aged 3 to 99 years) [27,28]. InBody technology divides the body into five components: two arms, two legs, and a trunk. Electrodes are placed under the subject's feet on the platform and on the palms and thumbs attached to the handles of the device. Age, height, and gender are entered manually after weight is determined using a scale placed inside the device. Body mass and impedance are automatically assessed using the manufacturer's software. Equations provided in the manufacturer's proprietary software calculated body composition characteristics [29]. Briefly, athletes stood barefoot and lightly clothed on the base components of a bioimpedance analyser with both feet and both thumbs placed on the electrodes and arms held away from the body at approximately 15° [30]. Once proper positioning of the device was achieved, the athlete was asked to remain still and quiet while the device completed the body composition measurement, which took an average of 30 s to one min. The researchers administered and monitored the entire test to ensure that the athlete maintained proper positioning and did not move [31,32].

2.3.7. Training Programme

Both groups participated in a 12-session (4-week) training programme with a duration of 90 min per session, which took place on three non-consecutive days (Monday, Wednesday, and Friday) and took into consideration a distribution of the training load, with an emphasis on technical–tactical development. Previously, both groups were instructed to use the scale of perceived exertion (RPE 0–10) to control the internal load during the application of the work protocols. Each training session started with 10 min of gentle jogging in a circle, joint mobility, and dynamic flexibility. Subsequently, for 20 min in pairs, all athletes performed a technical work sequence of front, spin, and circular kicks using a speed paddle. Then, for 30 min, all athletes performed adapted fights with technical specifications (i.e., task assignment), during which the coach intervened whenever necessary, giving tactical indications related to guarding, space distribution, technical gestures, and offensive and defensive situations. After 60 min, the experimental group (EG) was removed from the group of athletes to execute a technical-specific HIIT protocol with a volume of ≈10 min. Specifically, the EG performed a HIIT programme with 4 s of effort followed by 28 s of pause (effort: pause ratio 1:7) using alternating roundhouse kicks with both legs at maximum intensity (i.e., all-out) considering an RPE of 10 in front of a partner. This was followed by periods of active recovery mimicking the guard stance, which were distributed in three rounds of two min of activity for one minute of passive rest between rounds. During the passive rest, they hydrated and simulated receiving instructions from the coach and assistants. Meanwhile, the control group (CG) performed 10 min of technical kicking work using speed paddles and simulated sparring at moderate intensity (RPE 5–6). Finally, both groups concluded the sessions with a cool down consisting of static stretching exercises for 20 min. The total duration of all training sessions was one and a half hours (for details, see Table 1).

Table 1. Description of the load programming of the training protocols carried out.

	EG (*n* = 8)	CG (*n* = 8)
1st week	3 rounds of 4 repetitions of 4 s of work: 28 s rest/1 min recovery	Continuous roundhouse kick with partner with use of paddles for speed
2nd week	3 rounds of 5 repetitions of 4 s of work: 24 s rest/1 min recovery	Continuous bandal-tchagi kicks with partner with use of paddle for speed
3rd week	3 rounds of 5 repetitions of 4 s of work: 20 s rest/1 min recovery	Simulated combat with technical specifications
4th week	3 rounds of 6 repetitions of 4 s of work: 16 s rest/1 min recovery	Simulated combat with technical specifications

Simbolises: EG: experimental group; CG: control group.

2.4. Procedures

The CG was composed of eight taekwondo athletes, distributed in six males and two females. The EG was composed of eight taekwondo athletes, distributed in five males and three females. For randomisation, a block randomisation with a block size of four athletes was applied. Eligible athletes were randomly assigned, after completion of baseline assessments, to the control group or to HIIT training. The principal investigator coordinated the allocation sequence, and randomisation of the two study arms was electronically generated [33]. All athletes and study personal (including investigators and coach) were blinded to treatment allocation throughout the trial protocol. During the previous week, athletes completed a familiarisation session with the HIIT protocol and assessments to reduce the learning effect. Assessments were performed before and after the application of the training programme, with 48 h of rest between the first and the last training session. All assessments were scheduled between 9:00 h and 11:00 h, completed in the same order, in the same venue (gymnasium with wooden floor), with the same sports clothing and by the same pre- and post-intervention assessor, who was a qualified sports scientist blinded to the intervention group and assigned to the athletes. Previously, all athletes were instructed to (i) sleep for 7 to 8 h before each assessment session and (ii) not to modify their usual diet and hydration habits during the days prior to the assessments. The first session assessed chronological age, bipedal height, and body composition in the fasting state. The second assessment session considered the components of general and specific physical fitness, using the following assessments: squat jump (SJ), countermovement jump (CMJ), taekwondo specific agility test (TSAT), 5-metre linear sprint (5M), multiple frequency speed of kick test ($FSKT_{MULT}$), and 20-metre shuttle run (20MSR) (see details in Figure 2). A typical warm-up in this sport was performed, of 15 min duration, consisting of joint mobility, gentle jogging for five min, dynamic stretching (three min), three SJ and CMJ trials (two min), and low-intensity kicking (five min). Athletes were previously instructed to give their maximum effort during the assessments. The best of two attempts was considered for performance on all assessments, except for the $FSKT_{MULT}$ and 20MSR tests. A two-min pause interval between attempts was implemented and a rest interval of five to 10 min was applied between each assessment to reduce fatigue effects.

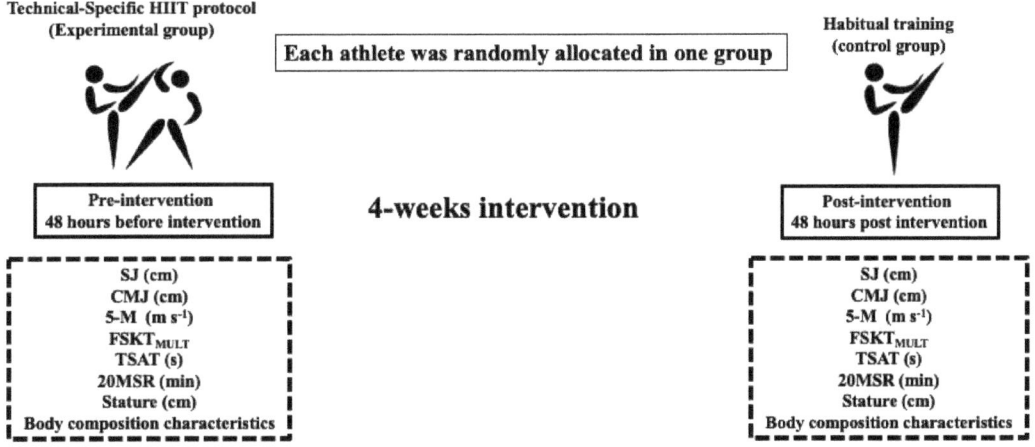

Figure 2. Training protocol. SJ: squat jump; CMJ: countermovement jump; 5M: linear sprint in 5 m; $FSKT_{MULT}$: multiple frequency speed of kick test; TSAT: taekwondo specific agility test; 20MSR: 20-metre shuttle run.

2.5. Statistical Analysis

Data analysis was performed with SPSS software version 24 (SPSS Institute, Chicago, IL, USA). All data are presented as mean ± standard deviation. Homoscedasticity of variance was verified using Levene's test. To quantify the reliability of SJ, CMJ, and 5M, an ICC with a 95% confidence interval (95%CI) was used. An acceptable reliability was determined with an ICC of 0.80 [34]. To determine possible differences in the characteristics on physical fitness and body composition components between the groups, an unpaired *t*-test was performed. Subsequently, two-way analysis of variance (ANOVA) for the factors group (EG vs. CG) and time (PRE intervention vs. POST intervention) was performed to examine the interaction effect of the characteristics on fitness and body composition components. If any significant interaction was observed, Tukey's post hoc test was applied to detect differences between groups. For ANOVA results, effect sizes were calculated using partial eta squared (η2p) and classified according to Cohen via the following interpretation scale: <0.2 [small]; 0.2 to < 0.8 [moderate]; > 0.8 [large]. Complementarily, post-intervention changes within and between groups were calculated via Cohen's d as effect size (ES). Threshold values for Cohen' d ES statistics were: < 0.20 [trivial], 0.20 [small], 0.60, [moderate], 1.20 [large], 2.0 [very large], and 4.0 [extremely large], respectively [35] using Hopkins' spreadsheets with the 90% interval confidence (90%CI). Following the end of the intervention, pre–post intervention differences in delta (Δ) were calculated for each variable, and the sample was classified into responders (Rs) and non-responders (NRs) using the two-technical error (TE) criterion, according to a previously established equation [16]. NRs were identified and defined as individuals who were unable to demonstrate an increase or decrease (in favour of beneficial changes) in body composition and fitness variables that was greater than twice the TE away from zero. For the current study, two replicates of all variables analysed were used to calculate TE. A change beyond twice the TE was representative of a high probability (i.e., 12 to 1 odds) that the observed response was a true physiological adaptation beyond what might be expected as a result of technical and/or biological variability [14]. In addition, Fisher's exact test was used to make comparisons between groups of subjects who were at $2 \times$ TE calculated at each outcome (NRs) or more than twice the TE (Rs) [14]. The TEs were as follows: [SJ 2.16 (cm) $\times$ 2; CMJ 2.36 (cm) $\times$ 2; TSAT 0.48 (s) $\times$ 2; 5M 0.06 (m s^{-1}) $\times$ 2; total kicks 3.93 kicks $\times$ 2; KDI 3. 60% $\times$ 2; 20MSR 0.44 (min) $\times$ 2; BM 0.94 (kg) $\times$ 2; %BM 2.24 (%) $\times$ 2; FM 1.34 (kg); MM 0.87 (kg) $\times$ 2]. Statistical significance was set at $p < 0.05$.

3. Results

3.1. Normality of the Results Analysed

The assumption of homoscedasticity of the results was verified in the totality of the results. Specifically, in general and specific physical fitness: SJ (F = 0.36; $p = 0.77$), CMJ (F = 2.23; $p = 0.88$), TSAT (F = 2.70; $p = 0.64$), 5M (F = 4.0; $p = 0.17$), total kicks (F = 0.39; $p = 0.69$), KDI (F = 1.21; $p = 0.32$), and 20MSR (F = 0.33; $p = 0.80$). In addition, in body composition, BM (F = 0.14; $p = 0.71$), FM% (F = 0.84; $p = 0.77$), FM (F = 0.64; $p = 0.80$), and MM (F = 0.05; $p = 0.81$).

3.2. Differences between Athletes in Both Groups at Baseline Assessments

No significant differences were documented in baseline assessments between groups in body composition characteristics: BM ($t = 0.18$; $p = 0.85$; ES = 0.09), FM% ($t = -0.48$; $p = 0.63$; ES = -0.24), FM ($t = -0.72$; $p = 0.47$; ES = -0.36), MM ($t = 0.06$; $p = 0.94$; ES = 0.33). Similarly, in the physical fitness components: SJ ($t = 0.80$; $p = 0.41$; ES = 0.41), CMJ ($t = 0.29$; $p = 0.77$; ES = 0.14), TSAT ($t = 0.24$; $p = 0.89$; ES = 0. 12), total kicks ($t = 0.26$; $p = 0.79$; ES = 0.13), KDI ($t = -1.54$; $p = 0.14$; ES = -0.77), 20MSR ($t = 0.10$; $p = 0.91$; ES = 0.05) with the exception of 5M ($t = 2.38$; $p = 0.03$; ES = 1.19).

3.3. Interaction between the Factors Analysed

Table 2 presents the summary of the interactions between the factors analysed for general and specific physical fitness and body composition.

Regarding the results of the two-factor ANOVA analysis: group (EG vs. CG) and time (PRE intervention and POST intervention), no significant differences were reported for the time factor, group factor, and interaction between the factors group by time. Specifically, general physical fitness presented the following results for SJ in the group factor (F = 0.78;

$p = 0.40$; $\eta^2_p = 0.02$) and in the time factor (F = 0.00; $p = 0.93$; $\eta^2_p = 0.00$), in CMJ for the group factor (F = 0.86; $p = 0.36$; $\eta^2_p = 0.02$) and time factor (F= 1.68; $p = 0.20$; $\eta^2_p = 0.05$), in 5M for the group factor (F = 1.05; $p = 0.31$; $\eta^2_p = 0.03$) and time factor (F = 2.37; $p = 0.01$; $\eta^2_p = 0.07$). In turn, specific fitness also exhibited no significant differences in TSAT for the group factor (F = 0.34; $p = 0.56$; $\eta^2_p = 0.00$) and time factor (F = 10.3; $p = 0.00$; $\eta^2_p = 0.26$), in total kicks for the group factor (F = 0.08; $p = 0.77$; $\eta^2_p = 0.00$) and time factor (F = 1.47; $p = 0.23$; $\eta^2_p = 0.05$), in KDI for the group factor (F = 4.06; $p = 0.05$; $\eta^2_p = 0.10$) and time factor (F = 6.74; $p = 0.01$; $\eta^2_p = 0.17$), and in 20MSR for the group factor (F = 0.08; $p = 0.76$; $\eta^2_p = 0.00$) and time factor (F = 1.80; $p = 0.19$; $\eta^2_p = 0.06$).

Table 2. Pre- and post-intervention differences between HIIT vs. traditional training protocols on physical fitness and body composition in taekwondo athletes ($n = 16$).

	PRE	POST	PRE	POST	F	p	η^2_p
Physical Fitness Components							
SJ (cm)	30 ± 6.8	29.2 ± 5.2	27.2 ± 6.2	28.3 ± 5.5	0.19	0.66	0.00
CMJ (cm)	33.3 ± 7.4	31.5 ± 6.4	32.3 ± 6.2	28.1 ± 6.44	0.25	0.61	0.09
5M (m s^{-1})	1.14 ± 0.07	1.24 ± 0.09	1.22 ± 0.05	1.23 ± 0.12	1.91	1.91	0.64
TSAT (s)	7.95 ± 1.11	5.0 ± 0.74	7.82 ± 1.04	6.78 ± 0.42	1.91	0.66	0.01
Total kicks (n)	95.3 ± 7.2	98.7 ± 7.3	96.3 ± 7.8	99.2 ± 6.5	0.09	0.92	0.00
KDI (%)	7.9 ± 3.9	5.2 ± 3.2	11.1 ± 4.3	7.1 ± 2.4	1.80	0.60	0.00
20MSR (min)	7.8 ± 2.6	8.8 ± 2.5	8.0 ± 2.1	9.2 ± 2.0	0.02	0.88	0.01
Anthropometric and Body Composition Characteristics							
BM (kg)	61.8 ± 11.5	60.6 ± 11.2	62.8 ± 11.1	61.43 ± 9.9	0.001	0.97	0.00
FM (kg)	10.6 ± 5.6	9.8 ± 5.5	12.7 ± 5.6	12 ± 5.1	0.20	0.92	0.01
FM (%)	17.0 ± 7.9	16.1 ± 8.2	19.3 ± 10.4	19.9 ± 8.6	0.23	0.63	0.00
MM (kg)	28.5 ± 6.2	28.6 ± 6.7	28.2 ± 7.3	27.6 ± 6.4	0.36	0.85	0.00

Data are presented as mean ± standard deviation. CG: control group EG: experimental group; PRE: before the intervention; POST: post-intervention. F: f-value interaction between factors time by group; p: p value; η^2_p: partial square eta; SJ: squat jump; CMJ: countermovement jump; TSAT: taekwondo specific agility test; KDI: kick decreased index; 20MSR: 20-metre shuttle run; BM: body mass; FM: fat mass; FM%: fat mass percentage; MM: muscle mass.

There were also no significant differences reported in body composition, specifically in BM for the group factor (F = 0.05; $p = 0.81$; $\eta^2_p = 0.00$) and time factor (F = 0.10; $p = 0.74$; $\eta^2_p = 0.00$), in FM% for the group factor (F = 0.92; $p = 0.35$; $\eta^2_p = 0.03$) and time factor (F= 0.00; $p = 0.95$; $\eta^2_p = 0.00$), in BF for group factor (F = 1.19; $p = 0.28$; $\eta^2_p = 0.04$) and time (F = 0.14; $p = 0.70$; $\eta^2_p = 0.00$), in MM for group factor (F = 0.06; $p = 0.80$; = $\eta^2_p = 0.02$) and time factor (F = 0.01; $p = 0.90$; $\eta^2_p = 0.00$). Similarly, no significant interaction was documented for the factors group by time.

3.4. Magnitude of Change Based on Inference

Following the intervention period, increases in TSAT physical performance were reported in both groups, moderately decreasing test performance times in the EG (-8.6%; ES = -1.07) and in the CG (-12.7%; ES = -0.87), with a trivial difference of 0.8% in favour of the EG (ES = 0.06). In the FSKT$_{MULT}$ test, an increase for total kicks was documented in the EG (4.4%; ES = 0.58) and in the CG (3.7%; ES = 0.36), with a trivial difference of 0.8% in favour of the EG (ES = 0.09). In addition, a moderate decrease in KDI in the EG (-32.5%; ES = -0.80) and a low decrease in the CG (-37.7%; ES = -0.48), with a trivial difference of -11.8% in favour of the CG (ES = -0.17). In relation to 20MSR performance, a moderate increase in time (min executed) was reported in EG (12.9%; ES = 1.07) and low in CG (9.2%; ES = 0.24) with a trivial difference of 2% in favour of the EG (ES = -0.06).

On the other hand, decreases in jump height were documented in SJ with a trivial decrease in the CG (-1.7%; ES = -0.07). In CMJ, a moderate decrease in jump height was documented in the EG (-10.4%; ES = -0.83) vs. a small decrease in the CG (-9.6%; ES = -0.36) with a low difference of 7.6% in favour of the EG (ES = 0.34). In turn, a moderate decrease in 5M performance was documented in the CG (7.5%; ES = 1.11) and moderate in the EG (−3.8%; ES = −0.52) with a trivial difference of 8.5% (ES = 1.27) between groups.

With respect to body composition characteristics, a small increase in FM% was documented in the EG (19.5%; ES = 0.45). Trivial decreases in MM were documented in the CG (−0.8%; ES = −0.02) and in the EG (−3.1%; ES = −0.17) with differences of 1.7% (ES = 0.06) in favour of the CG.

3.5. Inter-Individual Variability in Response to the Intervention

Regarding the inter-individual response of both groups, responders were documented for SJ (EG: n = 2, 25%), CMJ (CG: n = 1, 12.5%), TSAT (EG: n = 3, 37.5%; CG: 2, 25%), KDI (EG: n = 2, 25%; CG: n = 3, 37.5%), Total kicks (EG: n = 1, 12.5%; CG: n = 1, 12.5%), 20MSR (EG: n = 7, 87.5%; CG: n = 7, 87.5%), and BM (EG: n = 4, 50%; CG: n = 3, 37.5%), FM (EG: n = 1, 12.5%; CG: n = 1, 12.5%), FM% (EG: n = 1, 12.5%; CG: n = 1, 12.5%), and MM (CG: n = 1, 12.5%) outcomes, which are shown in detail in Table 3 and Figure 3.

Table 3. Differences and rates of responders and non-responders to HIIT and traditional training interventions.

	EG (n = 8)			CG (n = 8)			EG vs. CG	
	Δ % (90%CI)	ES (90%CI)	Rs, n (%)	Δ % (90%CI)	ES (90%CI)	Rs, n (%)	Δ % (90%CI)	ES (90%CI)
			Physical Fitness Components					
SJ (cm)	2.6 (0.1 to 5.3)	0.20 (0.01 to 0.40)	2 (25)	−1.7 (−8.8 to 5.9)	−0.07 (−0.35 to 0.22)	0 (0)	−5.2 (−15.7 to 6.6)	−0.20 (−0.64 to 0.24)
CMJ (cm)	−10.4 (−15.5 to −5.0)	−0.83 (−1.27 to −0.39)	0 (0)	−9.6 (−19.7 to 1.7)	−0.36 (−0.78 to 0.06)	1 (12.5)	11 (−0.7 to 24.2)	0.45 (−0.03 to 0.93)
TSAT (s)	−8.6 (−16.5 to 0.00)	−1.07 (−2.14 to 0.00)	3 (37.5)	−12.7 (−16 to −9.2)	−0.87 (−1.12 to −0.61)	2 (25)	0.8 (−6.9 to 9.1)	0.06 (−0.48 to 0.60)
5M (m s^{-1})	−3.8 (−9.0 to 1.8)	−0.52 (−1.28 to 0.24)	0 (0)	7.5 (1.8 to 13.5)	1.11 (0.27 to 1.94)	2 (25)	−8.5 (−13.6 to −3.0)	−1.27 (−2.10 to −0.44)
Total kicks (n)	4.4 (−3.6 to 13.0)	0.58 (−0.49 to 1.64)	1 (12.5)	3.7 (−1.6 to 9.4)	0.36 (−0.16 to 0.88)	1 (12.5)	0.8 (−4.5 to 6.3)	0.09 (−0.53 to 0.72)
KDI (%)	−32.5 (−56.4 to 4.5)	−0.80 (−1.69 to 0.09)	2 (25)	−37.7 (−79.8 to 92.1)	−0.48 (−1.63 to 0.67)	3 (37.5)	−11.8 (−66.4 to 131.8)	−0.17 (−1.48 to 1.14)
20MSR (min)	12.9 (4.0 to 22.6)	1.07 (0.34 to 1.79)	7 (87.5)	9.2 (3.4 to 15.3)	0.24 (0.09 to 0.39)	7 (87.5)	−2.0 (−10.9 to 7.7)	−0.06 (−0.34 to 0.22)
			Body Composition Characteristics					
BM (kg)	−2.1 (−4.7 a 0.4)	−0.12 (−0.26 to 0.02)	4 (50)	−1.7 (−3.4 to 0.1)	0.05 (−0.11 to 0.00)	3 (37.5)	0.3 (−1.6 to 2.4)	0.01 (−0.11 to 0.13)
FM (kg)	2.2 (−18.8 to 17.7)	0.05 (−0.48 to 0.38)	1 (12.5)	3.6 (−16.1 to 10.8)	0.04 (−0.22 to 0.13)	1 (12.5)	6.9 (−11.5 to 29.1)	0.11 (−0.20 to 0.42)
FM (%)	19.5 (−8.8 to 56.5)	0.45 (−0.23 to 1.12)	1 (12.5)	−2.0 (−13.8 to 11.5)	−0.03 (−0.20 to 0.15)	1 (12.5)	−10.0 (−24.8 to 7.8)	−0.17 (−0.46 to 0.12)
MM (kg)	−3.1 (−6.6 to 0.5)	−0.17 (−0.37 to 0.03)	0 (0)	−0.8 (−3.9 to 2.3)	−0.02 (−0.11 to 0.06)	1 (12.5)	0.8 (−2.5 to 4.2)	0.03 (−0.09 to 0.16)

Data are presented as mean ± standard deviation. EG: experimental group; CG: control group. Rs: responders; Δ %: change expressed as percentage delta; ES: effect size; 90%CI: 90% confidence interval. SJ: squat jump; CMJ: countermovement jump; TSAT: taekwondo specific agility test; total kicks; KDI: kick decreased index; 20MSR: 20-metre shuttle run; BM: body mass; FM: fat mass; FM%: percentage fat mass; MM: muscle mass.

On the other hand, non-responders were reported for SJ (CG: n = 6, 75%; EG: n = 8, 100%), CMJ (EG: n = 8, 100%; CG: n = 7, 87.5%), TSAT (EG: n = 2, 62.5%; CG: n = 6, 75%), 5M (EG: n = 8, 100%; CG: n = 6, 75%), total kicks (EG: n = 7, 87%; CG: n = 7, 87%), KDI (EG: n = 6, 75%; CG: n = 5, 62.5%), 20MSR (EG: n = 1, 12.5%; CG: n = 1, 12.5%), BM (EG: n = 4, 50%; CG n = 5, 62.5%), FM (EG: n = 7, 87.5%; CG: n = 7, 87.5%), FM% (EG: n = 7, 87.5%; CG: n = 7, 87.5%), and MM (EG: n = 8, 100%; CG: n = 7, 87.5%) outcomes, which are shown in detail in Table 3 and Figure 4.

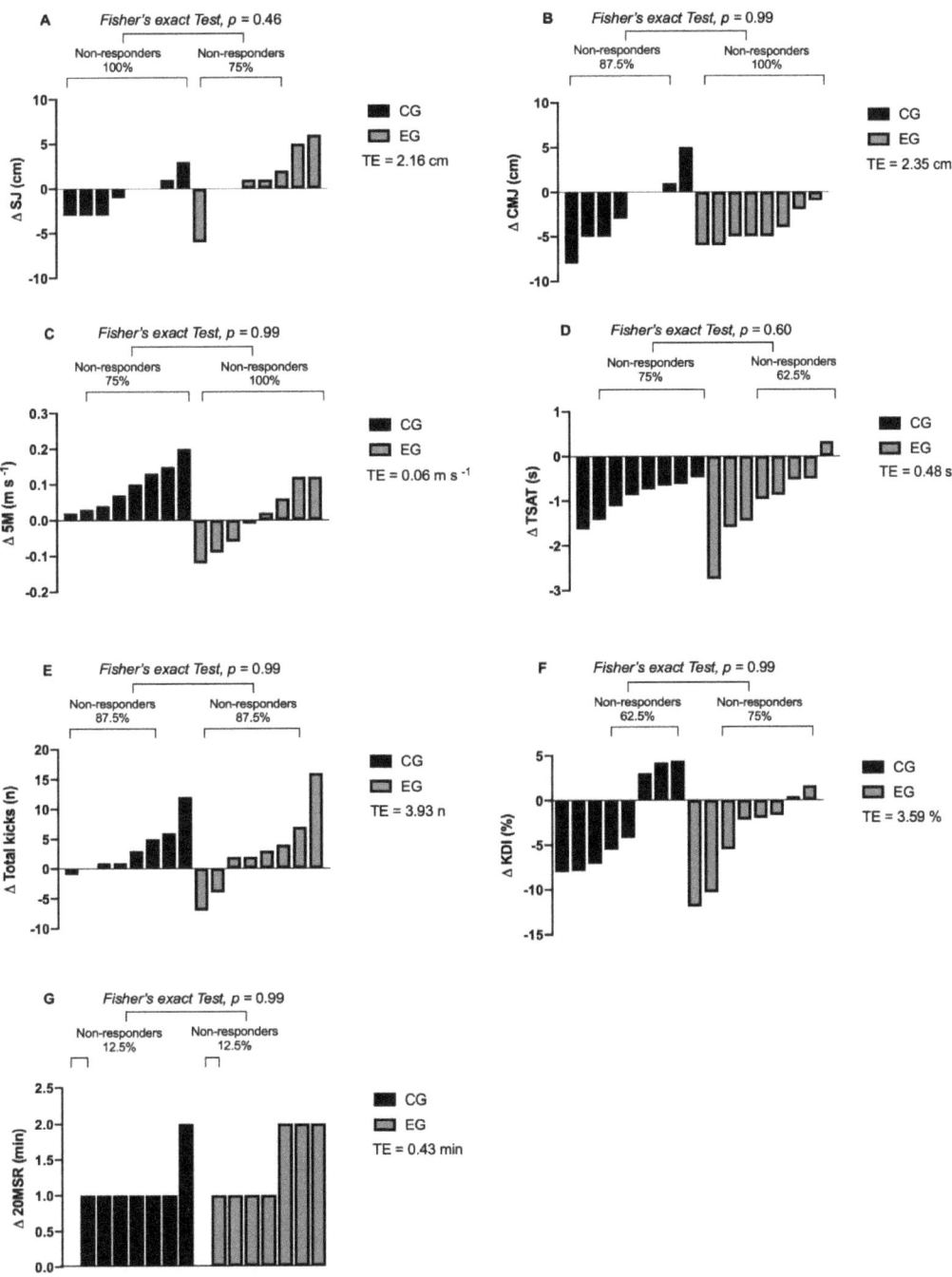

Figure 3. Inter-individual variability of the response of HIIT intervention and traditional training on the physical fitness of taekwondo athletes. Means: *p*: *p* value; TE: technical error; Δ: delta or change post-pre. Symbolises: (**A**) squat jump; (**B**) countermovement jump; (**C**) 5M linear sprint in 5 metre; (**D**) TSAT: taekwondo specific agility test; (**E**) total kicks; (**F**) KDI: kick decreased index; (**G**) 20MSR: 20-metre shuttle run.

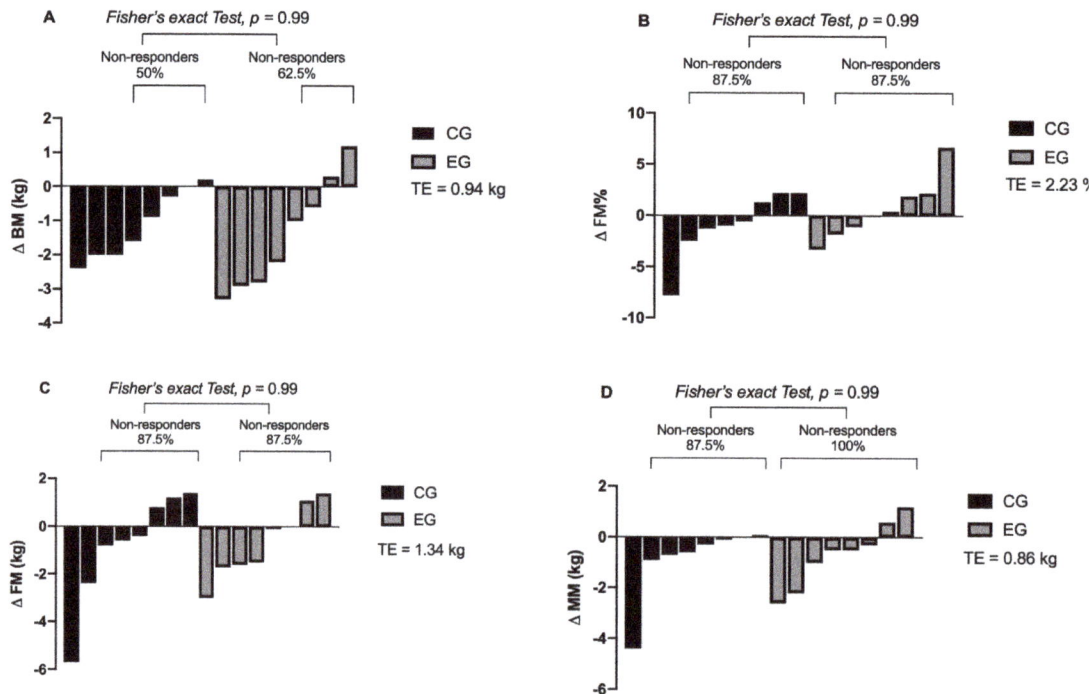

Figure 4. Inter-individual variability of the response of HIIT intervention and traditional training on body composition in taekwondo athletes. Means: *p*: *p*-value; TE: technical error; percentage change expressed as percentage delta. Symbolises: (**A**) BM: body mass, (**B**) FM%: fat mass percentage, (**C**) FM: fat mass; (**D**) MM: muscle mass.

4. Discussion

The main purpose of the present study was to compare the effects of a technique-specific HIIT protocol vs. traditional taekwondo training on general and specific physical fitness and body composition in taekwondo athletes and specifically, to analyse the inter-individual response of the athletes. Among the main findings, no significant differences ($p > 0.05$) were reported in the components analysed between the groups. Meanwhile, in the inter-individual response, responders and non-responders were observed in the EG and CG, although without statistically significant differences between the groups.

4.1. Changes in Jumping Performance

In relation to the jump ability results obtained through performance in SJ and CMJ, no significant interactions were documented between the groups by time factors. Although in SJ, EG improved by 2.6% (ES = 0.20), where 25% of athletes were classified as responders. However, these results contrast with the current evidence. In fact, significant increases in jump height in these components of physical fitness are observed after the application of HIIT protocols in taekwondo based on technique-specific movements [12] and also based on repeated sprinting [9,11]. In the study by Monks et al. [9], the authors applied two to three additional sessions per week using repeated 60 s sprints with two-minute breaks after four weeks of training. Similarly, in the study by Ouergui et al. [12], the technique-specific HIIT group performed two additional sessions of three sets of ten repetitions of six s with ten s of passive pause with three-min rests during four weeks of training. HIIT, through the application of sustained high-intensity efforts (>80–90% at VO2 max), stimulates the recruitment of fast fibres and the neuromuscular system, increasing performance in these components [36,37]. Therefore, it is likely that the volume of the HIIT protocol developed was insufficient to achieve significant results in these abilities.

4.1.1. TSAT and 5M

On the other hand, in relation to the results of specific agility assessed by the TSAT test, no significant interactions ($p > 0.05$) between the groups by time factors were reported. However, the EG improved by −8.6% (ES = −1.07) and the CG improved by −12.7% (ES = −0.87). In addition, both groups reported responders. This is important to analyse as, similarly, Ouergui et al. [12] recently reported significant increases in this skill following the application of technique-specific HIIT vs. traditional training for six weeks. In other agility tests—specifically change of direction as assessed by the T-test—significant increases in performance are also reported four weeks following the application of repeated four-week sprint-based HIIT protocols in taekwondo athletes [9]. Consequently, agility is considered a relevant complex skill in combat sports and a prerequisite in taekwondo for success in high performance, enabling technical–tactical movements in multiplanar directions [23,38]. This skill is characterised by the ability to maintain and control body position correctly while rapidly changing position through a series of movements [23]. In turn, this ability is dependent on other factors including balance, dynamic muscle actions, and cognitive factors [23]. Therefore, the trend towards a reduction in TSAT performance time exhibited by the taekwondo athletes in our study is auspicious, due to the specificity of the stimulus applied, which could influence the response observed for both groups [13].

4.1.2. FSKT$_{MULT}$

Continuing with the analysis of the components of the specific physical fitness, no significant interactions were reported between group-by-time factors. However, in the KDI score, the EG improved by −32.5% (ES = −0.80) and the CG improved by −37.7% (ES = −0.48). Similarly, in total kicks, the EG improved by 4.4% (ES = 0.58) and the CG improved by 3.7% (ES = 0.36). These results are partially similar to those reported by Aravena et al. [11], who after four weeks of applying an additional technique-specific HIIT protocol to training (3 blocks of 6 repetitions of 10 s of all-out effort with 10 s pause between sets and 1 min of passive rest interval between blocks) reported significant changes in this test. In this sense, the addition of HIIT sessions to the usual training reported by Aravena et al. [11] could explain these differences. In taekwondo, anaerobic fitness is an important characteristic to develop because punches and kicks are applied with high-intensity movement [39]. In addition, a decrease in KDI represents an increase in the ability to sustain high-intensity efforts [39]. In addition, an increase in total kicks is indicative of improved physical performance in this skill [39].

4.1.3. 20MSR

Regarding the 20MSR results, no significant interactions between group-by-time factors were reported. However, performance increases were reported in the EG by 12.9% (ES = 1.07) and in the CG by 9.2% (ES = 0.24). In addition, responders were observed in the majority of athletes in both groups. These results partially contrast with the study by Ouergui et al. [12], who report significant increases in the performance of this test after four weeks of application of a technique-specific HIIT protocol based on repeated sprinting, although without significant interactions with the control group, requiring further research to corroborate the effectiveness of this capacity.

Cardiorespiratory fitness is an important component of physical fitness for performance in combat sports due to the predominant contribution of the oxidative system [8,9,40,41]. Furthermore, according to Franchini et al. [8], this component is important for maintaining the volume and intensity of attacks during bouts, allowing a rapid resynthesis of creatine phosphate during the short pauses between the high-intensity actions performed, which allows a faster recovery between successive bouts. On the other hand, HIIT is characterised by the use of high-intensity stimuli with the purpose of spending most of the time of the protocol at high VO2max, this being a powerful stimulus to develop central adaptations (oxygen transport) and peripheral adaptations (oxygen utilisation) [18,42].

4.1.4. Changes in Body Composition

In relation to body composition, no significant group-by-time factor interactions were reported, although inter-individual differences were found in both groups independently. The low effectiveness of the HIIT intervention on body composition is consistent with previous reports in combat sports. Specifically, in taekwondo athletes, Monks et al. [9] reported no significant differences in FM% after comparing a repeated sprint-based HIIT protocol (3 sets of 60 s at 85–100% HRmax with 120 s) with a continuous moderate-intensity training (5 km at 85% of HRmax). Similarly, using technique-specific HIIT protocols in judo after four weeks [43] and in boxing after one month of intervention [44], no significant differences were found with the control groups. In this regard, it is important to consider that these studies did not establish a nutritional intervention, which is a limitation that is also present in our study. However, these results are supported by evidence from high-level combat sports athletes, indicating that no body composition adaptations are generated in short periods of intervention (4–12 weeks) [8]. In this regard, Keating et al. [45] through a systematic review with meta-analysis have determined that HIIT is no more efficient than moderate training in reducing FM, FM%, and visceral fat. On the other hand, in overweight and obese populations, HIIT seems to be more efficient in reducing FM% and FM [46]. In this context, evidence suggests that in addition to the energy expenditure of physical exercise, it is important to maintain a negative energy balance, i.e., a caloric intake that does not exceed total energy expenditure, in order to modulate body composition [45–47]. This is still a controversial issue [48].

4.2. Limitations

Possible limitations of the study include the following: (i) the lack of control of intensity by physiological measures. In this sense, although the HIIT all-out format is accepted in the scientific literature, taekwondo athletes may have underestimated the intensity of the work performed; (ii) the lack of control of dietary habits that could have influenced the reported changes in body composition; (iii) the lack of progression of the training load applied in HIIT; (iv) the evaluation by bioimpedance, which could have overestimated the body composition; and (v) the small number of athletes analysed. In addition, potential biases that could have influenced the results of this study include the following: (i) the variability of the response according to the sex of the athletes [49–51]; (ii) the absence of analysis and subsequent distribution of the athletes according to their biological age [52,53]; (iii) the variation of physical performance according to the time of day [54]; and (vi) the possible variability of the body composition due to the use of bioimpedance [55].

To address the limitations and biases of this study, future research could (i) use heart monitors or other physiological monitoring methods to verify compliance with training intensity; (ii) monitor dietary habits; (iii) apply more physiological stress by increasing the training load (e.g., increased number of sets, duration of bouts) [56]; (iv) consider studying a larger number of athletes; (v) perform independent statistical analyses by gender; (vi) assess biological age in addition to chronological age; (vii) homogenise the assessment and application of training protocols by time of day; and (viii) use the four-compartment model to assess body composition including air plethysmography, Dual X-ray Absorptiometry, and dilution techniques [57,58].

4.3. Highlights

In accordance with the above, it is relevant to point out that to the best of our knowledge, this is the first randomised controlled trial to apply a technique-specific HIIT protocol that adhered to the regular taekwondo training session, using the total duration of the bout and analysing the inter-individual response on general and specific physical fitness and body composition in athletes. Although no significant differences were found, this study reveals the need for further research in this area. In fact, most of the studies with HIIT in combat sports [8], which report significant differences in the aforementioned variables, complement the training with an extra HIIT session [9–12].

Although requiring further study, HIIT protocols based on taekwondo-specific technical movements and using the temporal structure of combat could be an alternative to incorporate as part of the training session. Since, in a short period of time, coaches could maintain or improve fitness components, which would help in pre- and inter-competition training (i.e., shock microcycle), due to the limited time available for athletes to cope with the demands of this period.

Although, in particular, this trial addresses three questions that may be important to develop in future research: (i) the potential efficacy of using technique-specific work stimuli during HIIT; (ii) the use of the appropriate time structure of the bout as a work interval during HIIT; (iii) the efficacy of the application of HIIT during the training session.

Moreover, coaches could use inter-individual response analysis as a practical monitoring tool to track each athlete's progress against the training programme in order to understand and document individual response, which would assist in modifications or remediation to improve performance. Therefore, researchers are encouraged to conduct further studies on this research topic.

5. Conclusions

A four-week HIIT protocol based on taekwondo-specific technical movements does not report significant differences in general and specific physical fitness and body composition compared to traditional training in taekwondo athletes. However, there was a higher percentage of responders in the EG compared to the CG, which is promising for future research.

Author Contributions: Conception: A.O.-A.; T.H.-V. Implementation of the work: T.H.-V., P.V.-B., J.C.-L., J.Z.-B. and J.M.G.-G. Data interpretation or analysis: A.O.-A., T.H.-V. Manuscript preparation: A.O.-A., P.V.-B., T.H.-V., J.C.-L., J.Z.-B. and J.M.G.-G. Proofreading of important intellectual content: A.O.-A., T.H.-V., P.V.-B., J.C.-L., J.Z.-B. and J.M.G.-G. Supervision: A.O.-A., T.H.-V., P.V.-B., J.C.-L., J.Z.-B. and J.M.G.-G. All authors have read and agreed to the published version of the manuscript.

Funding: The authors declare that the present study was not funded.

Institutional Review Board Statement: The study was conducted according to the guidelines of the Declaration of Helsinki and approved by the Ethics Committee of Universidad Autónoma (Code: N° 080-18, Date: 10-05-2018).

Informed Consent Statement: Informed consent was obtained from all subjects involved in the study.

Data Availability Statement: The data presented in this study are available on request from the corresponding author.

Acknowledgments: The authors are grateful for the support of coach Erwin Gonzalez and his athletes in carrying out this study.

Conflicts of Interest: The authors declare that they have no conflict of interest.

References

1. Janowski, M.; Zieliński, J.; Ciekot-Sołtysiak, M.; Schneider, A.; Kusy, K. The Effect of Sports Rules Amendments on Exercise Intensity during Taekwondo-Specific Workouts. *Int. J. Environ. Res. Public Health* **2020**, *17*, 6779. [CrossRef]
2. da Silva Santos, J.F.; Wilson, V.D.; Herrera-Valenzuela, T.; Machado, F.S.M. Time-Motion Analysis and Physiological Responses to Taekwondo Combat in Juvenile and Adult Athletes: A Systematic Review. *Strength Cond. J.* **2020**, *42*, 103–121. [CrossRef]

3. Bridge, C.A.; da Silva Santos, J.F.; Chaabene, H.; Pieter, W.; Franchini, E. Physical and Physiological Profiles of Taekwondo Athletes. *Sports Med.* **2014**, *44*, 713–733. [CrossRef] [PubMed]
4. Campos, F.A.D.; Bertuzzi, R.; Dourado, A.C.; Santos, V.G.F.; Franchini, E. Energy Demands in Taekwondo Athletes during Combat Simulation. *Eur. J. Appl. Physiol.* **2012**, *112*, 1221–1228. [CrossRef] [PubMed]
5. Ojeda-Aravena, A.; Azocar-Gallardo, J.; Galle, F.; García-García, J.M. Relación Entre Las Características de La Composición Corporal y El Rendimiento Físico General y Específico En Competidores de Taekwondo Chilenos de Nivel Nacional de Ambos Sexos: Un Estudio Observacional. *Rev. Esp. Nutr. Hum. Diet.* **2020**, *24*, 154–164. [CrossRef]
6. Andreato, L.V. High-Intensity Interval Training: Methodological Considerations for Interpreting Results and Conducting Research. *Trends Endocrinol. Metab.* **2020**. [CrossRef]
7. Vasconcelos, B.B.; Protzen, G.V.; Galliano, L.M.; Kirk, C.; Del Vecchio, F.B. Effects of High-Intensity Interval Training in Combat Sports: A Systematic Review with Meta-Analysis. *J. Strength Cond. Res.* **2020**, *34*, 888–900. [CrossRef]
8. Franchini, E.; Cormack, S.; Takito, M.Y. Effects of High-Intensity Interval Training on Olympic Combat Sports Athletes' Performance and Physiological Adaptation: A Systematic Review. *J. Strength Cond. Res.* **2019**, *33*, 242–252. [CrossRef]
9. Monks, L.; Seo, M.-W.; Kim, H.-B.; Jung, H.C.; Song, J.K. High-Intensity Interval Training and Athletic Performance in Taekwondo Athletes. *J. Sports Med. Phys. Fit.* **2017**, *57*, 1252–1260. [CrossRef]
10. Seo, M.-W.; Lee, J.-M.; Jung, H.C.; Jung, S.W.; Song, J.K. Effects of Various Work-to-Rest Ratios during High-Intensity Interval Training on Athletic Performance in Adolescents. *Int. J. Sports Med.* **2019**, *40*, 503–510. [CrossRef]
11. Aravena, D.E.A.; Barrera, V.R.; Santos, J.F.D.S.; Franchini, E.; Badilla, P.V.; Orihuela, P.; Valenzuela, T.H. High-Intensity Interval Training Improves Specific Performance in Taekwondo Athletes. *Rev. Artes Marciales Asiát.* **2020**, *15*, 4–13. [CrossRef]
12. Ouergui, I.; Messaoudi, H.; Chtourou, H.; Wagner, M.O.; Bouassida, A.; Bouhlel, E.; Franchini, E.; Engel, F.A. Repeated Sprint Training vs. Repeated High-Intensity Technique Training in Adolescent Taekwondo Athletes—A Randomized Controlled Trial. *Int. J. Environ. Res. Public Health* **2020**, *17*, 4506. [CrossRef] [PubMed]
13. Franchini, E. High-Intensity Interval Training Prescription for Combat-Sport Athletes. *Int. J. Sports Physiol. Perform.* **2020**, *15*, 767–776. [CrossRef]
14. Ramirez-Campillo, R.; Alvarez, C.; Gentil, P.; Moran, J.; García-Pinillos, F.; Alonso-Martínez, A.M.; Izquierdo, M. Inter-Individual Variability in Responses to 7 Weeks of Plyometric Jump Training in Male Youth Soccer Players. *Front. Physiol.* **2018**, *9*, 1156. [CrossRef] [PubMed]
15. Bonafiglia, J.T.; Nelms, M.W.; Preobrazenski, N.; LeBlanc, C.; Robins, L.; Lu, S.; Lithopoulos, A.; Walsh, J.J.; Gurd, B.J. Moving beyond Threshold-Based Dichotomous Classification to Improve the Accuracy in Classifying Non-Responders. *Physiol. Rep.* **2018**, *6*, e13928. [CrossRef] [PubMed]
16. Bonafiglia, J.T.; Rotundo, M.P.; Whittall, J.P.; Scribbans, T.D.; Graham, R.B.; Gurd, B.J. Inter-Individual Variability in the Adaptive Responses to Endurance and Sprint Interval Training: A Randomized Crossover Study. *PLoS ONE* **2016**, *11*. [CrossRef]
17. Dolci, F.; Kilding, A.E.; Chivers, P.; Piggott, B.; Hart, N.H. High-Intensity Interval Training Shock Microcycle for Enhancing Sport Performance: A Brief Review. *J. Strength Cond. Res.* **2020**, *34*, 1188–1196. [CrossRef]
18. Laursen, P.B.; Buchheit, M. *Science and Application of High-Intensity Interval Training*; Human Kinetics: Champaign, IL, USA, 2018; ISBN 978-1-4925-5212-3.
19. World Medical Association World Medical Association Declaration of Helsinki: Ethical Principles for Medical Research Involving Human Subjects. *JAMA* **2013**, *310*, 2191–2194. [CrossRef]
20. Groeber, M.; Stafilidis, S.; Seiberl, W.; Baca, A. Contribution of Stretch-Induced Force Enhancement to Increased Performance in Maximal Voluntary and Submaximal Artificially Activated Stretch-Shortening Muscle Action. *Front. Physiol.* **2020**, *11*, 592183. [CrossRef] [PubMed]
21. Ramírez-Campillo, R.; Andrade, D.C.; Izquierdo, M. Effects of Plyometric Training Volume and Training Surface on Explosive Strength. *J. Strength Cond. Res.* **2013**, *27*, 2714–2722. [CrossRef]
22. Moran, J.; Sandercock, G.R.; Ramírez-Campillo, R.; Todd, O.; Collison, J.; Parry, D.A. Maturation-Related Effect of Low-Dose Plyometric Training on Performance in Youth Hockey Players. *Pediatr. Exerc. Sci.* **2017**, *29*, 194–202. [CrossRef]
23. Chaabene, H.; Negra, Y.; Capranica, L.; Bouguezzi, R.; Hachana, Y.; Rouahi, M.A.; Mkaouer, B. Validity and Reliability of a New Test of Planned Agility in Elite Taekwondo Athletes. *J. Strength Cond. Res.* **2018**, *32*, 2542–2547. [CrossRef]
24. da Silva Santos, J.F.; Loturco, I.; Franchini, E. Relationship between Frequency Speed of Kick Test Performance, Optimal Load, and Anthropometric Variables in Black-Belt Taekwondo Athletes. *Ido Mov. Cult. J. Martial Arts Anthropol.* **2018**, *18*, 39–44. [CrossRef]
25. Leger, L.A.; Mercier, D.; Gadoury, C.; Lambert, J. The Multistage 20 Metre Shuttle Run Test for Aerobic Fitness. *J. Sports Sci.* **1988**, *6*, 93–101. [CrossRef] [PubMed]
26. Caballero, P.G.; Díaz, J.C. *Manual de Antropometría*; Instituto Superior De Cultura Física: La Habana, Cuba, 2003.
27. Lee, L.-W.; Liao, Y.-S.; Lu, H.-K.; Hsiao, P.-L.; Chen, Y.-Y.; Chi, C.-C.; Hsieh, K.-C. Validation of Two Portable Bioelectrical Impedance Analyses for the Assessment of Body Composition in School Age Children. *PLoS ONE* **2017**, *12*. [CrossRef] [PubMed]
28. Montgomery, M.M.; Marttinen, R.H.; Galpin, A.J. Comparison of Body Fat Results from 4 Bioelectrical Impedance Analysis Devices vs. Air Displacement Plethysmography in American Adolescent Wrestlers. *Int. J. Kinesiol. Sports Sci.* **2017**, *5*, 18–25. [CrossRef]

29. Miller, R.M.; Chambers, T.L.; Burns, S.P.; Godard, M.P. Validating Inbody®570 Multi-Frequency Bioelectrical Impedance Analyzer versus DXA for Body Fat Percentage Analysis. *Med. Sci. Sports Exerc.* **2016**, *48*, 991. [CrossRef]
30. An, K.H.; Han, K.A.; Sohn, T.S.; Park, I.B.; Kim, H.J.; Moon, S.D.; Min, K.W. Body Fat Is Related to Sedentary Behavior and Light Physical Activity but Not to Moderate-Vigorous Physical Activity in Type 2 Diabetes Mellitus. *Diabetes Metab. J.* **2019**, *44*, 316–325. [CrossRef] [PubMed]
31. Marenco, R.G.; Escobedo, M.M.; Balam, M.G.; Zapata, J.E.; Barreiro, A.C.; Poot, P.V.; Martín, K.C. Concordancia entre la composición corporal medida con un inbody 120 y un skulpt chisel en atletas de combate adolescentes. *Rev. Digit. Act. Fís. Deporte* **2021**, *7*, 1–12. [CrossRef]
32. Antonio, J.; Kenyon, M.; Ellerbroek, A.; Carson, C.; Burgess, V.; Tyler-Palmer, D.; Mike, J.; Roberts, J.; Angeli, G.; Peacock, C. Comparison of Dual-Energy X-Ray Absorptiometry (DXA) Versus a Multi-Frequency Bioelectrical Impedance (InBody 770) Device for Body Composition Assessment after a 4-Week Hypoenergetic Diet. *J. Funct. Morphol. Kinesiol.* **2019**, *4*, 23. [CrossRef]
33. Research Randomizer. Available online: https://www.randomizer.org (accessed on 1 March 2019).
34. Hopkins, W.G. Measures of Reliability in Sports Medicine and Science. *Sports Med.* **2000**, *30*, 1–15. [CrossRef]
35. Hopkins, W.G.; Marshall, S.W.; Batterham, A.M.; Hanin, J. Progressive Statistics for Studies in Sports Medicine and Exercise Science. *Med. Sci. Sports Exerc.* **2009**, *41*, 3–13. [CrossRef]
36. Buchheit, M.; Laursen, P.B. High-Intensity Interval Training, Solutions to the Programming Puzzle. Part II: Anaerobic Energy, Neuromuscular Load and Practical Applications. *Sports Med.* **2013**, *43*, 927–954. [CrossRef]
37. Kinnunen, J.-V.; Piitulainen, H.; Piirainen, J.M. Neuromuscular Adaptations to Short-Term High-Intensity Interval Training in Female Ice-Hockey Players. *J. Strength Cond. Res.* **2019**, *33*, 479–485. [CrossRef]
38. de Quel, Ó.M.; Ara, I.; Izquierdo, M.; Ayán, C. Does Physical Fitness Predict Future Karate Success? A Study in Young Female Karatekas. *Int. J. Sports Physiol. Perform.* **2020**, *15*, 868–873. [CrossRef] [PubMed]
39. da Silva Santos, J.F.; Franchini, E. Frequency Speed of Kick Test Performance Comparison between Female Taekwondo Athletes of Different Competitive Levels. *J. Strength Cond. Res.* **2018**, *32*, 2934–2938. [CrossRef] [PubMed]
40. Ravier, G.; Dugué, B.; Grappe, F.; Rouillon, J.D. Impressive Anaerobic Adaptations in Elite Karate Athletes Due to Few Intensive Intermittent Sessions Added to Regular Karate Training. *Scand. J. Med. Sci. Sports* **2009**, *19*, 687–694. [CrossRef] [PubMed]
41. Farzad, B.; Gharakhanlou, R.; Agha-Alinejad, H.; Curby, D.G.; Bayati, M.; Bahraminejad, M.; Mäestu, J. Physiological and Performance Changes from the Addition of a Sprint Interval Program to Wrestling Training. *J. Strength Cond. Res.* **2011**, *25*, 2392–2399. [CrossRef]
42. Wen, D.; Utesch, T.; Wu, J.; Robertson, S.; Liu, J.; Hu, G.; Chen, H. Effects of Different Protocols of High Intensity Interval Training for VO2max Improvements in Adults: A Meta-Analysis of Randomised Controlled Trials. *J. Sci. Med. Sport* **2019**, *22*, 941–947. [CrossRef]
43. Franchini, E.; Julio, U.F.; Panissa, V.L.; Lira, F.S.; Gerosa-Neto, J.; Branco, B.H. High-Intensity Intermittent Training Positively Affects Aerobic and Anaerobic Performance in Judo Athletes Independently of Exercise Mode. *Front. Physiol.* **2016**, *7*, 268. [CrossRef]
44. Kamandulis, S.; Bruzas, V.; Mockus, P.; Stasiulis, A.; Snieckus, A.; Venckunas, T. Sport-Specific Repeated Sprint Training Improves Punching Ability and Upper-Body Aerobic Power in Experienced Amateur Boxers. *J. Strength Cond. Res.* **2018**, *32*, 1214–1221. [CrossRef] [PubMed]
45. Keating, S.E.; Johnson, N.A.; Mielke, G.I.; Coombes, J.S. A Systematic Review and Meta-Analysis of Interval Training versus Moderate-Intensity Continuous Training on Body Adiposity. *Obes. Rev.* **2017**, *18*, 943–964. [CrossRef] [PubMed]
46. Maillard, F.; Pereira, B.; Boisseau, N. Effect of High-Intensity Interval Training on Total, Abdominal and Visceral Fat Mass: A Meta-Analysis. *Sports Med.* **2018**, *48*, 269–288. [CrossRef]
47. Cox, C.E. Role of Physical Activity for Weight Loss and Weight Maintenance. *Diabetes Spectr.* **2017**, *30*, 157–160. [CrossRef] [PubMed]
48. Gentil, P.; Viana, R.B.; Naves, J.P.; Del Vecchio, F.B.; Coswig, V.; Loenneke, J.; de Lira, C.A.B. Is It Time to Rethink Our Weight Loss Paradigms? *Biology* **2020**, *9*, 70. [CrossRef] [PubMed]
49. Ransdell, L.B.; Wells, C.L. Sex Differences in Athletic Performance. *Women Sport Phys. Act. J.* **1999**, *8*, 55–81. [CrossRef]
50. Courtright, S.H.; McCormick, B.W.; Postlethwaite, B.E.; Reeves, C.J.; Mount, M.K. A Meta-Analysis of Sex Differences in Physical Ability: Revised Estimates and Strategies for Reducing Differences in Selection Contexts. *J. Appl. Psychol.* **2013**, *98*, 623. [CrossRef]
51. Schmitz, B.; Niehues, H.; Thorwesten, L.; Klose, A.; Krüger, M.; Brand, S.-M. Sex Differences in High-Intensity Interval Training–Are HIIT Protocols Interchangeable Between Females and Males? *Front. Physiol.* **2020**, *11*. [CrossRef]
52. Mirwald, R.L.; Baxter-Jones, A.D.; Bailey, D.A.; Beunen, G.P. An Assessment of Maturity from Anthropometric Measurements. *Med. Sci. Sports Exerc.* **2002**, *34*, 689–694. [CrossRef]
53. Malina, R.M.; Rogol, A.D.; Cumming, S.P.; de Silva, M.J.C.; Figueiredo, A.J. Biological Maturation of Youth Athletes: Assessment and Implications. *Br. J. Sports Med.* **2015**, *49*, 852–859. [CrossRef]
54. Chtourou, H.; Souissi, N. The Effect of Training at a Specific Time of Day: A Review. *J. Strength Cond. Res.* **2012**, *26*, 1984–2005. [CrossRef] [PubMed]

55. McLester, C.N.; Nickerson, B.S.; Kliszczewicz, B.M.; McLester, J.R. Reliability and Agreement of Various InBody Body Composition Analyzers as Compared to Dual-Energy X-Ray Absorptiometry in Healthy Men and Women. *J. Clin. Densitom.* **2020**, *23*, 443–450. [CrossRef] [PubMed]
56. Chaabene, H.; Negra, Y.; Bouguezzi, R.; Capranica, L.; Franchini, E.; Prieske, O.; Hbacha, H.; Granacher, U. Tests for the Assessment of Sport-Specific Performance in Olympic Combat Sports: A Systematic Review with Practical Recommendations. *Front. Physiol.* **2018**, *9*, 386. [CrossRef] [PubMed]
57. Marini, E.; Campa, F.; Buffa, R.; Stagi, S.; Matias, C.N.; Toselli, S.; Sardinha, L.B.; Silva, A.M. Phase Angle and Bioelectrical Impedance Vector Analysis in the Evaluation of Body Composition in Athletes. *Clin. Nutr.* **2020**, *39*, 447–454. [CrossRef] [PubMed]
58. Campa, F.; Matias, C.N.; Marini, E.; Heymsfield, S.B.; Toselli, S.; Sardinha, L.B.; Silva, A.M. Identifying Athlete Body Fluid Changes during a Competitive Season with Bioelectrical Impedance Vector Analysis. *Int. J. Sports Physiol. Perform.* **2020**, *15*, 361–367. [CrossRef] [PubMed]

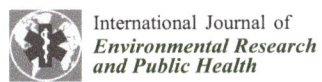

Brief Report

Exercise-Induced Release of Cardiac Troponins in Adolescent vs. Adult Swimmers

Rafel Cirer-Sastre [1,*], Francisco Corbi [1], Isaac López-Laval [2], Luis Enrique Carranza-García [3] and Joaquín Reverter-Masià [4]

[1] Institut Nacional d'Educació Física de Catalunya (INEFC), Universitat de Lleida (UdL), 25192 Lleida, Spain; fcorbi@inefc.es
[2] Facultad de Ciencias de la Salud y del Deporte, Universidad de Zaragoza, 50009 Zaragoza, Spain; isaac@unizar.es
[3] Facultad de Organización Deportiva (FOD), Universidad Autónoma de Nuevo León (UANL), San Nicolás de los Garza 66550, Mexico; luis.carranzagr@uanl.edu.mx
[4] Departament de Didàctiques Específiques, Universitat de Lleida (UdL), 25003 Lleida, Spain; joaquim.reverter@udl.cat
* Correspondence: rcirer@inefc.es; Tel.: +34-973-27-20-22

Abstract: To examine the exercise-induced release of cardiac troponin T (cTnT) in adolescent and adult swimmers. Thirty-two trained male (18 adolescents, 14 adults) swam at maximal pace in a 45 min distance trial, and blood samples were drawn before, immediately and 3 h after exercise for subsequent cTnT analysis and comparison. Having comparable training experience and baseline values of cTnT ($p = 0.78$ and $p = 0.13$), adults exercised at lower absolute and relative intensity ($p < 0.001$ and $p < 0.001$, respectively), but presented higher immediate cTnT after exercise than adolescents ($p < 0.001$). Despite that, peak concentrations were observed at 3 h post exercise and peak elevations were comparable between groups ($p = 0.074$). Fourteen (44%) apparently healthy subjects exceeded the cutoff value for myocardial infarction (MI). Adolescents presented a delayed elevation of cTnT compared with adults, but achieved similar peak values.

Keywords: biomarkers; heart damage; swimming; growth

Citation: Cirer-Sastre, R.; Corbi, F.; López-Laval, I.; Carranza-García, L.E.; Reverter-Masià, J. Exercise-Induced Release of Cardiac Troponins in Adolescent vs. Adult Swimmers. *Int. J. Environ. Res. Public Health* **2021**, *18*, 1285. https://doi.org/10.3390/ijerph18031285

Academic Editor: Tadeusz Ambroży
Received: 28 December 2020
Accepted: 26 January 2021
Published: 1 February 2021

Publisher's Note: MDPI stays neutral with regard to jurisdictional claims in published maps and institutional affiliations.

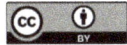

Copyright: © 2021 by the authors. Licensee MDPI, Basel, Switzerland. This article is an open access article distributed under the terms and conditions of the Creative Commons Attribution (CC BY) license (https://creativecommons.org/licenses/by/4.0/).

1. Introduction

Elevations of serum cardiac troponin (cTn) are the preferred criteria to diagnose myocardial injury [1]. Concretely, the release of cTn into the bloodstream has been related to different clinical scenarios and explained by mechanisms of release such as myocardial ischemia, inflammatory and immunological processes, trauma, drugs or toxins [1,2]. It is of particular interest though that exercise frequently evokes elevations of serum cardiac troponin (cTn), that peak approximately 3 h after exercise and return to basal concentrations within the subsequent 24 h [3]. Furthermore, a growing body of evidence suggests that cTn elevations induced by exercise occur in apparently healthy athletes and might respond to a physiological acute response to exercise rather than pathological sign [2–4]. Although the mechanisms underlying the release of cTn following exercise in apparently healthy individuals are not completely understood, previous research suggested potential mechanisms, among them: changes in membrane permeability allowing unbound cTn from cytosol to diffuse outside the cells, normal turnover of myocardial cells, cTn degradation producing cellular release, membranous blebs, myocyte apoptosis/necrosis resulting in genuine cardiac injury or cross-reaction with skeletal troponin [3,5].

Post-exercise elevations of cTn have been noted also in adolescent athletes [6]. However, differences between adolescents and adults are inconsistent [4,6–8]. In this regard, it has been previously suggested that higher exercise-induced elevations of cTn in the younger might be attributable to the immaturity of adolescents myocardium, since it would experience greater stress in response to an increased myocardial workload compared with the adults [9]. Based on this hypothesis, it is possible that younger athletes respond to exercise with higher elevations of this biomarker than adults. Notwithstanding that, prior literature has also linked exercise-induced elevations of cTn above the upper reference limit to higher mortality and cardiovascular events in older athletes [10]. In this case, higher elevations in the older might be related to underlying, subclinical, cardiac pathology [11].

Understanding how, when, and why cTn elevates after exercise is relevant for the triage of athletes who develop chest pain that mimics cardiac injury after exercise, and who might have serum cTn drawn in the emergency departments (EDs). Furthermore, a better knowledge of the relationship between exercise-induced elevations of cTn and participants' age might contribute to a better understanding of the phenomenon and its mechanisms. For these reasons, the purpose of this study was to compare the release of cTnT after a distance-trial test of 45 min swimming between two cohorts of adolescent and adult swimmers. Based on previous studies, our hypothesis was that adolescents would respond to exercise with higher peak elevations of cTn, supporting the theory that the immature myocardium experiences higher workload compared with the adults.

2. Materials and Methods

2.1. Participants

A convenience sample of thirty-two trained male swimmers were recruited for this study. All participants and parents of those under the age of 18 provided their informed consent. All swimmers trained in the same club and competed at the regional level. Participants were divided into adolescent (<18 years) and adult (≥18 years) groups (see participant characteristics in Table 1). The study was approved by the Ethical Committee of Clinical Research of Sports Administration of Catalonia (02/2018/CEICGC).

Table 1. Summary of participants' characteristics and exercise load.

	Adolescents (n = 18)	Adults (n = 14)	Between-Groups
Participant Characteristics			
Age (years)	14 ± 3 [11–17]	35 ± 9 [23–52]	$p < 0.001$
Training experience (years)	7 ± 2 [2–11]	6 ± 2 [4–9]	$p = 0.78$
Body height (cm)	172.3 ± 9.6 [151–187]	177.4 ± 5.5 [169–187]	$p = 0.065$
Body mass (kg)	60.6 ± 10.2 [44.5–77.8]	71 ± 4.4 [66–81]	$p < 0.001$
Body mass index	20.3 ± 2.2 [16.9–24.3]	26.6 ± 1.3 [20–24.8]	$p = 0.001$
Exercise Load			
Distance (m)	1862 ± 276 [1250–2300]	1650 ± 239 [1320–2060]	$p = 0.027$
Mean relative heart rate (% HRmax)	89 ± 5 [75–99]	82 ± 4 [75–88]	$p < 0.001$
Peak relative heart rate (% HRmax)	95 ± 6 [82–110]	91 ± 4 [82–96]	$p = 0.037$
Rating of perceived exertion	7 ± 2 [3–10]	8 ± 1 [6–10]	$p = 0.24$
Cardiac Troponin			
Basal cTnT (ng/L)	5.39 (2.15) [1.5–8.09]	3.93 (3.97) [1.5–6.07]	$p = 0.13$
Δ 0 h post-exercise cTnT (ng/L)	0.38 (0.62) [−0.46–2.41]	3.69 (2.78) [0.57–9.25]	$p < 0.001$
Δ 3 h post-exercise cTnT (ng/L)	5.08 (6.37) [1.07–34.67]	11.64 (13.62) [2.83–38.84]	$p = 0.074$

Participant characteristics and exercise load data are described as mean ± standard deviation [range], whereas cTn data are described as median (interquartile range) [range]. Δ 0 h post-exercise cTnT, absolute change from baseline to immediately after exercise; Δ 3 h post-exercise cTnT, absolute change from baseline to 3 h post-exercise.

2.2. Procedures

Before the intervention, participants underwent anthropometric assessment and a resting 12-lead electrocardiogram (Click ECG BT 12 channel, Milano, Italy). Swimmers performed a self-paced 5 min swimming warm-up (<60% of %HRmax) [6], followed by a distance-trial test of 45 min continuous swimming, and venous blood samples were drawn before, immediately and at 3 h after exercise. Participants were asked to avoid vigorous exercise during the 48 h prior to the intervention. Serum cTnT was determined using a Troponin T hs STAT immunoassay in a Cobas E 601 analyzer (Roche Diagnostics, Penzberg, Germany, range 3–10,000 ng/L). The upper reference limit for cTnT was 13.5 ng/L [11]. Concentrations below the limit of detection were set to 1.5 ng/L for statistical analyses. Heart rate during the test was recorded using Polar OH1™ optical heart rate sensors (Polar Electro Oy, Kempele, Finland). Maximum heart rate for relative intensities was calculated using Tanaka's formula of 208 − (0.7 × Age). A year after the intervention, participants were interviewed to identify cases of cardiac signs or symptoms.

2.3. Statistical Analysis

Analyses were performed using R version 3.5.1 (R Foundation for Statistical Computing, Vienna, Austria). Data were visually inspected to detect abnormal values, and Shapiro-Wilk test was used to assess normality. Accordingly, data were presented as mean ± SD [range] or median (interquartile range) [range], as appropriate. Participant characteristics and exercise load were compared among groups using t-test for independent samples. Then, time differences within each group were compared using non-parametric Friedman test for repeated measures and pairwise comparisons between moments were made with Wilcoxon signed rank tests applying Bonferroni corrections. Differences between groups in absolute cTn and its changes (Δ 0 h and Δ 3 h) were analyzed using Kruskal-Wallis rank sum test. Associations between cTn elevations and the rest of the variables were assessed using Spearman correlation coefficients (ρ). Statistical significance in all comparisons was assumed when $p < 0.05$.

3. Results

Participant characteristics and exercise load during the distance trial are summarized in Table 1. There were group differences in age, body mass, body mass index and maximal heart rate, and training experience was comparable between groups. During the distance trial, adolescents covered more distance and achieved higher cardiac intensity than adults, though the rating of perceived exertion was comparable between groups.

Concentrations of cTnT changed significantly over time ($\chi^2 = 59.5$, $p < 0.001$). Concretely, baseline concentrations were comparable between adolescents and adults ($\chi^2 = 2.2$; $p = 0.13$), and in both groups it raised immediately after and at 3 h post exercise. Furthermore, immediate changes (Δ0 h) were different between groups ($\chi^2 = 18.1$; $p < 0.001$), slightly higher in the adults (Figure 1). Peak changes (Δ3 h), however, were comparable between groups ($\chi^2 = 3.2$; $p = 0.074$). Peak cTnT concentrations were observed at 3 h post-exercise in all participants, and 14 (44%) subjects exceeded the cutoff value for myocardial infarction (MI) (6 (33%) adolescents, 8 (57%) adults). Peak changes (Δ3 h) were uncorrelated with age ($\rho = 0.19$, $p = 0.29$), training experience ($\rho = -0.21$, $p = 0.24$), body mass index ($\rho = 0.05$, $p = 0.8$), distance ($\rho = -0.1$, $p = 0.59$), peak heart rate ($\rho = 0.06$, $p = 0.74$), and mean heart rate ($\rho = 0.06$, $p = 0.73$).

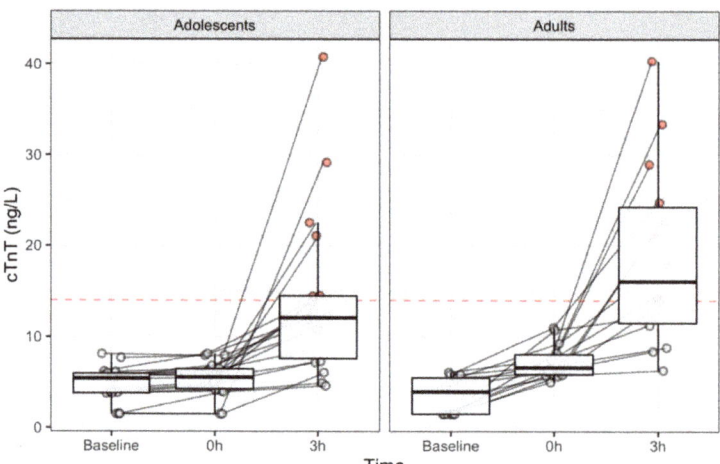

Figure 1. Individual points of cTnT by group. Red horizontal line and red dots denote the cutoff value for myocardial infarction (MI) of 13.5 ng/L and above values, respectively.

4. Discussion

The purpose of this study was to compare the exercise-induced release of cTnT between adolescents and adults. Our main finding was that, although having comparable training experience and baseline values of cTnT, adults exercised at lower absolute and relative intensity, but presented higher immediate concentrations of cTnT after exercise than adolescents. However, peak concentrations were observed at 3 h post exercise in all participants and were comparable between groups.

Reference values of cTn seem to be lower in the young, and this might be explained by a positive association between age and the prevalence of cardiovascular diseases [4,11]. However, our results did not support those previous statements since swimmers had comparable basal concentrations of cTnT. Even though this study was limited by a small sample size, it is not the first research finding no age-differences in apparently healthy, trained, young participants [7]. Interestingly though, although peak cTnT was found in all participants at 3 h post exercise, we detected higher elevations immediately after exercise in the adults. Since peak elevations were comparable among groups, this suggests that serological cTnT elevations might appear earlier after exercise in adults compared with adolescents.

It has been suggested that higher concentrations of post-exercise cTn in the older may represent myocardial injury because of underlying, subclinical, cardiac pathology [11]. However, all participants in this study had normal resting ECG at the beginning of the study. Furthermore, one year after the intervention, none of them reported to have had cardiac symptoms or events during this period. Assuming that our participants were healthy, these evidences align with the theory of transient elevations of cTnT after exercise being a physiological acute response to exercise rather than a sign of myocardial injury [3]. However, this study did not include other examinations of myocardial health such as echocardiographies or other biomarker assessments such as N-terminal prohormone of brain natriuretic peptide (NT-proBNP), creatine kinase myocardial band (CK-MB), or c-reactive protein (CRP). Due to this limitation, we cannot be certain to discard a possible role of underlying, undetected scenarios such as cardiac hypertrophy and thyroid dysfunction [12].

In the present study, cTnT raised in all participants after exercise, and peak elevations at 3 h post exercise were comparable among groups. This is contrary to our expectations, since previous authors suggested that the less mature myocardium in the younger might be more susceptible to exercise-induced elevations of cTn [8,9]. Interestingly though, a recent study reported higher exercise-induced elevations of cTnT in late puberty, suggesting that this might be explained by the higher relative intensities during exercise achieved in this group [13]. In line with this study, our adolescents group also achieved higher cardiac intensities during the test. In spite of that, we found no association between exercise intensity and peak elevations of cTnT. This finding seems interesting, since we expected post-exercise cTnT concentrations to be directly associated with exercise intensity, as has been reported in previous studies [4]. Thus, our results not only suggest that adults elevate cTn before adolescents, but also that the association between cTnT elevations and exercise intensity might not depend on age.

Almost one-half of the participants in this study (44%) exceeded the upper reference limit for cTnT in the third blood extraction. Previous studies involving similar assessments and exercise exposures also found high rates of positive detection in both young and adult trained participants [4,6–8,13]. This is particularly relevant for the triage of athletes who develop chest pain that mimics cardiac injury after exercise, and who might have serum cTn drawn in the EDs. For these reasons, future studies should address the limitations present in this research, including a more exhaustive clinical screening of the participants in order to discard or identify a potential role of underlying pathology.

Finally, in the authors' opinion, the main strength of this study is that that we could compare the elevations of cTnT in a cohort of trained swimmers that allowed comparisons between age groups, and this made it possible for us to identify an earlier elevation in the adults compared with the adolescents. The main limitations in this study, by contrast, have been mentioned in the above paragraphs. We could not perform an exhaustive cardiac screening including echocardiography, additional biochemical analyses, or assessments of maturational status, as has been done or mentioned in some previous studies [6,12,13]. Additionally, we did not perform cTnT measurements beyond the 3 h post exercise. Consequently, the limited sampling points in our design imply a potential under-estimation error in the peak cTnT concentrations, as has been previously suggested by others [14,15].

5. Conclusions

In conclusion, in this study we observed age differences in the immediate elevation of cTnT after exercise, but not in its peak elevations, at 3 h post exercise. Although participants were apparently healthy based on resting ECG and a 1 year term follow-up, future works might continue this line of research and explore the association between immediate elevations of cTnT, age, and health.

Author Contributions: Conceptualization, R.C.-S., F.C. and J.R.-M.; Data curation, R.C.-S. and I.L.-L.; Formal analysis, R.C.-S.; Funding acquisition, F.C. and J.R.-M.; Investigation, R.C.-S., I.L.-L., and L.E.C.-G.; Methodology, R.C.-S. and F.C.; Project administration, R.C.-S. and J.R.-M.; Resources, R.C.-S., F.C. and I.L.-L.; Software, R.C.-S.; Supervision, F.C. and J.R.-M.; Validation, R.C.-S. and L.E.C.-G.; Visualization, R.C.-S.; and Writing—review and editing, R.C.-S., L.E.C.-G., F.C., and J.R.-M. All authors have read and agreed to the published version of the manuscript.

Funding: This research was funded by the National Institute of Physical Education of Catalonia, grant number 2016-PINEF-00007 and Institut de Desenvolupament Social i Territorial (INDEST), grant number 2018CRINDESTABC.

Institutional Review Board Statement: The study was conducted according to the guidelines of the Declaration of Helsinki, and approved by the Ethical Committee of Clinical Research of Sports Administration of Catalonia (02/2018/CEICGC).

Informed Consent Statement: Informed consent was obtained from all subjects involved in the study.

Data Availability Statement: The data presented in this study are available on request to the authors. Some variables are restricted to preserve the anonymity of study participants.

Conflicts of Interest: The authors declare no conflict of interest.

References

1. Thygesen, K.; Alpert, J.S.; Jaffe, A.S.; Chaitman, B.R.; Bax, J.J.; Morrow, D.A.; White, H.D. Fourth Universal Definition of Myocardial Infarction (2018). *J. Am. Coll. Cardiol.* **2018**, *33*, 2551–2567. [CrossRef]
2. Mair, J.; Lindahl, B.; Hammarsten, O.; Müller, C.; Giannitsis, E.; Huber, K.; Möckel, M.; Plebani, M.; Thygesen, K.; Jaffe, A.S. How is Cardiac Troponin Released from Injured Myocardium? *Eur. Heart J. Acute Cardiovasc. Care* **2018**, *7*, 553–560. [CrossRef] [PubMed]
3. Baker, P.; Leckie, T.; Harrington, D.; Richardson, A. Exercise-Induced Cardiac Troponin Elevation: An Update on the Evidence, Mechanism and Implications. *Int. J. Cardiol. Heart Vasc.* **2019**, *22*, 181–186. [CrossRef] [PubMed]
4. Cirer-Sastre, R.; Legaz-Arrese, A.; Corbi, F.; George, K.; Nie, J.; Carranza-García, L.E.; Reverter-Masià, J. Cardiac Biomarker Release After Exercise in Healthy Children and Adolescents: A Systematic Review and Meta-Analysis. *Pediatr. Exerc. Sci.* **2019**, *31*, 28–36. [CrossRef] [PubMed]
5. Klinkenberg, L.J.J.; Luyten, P.; van der Linden, N.; Urgel, K.; Snijders, D.P.C.; Knackstedt, C.; Dennert, R.; Kietselaer, B.L.J.H.; Mingels, A.M.A.; Cardinaels, E.P.M.; et al. Cardiac Troponin T and I Release After a 30-Km Run. *Am. J. Cardiol.* **2016**, *118*, 281–287. [CrossRef] [PubMed]
6. Legaz-Arrese, A.; Carranza-García, L.E.; Navarro-Orocio, R.; Valadez-Lira, A.; Mayolas-Pi, C.; Munguía-Izquierdo, D.; Reverter-Masía, J.; George, K. Cardiac Biomarker Release after Endurance Exercise in Male and Female Adults and Adolescents. *J. Pediatr.* **2017**, *191*, 96–102. [CrossRef] [PubMed]
7. López-Laval, I.; Legaz-Arrese, A.; George, K.; Serveto-Galindo, O.; González-Rave, J.M.; Reverter-Masia, J.; Munguía-Izquierdo, D. Cardiac Troponin I Release after a Basketball Match in Elite, Amateur and Junior Players. *Clin. Chem. Lab. Med. CCLM* **2016**, *54*, 333–338. [CrossRef] [PubMed]
8. Tian, Y.; Nie, J.; Huang, C.; George, K.P. The Kinetics of Highly Sensitive Cardiac Troponin T Release after Prolonged Treadmill Exercise in Adolescent and Adult Athletes. *J. Appl. Physiol.* **2012**, *113*, 418–425. [CrossRef] [PubMed]
9. Fu, F.; Nie, J.; Tong, T. Serum Cardiac Troponin T in Adolescent Runners: Effects of Exercise Intensity and Duration. *Int. J. Sports Med.* **2009**, *30*, 168–172. [CrossRef] [PubMed]
10. Aengevaeren, V.L.; Hopman, M.T.E.; Thompson, P.D.; Bakker, E.A.; George, K.P.; Thijssen, D.H.J.; Eijsvogels, T.M.H. Exercise-Induced Cardiac Troponin I Increase and Incident Mortality and Cardiovascular Events. *Circulation* **2019**, *140*, 804–814. [CrossRef] [PubMed]
11. Giannitsis, E.; Kurz, K.; Hallermayer, K.; Jarausch, J.; Jaffe, A.S.; Katus, H.A. Analytical Validation of a High-Sensitivity Cardiac Troponin T Assay. *Clin. Chem.* **2010**, *56*, 254–261. [CrossRef] [PubMed]
12. Żebrowska, A.; Waśkiewicz, Z.; Nikolaidis, P.T.; Mikołajczyk, R.; Kawecki, D.; Rosemann, T.; Knechtle, B. Acute Responses of Novel Cardiac Biomarkers to a 24-h Ultra-Marathon. *J. Clin. Med.* **2019**, *8*, 57. [CrossRef] [PubMed]
13. Cirer-Sastre, R.; Legaz-Arrese, A.; Corbi, F.; López-Laval, I.; George, K.; Reverter-Masia, J. Influence of Maturational Status in the Exercise-Induced Release of Cardiac Troponin T in Healthy Young Swimmers. *J. Sci. Med. Sport* **2020**, *24*, 116–121. [CrossRef] [PubMed]
14. Nie, J.; George, K.P.; Tong, T.K.; Gaze, D.; Tian, Y.; Lin, H.; Shi, Q. The Influence of a Half-Marathon Race upon Cardiac Troponin T Release in Adolescent Runners. *Curr. Med. Chem.* **2011**, *18*, 3452–3456. [CrossRef] [PubMed]
15. Nie, J.; Tong, T.K.; Shi, Q.; Lin, H.; Zhao, J.; Tian, Y. Serum Cardiac Troponin Response in Adolescents Playing Basketball. *Int. J. Sports Med.* **2008**, *29*, 449–452. [CrossRef] [PubMed]

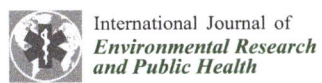

Article

Evaluation of the Body Composition and Selected Physiological Variables of the Skin Surface Depending on Technical and Tactical Skills of Kickboxing Athletes in K1 Style

Łukasz Rydzik [1,*], Tadeusz Ambroży [1], Zbigniew Obmiński [2], Wiesław Błach [3] and Ibrahim Ouergui [4]

1. Institute of Sports Sciences, University of Physical Education, 31-571 Krakow, Poland; tadek@ambrozy.pl
2. Department of Endocrinology, Institute of Sport-National Research Institute, 01-982 Warsaw, Poland; zbigniew.obminski@insp.pl
3. Faculty of Physical Education & Sport, University School of Physical Education, 51-612 Wroclaw, Poland; wieslaw.blach@awf.wroc.pl
4. High Institute of Sport and Physical Education of Kef, University of Jendouba, Jendouba 8189, Tunisia; ouergui.brahim@yahoo.fr
* Correspondence: lukasz.gne@op.pl

Abstract: Background: Kickboxing is a combat sport with high demands on fitness and coordination skills. Scientific research shows that kickboxing fights induce substantial physiological stress. Therefore, it is important to determine the body composition of athletes before competitions and to analyze the skin temperature and skin pH during the fight. Methods: This study aimed to determine the body composition, skin temperature, and skin pH in kickboxers during a fight according to K1 rules. A total of 24 kickboxers (age range: 19 to 28 years) competing in a local K1 kickboxing league participated in the present study. Results: Changes in skin temperature and pH were observed and significant correlations were found between body composition and weight category. Conclusions: Changes in skin temperature and pH were demonstrated after each round of the bout. Level of body fat and muscle tissue significantly correlates with technical-tactical skills of the K1 athletes studied.

Keywords: skin temperature; skin pH; kickboxing contest; body composition

1. Introduction

Kickboxing is a physically demanding combat sport with a high focus on coordination skills, with many systems and organs of the human body involved during the fight [1]. To score points and defeat the opponent, kickboxers use both upper limbs, in an attempt to deliver punches, and lower limbs, used to perform kicks [2]. The K1 formula places the least restrictions on the techniques used and the strength of their execution. It allows for all kickboxing techniques to be performed without any restrictions on the strength of the blows. The competitors fight with naked torsos in shorts, wearing helmets on their heads, gloves on hands, and shin and feet guards. Fights, according to the regulations of the World Association of Kickboxing Federation (WAKO), last 3 × 2 min. A bout can be won by knockout or point advantage [3]. Kickboxers are, therefore, required to have an optimal motor and technical skills level and be able to perform specific tactical actions during the fight [4]. However, an important element in sports competition is the body mass and body composition of the athletes and the correct ratios of anthropometric characteristics [5]. These aspects do not only determine the competition with opponents of a similar level of somatic predispositions (i.e., division into weight classes), but also ensure an optimal basis for mastering and using fighting techniques during competition [6]. The adequate level of body composition (i.e., low body fat with the body mass close to the upper threshold for the given class) and the right length ratios may indicate the athlete's aptitudes and determine his or her sports success [6,7]. In the world of modern sport, body composition monitoring is a basic activity that allows for the evaluation of body changes resulting from practicing a particular sport and determining its participation as the basis for sports selection [8]. The necessity to compete in a sport with weight classes such as K1 rules also requires kickboxers to regularly control their weight and body composition. Based on the diagnosed parameters of body composition, it is possible to precisely determine training (e.g., to develop the range of techniques used and the tactical way of fighting) and a nutritional plan (i.e., to optimize body mass and composition) for kickboxers [8]. Before taking part in sports competition, athletes often strive to gain the lowest possible body mass in order to qualify for a lower weight category in relation to their individual potential depending on body build [9]. In combat sports, athletes often dehydrate to quickly reduce weight during a pre-tournament weigh-in [10].

A K1 kickboxing fight has been reported to induce high physiological stress [11]. Kickboxers are prone to injuries, especially to the head and neck [12]. A longer kickboxing practice creates a risk of pituitary hormone-secretion impairment (hypopituitarism), which manifests itself in decreased concentrations of growth hormone, ACTH, and IGF-I [13]. A single fight in kickboxing, just as in boxing, is an effort in which anaerobic and glycolytic processes are the source of energy, which is indicated by the high concentration of blood lactate [14,15]. Apart from the significant acidification after a kickboxing fight, large changes in hormone concentrations, especially cortisol and growth hormone, similar in winning and losing competitors, have also been reported [16]. During exercise, about 75% of the energy expended is heat and 25% is mechanical work. As a result, mechanical work is accompanied by an increase in body temperature, which depends on the intensity, duration of work, and external conditions and the possibility of heat release into the environment. The energy expended for heat production during the competitive effort has been estimated in athletes of different sports. In boxers, the level of this energy exceeds 1000 watts [17]. The heat exchange during a short but very intensive effort such as a kickboxing bout can be one of the determinants of the level of cognitive abilities and, consequently, the course of the fight. For this reason, it may, therefore, be important to determine skin temperature and pH during kickboxing bouts, as these parameters have not yet been determined for kickboxing in the K1 style. The results of the examination may provide answers regarding the cutaneous changes and body responses caused by the kickboxing bout and the related punches and kicks. The human body is warm-blooded and, through thermoregulatory processes, maintains a constant temperature regardless of changes in the ambient temperature [18,19]. Maintaining a relatively constant body core temperature is a prerequisite for the efficient functioning of the organs, including the activity of enzymes that control metabolism. The most constant temperature is in the right ventricle, while the highest temperature, apart from the heart, is in the liver, brain, and brown adipose tissue [20]. The thermal balance in skeletal muscles varies over a very wide range, with the amount of heat released increasing during work and decreasing at rest [21]. At rest, muscles generate heat depending on their contraction maintained by nerve impulses [22]. Skin temperature (ST) varies over a wide range on the body surface, especially in cold environments and during exercise [23]. Hot water, surfactants, or mechanical actions lead to the damage to the skin's protective barrier or disturbance of the pH level [24]. The skin is protected and, therefore, it can effectively protect the inside of the human body when its pH remains at its natural level, allowing for a healthy balance of bacterial flora to be maintained [25].

The pH of the skin ranges between 4.5 and 5.5 [26]. In resting conditions, it was around two, but increased up to above five as a response to exercise [27,28]. In contrast, blood pH values are always much higher, even following intensive exercise. This is due to the buffer system that neutralizes the effects of lactic acidosis [28]. An alkaline pH facilitates the spread of bacteria throughout the epidermis, promotes the growth of pathogenic strains, and encourages the growth of bacteria that contribute to the unpleasant smell of sweat [29]. An acidic pH helps to keep the number of microorganisms at an appropriate level, increases the activity of bactericidal proteins and lipids, and facilitates proper skin keratinization and exfoliation, and wound healing [30]. Therefore, it is important to determine the local temperature at specific locations on the body surface and the pH level. An interesting issue is also the search for relations between skin temperature and its pH and the values of indicators of technical preparation.

A review of the literature on body composition and physiological variables in martial arts and combat sports reveals a lack of comprehensive analyses of body composition and cutaneous responses during fights in martial arts and combat sports. Research is often devoted to the aspects of proper hydration and the consequences of dehydration in sports [31]. The limits of dehydration and its consequences have also been explored [32]. Silva et al. [33] determined the body composition and power changes in elite judo athletes and confirmed the important role of proper hydration in judo competitions. The anthropometric characteristics and body composition of karate players at different sports skill levels have been also determined [34]. Scientific research on kickboxing has been mainly concerned with physiological and biochemical aspects [35–37]. Partial time-motion analyses of a kickboxing fight have also been conducted [38]. Previous research suggests that in addition to body mass, body composition may also be related to performance during athletic competition [39]. Additionally, the level of technical skills can be affected, to some extent, by the physique and body proportions of the athletes. For example, athletes with long limbs gain an advantage over their rivals by increasing the range of their attacks [6,40]. The literature review revealed the lack of studies in the context of measuring skin temperature and acidity during kickboxing competitions and linking body composition to indices of technical and tactical skill levels.

Thus, the present study aimed to verify the body composition of athletes, their skin temperature and its acidity during a kickboxing K1 rules competition and also the level of the technical and tactical skills of the athletes in relation to body composition, weight category, and skin pH and temperature. We hypothesized that the temperature and pH of the skin change with each round of combat as a result of direct skin contact with blows delivered by the opponent.

2. Materials and Methods
2.1. Participants

Twenty-four male kickboxers (Age range: 19 to 28 years), from different weight classes −71, −75, −81, −86, −91, and +91 kg, competing in a K1 kickboxing league volunteered to participate in the study. The inclusion criterion was primarily the sports' skill level, which was determined based on training experience of at least 6 years including 4 years of active participation in competitions and informed consent to participate in the study. A detailed description of the participants divided into weight categories is presented in Table 1. The athletes were participating regularly in kickboxing tournaments for more than 2 years. The rank of the tournaments is varied. The athletes compete both at a low level (category C), a middle level (category B), and a high level (category A). For the purpose of this study, category A athletes were analyzed. They were also all assigned to the same training regimen four times per week (1.5 h per session). Athletes did not present any medical restrictions during the experimental period and refrained from any strenuous exercises for 48 h before the experimental sessions started. Furthermore, subjects were not advised to follow a special diet and were asked to refrain from all forms of additional supplementation. The dietary assessment of the experimental group was based on the interview method. The respondents kept records in a notebook where they noted the foods, dishes, and drinks consumed on a daily basis. Without weighing, they recorded portion sizes using home measures based on a photo album of produce and dishes provided. The recording procedure was performed for 3 days: 2 working days, 1 day off [41].

Table 1. Characteristics of athletes in each weight category.

Weight Classes of Athletes	N	Age	Body Mass	BMI	%
−71 kg	4	23.0 ± 4.24	68.9 ± 1.09	21.37 ± 0.21	16.7%
−75 kg	4	21.75 ± 2.75	73.9 ± 0.44	22.26 ± 0.49	16.7%
−81 kg	4	21.25 ± 2.21	78.92 ± 1.35	24.89 ± 0.53	16.7%
−86 kg	4	21.5 ± 2.65	85.05 ± 1.18	25.8 ± 0.29	16.7%
−91 kg	4	21.3 ± 2.21	89.0 ± 1.20	26.03 ± 0.32	16.7%
+91 kg	4	23.0 ± 3.74	91.92 ± 0.58	26.58 ± 1.20	16.7%
Total	24	21.95 ± 2.82	81.28 ± 8.39	25.99 ± 2.04	100.0%

N—number of observations; %—percentage. Source: author's own elaboration.

Analysis of dietary records showed no special diets or use of nutrients and supplements to enhance exercise in the training groups. Control of diet and supplementation helped exclude factors that could significantly interfere with the results of the experiment. The body mass of the participants ranged from 67.9 to 92.6 kg (mean: 81.3 ± 8.38 kg). Body fat percentage measured for the participants was estimated at a mean level of 14.09% and ranged from 5.8 to 27.0%. Furthermore, the level of muscle tissue of the participants ranged from 55.8 to 75.0 kg, with a mean of 65.12 kg. The mean bone mass was 3.46 kg, and its variation was found to be between 2.9 and 3.9 kg. Body mass index (BMI) of the participants ranged from 21.4 to 27.17 kg/m^2, with a mean of 24.59 kg/m^2. Body water content in the athletes studied was determined at a mean level of 63.46%, with the obtained values ranging from 56.1 to 69.4%.

Prior to participation in the tests, the competitors were informed about the research procedures, which were in accordance with the recent ethical principles of the Declaration of Helsinki (WMA, 2013). Athletes provided written informed consent after the explanation of the aims, benefits, and risks of the study. The research was approved by the Bioethics Committee at the Regional Medical Chamber (No. 287/KBL/OIL/2020).

2.2. Procedures

The examinations were conducted during a local kickboxing tournament that was refereed. The bouts were held based on K1 rules in accordance with the regulations of the World Association of Kickboxing Organizations (WAKO) and lasted for three rounds of 2 min each. The breaks between rounds lasted 1 min, and the measurements were made during this time (Figure 1). The tournament hall was equipped with an air conditioning system to keep a constant ambient temperature (20–21 °C) and humidity (50–52%) throughout the study.

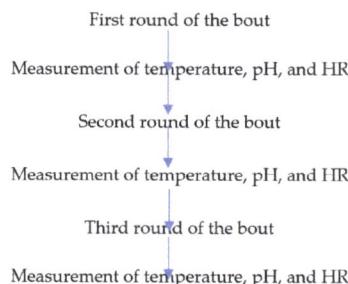

Figure 1. Research design.

2.3. Sparring Bout Analysis

The analysis of the sports fight was performed by two champion-level kickboxing coaches and one referee based on digital video recordings of the examined athlete. The recording was made with three cameras. Movavi Video Editor 14 software (Movavi, Wildwood, MO, USA) was used to merge the images. The setting of cameras allowed continuous observation of the athletes, referees, and the scoreboard. After the competition, the indices of attack activeness (A_a), which represents the ratio of all offensive actions used during the fight, attack effectiveness (E_a), which is the ratio of scoring techniques to all attacks used, and attack efficiency (S_a), which is the number of attacks scored, were calculated using established equations from the literature [2,4,42].

Activeness of the attack (A_a)

$$A_a = \frac{\text{number of all registered offensive actions of a kickboxer}}{\text{number of bouts fought by a kickboxer}}$$

Effectiveness of the attack (E_a)

$$E_a = \frac{\text{number of efective attacks}}{\text{number of all attacks}} \times 100$$

An effective attack is a technical action awarded a point.
Number of all attacks is a number of all offensive actions.
Efficiency of the attack (S_a)

$$S_a = \frac{n}{N}$$

n—number of attacks awarded 1 pt.
In K1 formula, each fair hit is awarded 1 pt.
N—number of bouts.

2.4. Biomedical Measurements

2.4.1. Skin Temperature Measurement

Skin temperature was measured using a professional Skin-Thermometer ST 500 (Khazaka Electronic Germany) in degrees Celsius (°C). The measurement was performed using a special lens and an IR detector by measuring the infrared radiation (IR) emitted by the skin. Measurements were taken before the bout, and after the first, second, and third rounds. The measurement site was previously wiped with a dry towel. The single measurement time was 2 s.

2.4.2. Skin/Sweat pH Measurement

Skin surface acidity was measured using the Skin-pH- Meter PH 905 (Khazaka Electronic Germany). Both skin temperature and pH measurements were taken at the following locations: forehead, chest, arm, hand, thigh, shank, and foot. After the measurements were completed for an individual, the probe was cleaned. The measurement time was one second.

2.4.3. Heart Rate Measurement

Heart rate (HR) during a bout was also measured using a chest strap (Garmin HRM-PRO) and a specialized watch Garmin Fenix 6x pro (Garmin, Olathe, KS, USA). The strap was worn after each round of the fight to determine the heart rate at the end of the round.

2.5. Body Composition Analysis

Body composition was determined using the electrical bioimpedance technique using the Tanita Bc 601 body composition analyzer before the tournament, from 6 to 8 am during the weigh-in before the competition. Body mass, body fat, muscle tissue, bone mass, BMI, DCI, metabolic age, and body water content were determined. All parameters were automatically calculated using the measuring device.

2.6. Statistical Analysis

Descriptive statistics (mean, median, minimum and maximum values, first and third quartile values, and standard deviation) were calculated for all variables. Statistical analysis was performed using the statistical software package Statistica for Windows (version 13.1; Tulsa, OK, USA). The normality of data sets was checked and confirmed using the Shapiro–Wilk W test. The correlations between two variables with normal distribution (activeness of the attack, effectiveness of the attack, body mass, muscle tissue level, DCI) were determined using Pearson's linear correlation coefficient, whereas for variables not meeting the criterion of normal distribution (efficiency of the attack, body fat %, bone mass, BMI, metabolic age, body water %), Spearman's rank correlation coefficient was calculated. Changes in skin temperature, HR, and pH over time were evaluated using Friedman's ANOVA. The level of statistical significance was set at $p < 0.05$. To control type-I error for multiple comparisons, Bonferroni procedure for correction of p-value has been used.

3. Results

The activeness of the attack in the athletes studied was estimated to range from 61 to 129 points, with a mean of 100.04 points. The efficiency of the attack was between 43 and 69 points, with a mean of 53.63 points. The effectiveness of the attack was at a mean level of 54.42 points, and it ranged from 40 to 69 points (Table 2).

Table 2. Level of indices of technical and tactical skills of athletes.

Index	Descriptive Statistics							
	N	Mean	Med.	Min.	Max.	Lower Quartile	Upper Quartile	Std. Deviation
Activeness of the attack	24	100.04	100.50	61.00	129.00	89.50	116.50	18.36
Efficiency of the attack	24	53.63	50.50	43.00	69.00	46.50	60.50	8.07
Effectiveness of the attack	24	54.42	56.00	40.00	69.00	47.50	59.50	8.09

N—number of observations; $\bar{x}$—arithmetic mean; Me—median; Min—minimum; Max—maximum; Q1—lower quartile; Q3—lower quartile; SD—standard deviation.

Statistical analysis confirmed the presence of statistically significant relationships between the activeness, effectiveness, and efficiency of the attack, and most anthropometric characteristics of the athletes (Table 3). For other correlations, the higher activeness, efficiency, and effectiveness of the attack correlated with a lower body mass of athletes, lower body fat percentage, lower body fat, lower BMI, DCI, metabolic age, and higher body water percentage (all $p < 0.05$) (Table 3). There was an unexpected positive correlation between the effectiveness of attack and the variable obtained from the aggregation of the individual pH involving four time points and seven places on the body's surface. This suggests that the more alkaline the skin is, the higher the index of effectiveness of attack is (Table 3).

Significant correlations were found between the selected anthropometric characteristics and the weight classes. There were positive relationships of weight class with body mass, body fat percentage, muscle tissue level, BMI, DCI, and metabolic age (Table 4). The value of the above-mentioned parameters increased in the athletes with the higher weight class. There was a statistically significant, negative correlation between the weight class and body water content in the athletes studied. Those performing in the higher weight classes had a lower body water percentage. Furthermore, there were also negative relationships of the activeness, efficiency, and effectiveness of the attack with weight class (Table 4).

Table 3. Evaluation of relationships between indices of technical and tactical skills and anthropometric characteristics (n = 24).

Variables	Activeness of the Attack		Efficiency of the Attack		Effectiveness of the Attack	
	r/R	p	r/R	p	r/R	p
Body mass	−0.88	<0.001	−0.87	<0.001	−0.82	<0.001
Body fat %	−0.67	<0.001	−0.80	<0.001	−0.75	<0.001
Muscle tissue	−0.80	<0.001	−0.66	<0.001	−0.60	0.002
Bone mass	−0.33	0.110	−0.13	0.556	−0.16	0.462
BMI	−0.94	<0.001	−0.83	<0.001	−0.75	<0.001
DCI	−0.59	0.003	−0.27	0.195	−0.45	0.029
Metabolic age	−0.62	0.001	−0.66	<0.001	−0.67	<0.001
Body water content (%)	0.61	0.001	0.69	<0.001	0.65	0.001
Mean skin pH	0.28	0.284	0.42	0.039	0.43	0.043
Mean skin temperature	0.17	0.424	0.14	0.051	0.5	0.813

BMI: body mass index, DCI: daily calorie intake, r—Pearson linear correlation; R—Spearman's rank correlation; p—test probability; values in bold are statistically significant. Source: author's own elaboration.

Table 4. Evaluation of the relationship of effectiveness and anthropometric characteristics with weight class (n = 24).

Variables	R	p
Body mass vs. weight class	0.99	<0.001
Body fat % vs. weight class	0.78	<0.001
Muscle tissue vs. weight class	0.73	<0.001
Bone mass vs. weight class	0.26	0.218
BMI vs. weight class	0.93	<0.001
DCI vs. weight class	0.53	0.008
Metabolic age vs. weight class	0.74	<0.001
Body water % vs. weight class	−0.73	<0.001
Activeness of the attack vs. weight class	−0.94	<0.001
Efficiency of the attack vs. weight class	−0.87	<0.001
Effectiveness of the attack vs. weight class	−0.84	<0.001

R—Spearman's rank correlation; p—test probability; values in bold are statistically significant. Source: author's own elaboration.

The mean temperature dropped with each round of the bout on the chest, arm, and thigh. On the hand and foot, the skin temperature increased with each round (Table 5).

Table 5. Descriptive statistics for temperature after warming up (WU) and three successive rounds.

Temperature	N	Mean	Confidence: −95%	Confidence: +95%	Med.	Min.	Max.	Lower Quartile	Upper Quartile	Std. Deviation
Forehead (WU)	24	31.92	31.35	32.49	32.50	30.00	33.40	30.00	32.99	1.34
1	24	30.52	29.87	31.16	30.60	27.40	32.80	29.70	31.00	1.53
2	24	30.73	30.11	31.34	31.40	28.30	32.30	29.40	32.10	1.45
3	24	31.13	30.68	31.58	31.10	29.20	32.60	30.45	31.80	1.07
p			Chi^{2}Anova = 20.35, $p < 0.001$, η square = 0.988							
Chest (WU)	24	29.53	29.07	29.98	30.00	27.40	31.00	28.85	30.20	1.09
1	24	27.34	26.92	27.75	27.80	25.40	28.60	26.75	27.90	0.98
2	24	26.38	26.08	26.67	26.70	25.10	27.30	25.90	26.80	0.70
3	24	25.85	25.29	26.41	26.00	24.10	28.00	24.20	27.00	1.32
p			Chi^{2}Anova = 56.60 $p < 0.001$, η square = 0.998							

Table 5. Cont.

Temperature	N	Mean	Confidence: −95%	Confidence: +95%	Med.	Min.	Max.	Lower Quartile	Upper Quartile	Std. Deviation
Arm (WU)	24	29.23	28.86	29.60	29.50	27.70	30.40	28.55	30.00	0.88
1	24	27.85	27.31	28.38	28.10	26.10	29.80	26.30	28.60	1.27
2	24	26.96	26.31	27.61	27.30	24.70	28.80	25.20	28.70	1.54
3	24	26.71	26.23	27.19	26.70	24.70	28.10	26.00	28.10	1.13
p				Chi^{2}Anova = 53.69 p < 0.001, η square = 0.987						
Hand (WU)	24	30.17	29.43	30.91	30.40	28.00	32.60	28.10	31.90	1.75
1	24	30.23	29.52	30.94	31.50	28.10	31.90	28.60	31.80	1.68
2	24	30.73	30.12	31.35	31.50	28.90	32.40	29.20	32.30	1.45
3	24	31.41	30.75	32.08	30.70	29.70	34.10	30.00	32.70	1.57
p				Chi^{2}Anova = 28.29 p < 0.001, η square = 0.991						
Thigh (WU)	24	29.58	29.25	29.92	29.70	28.20	30.70	29.00	30.20	0.79
1	24	27.78	27.38	28.18	27.90	25.80	28.90	27.30	28.70	0.95
2	24	27.34	26.72	27.95	27.30	25.20	30.00	26.10	27.60	1.45
3	24	27.06	26.44	27.68	26.80	25.30	29.50	25.70	28.20	1.46
p				Chi^{2}Anova = 49.05 p < 0.001, η square = 0.997						
Shank (WU)	24	29.14	28.86	29.43	29.20	27.70	30.10	29.00	29.50	0.67
1	24	27.68	27.36	28.01	27.90	26.30	28.90	27.20	28.20	0.77
2	24	27.10	26.78	27.43	27.00	25.50	28.10	26.90	27.75	0.77
3	24	27.21	26.91	27.52	27.20	25.80	28.20	26.80	28.00	0.73
p				Chi^{2}Anova = 57.88 p < 0.001, η square = 0.999						
Foot (WU)	24	24.98	24.03	25.92	24.00	23.10	29.70	23.20	26.90	2.24
1	24	25.06	24.19	25.93	25.00	23.00	29.60	23.35	25.90	2.07
2	24	25.74	24.54	26.93	26.00	21.30	30.00	23.20	27.60	2.83
3	24	26.03	25.05	27.00	25.30	22.50	29.50	24.90	28.50	2.30
p				Chi^{2}Anova = 6.85 p = 0.077, η square = 0.108						

p—test probability; values in bold are statistically significant η square-effect size.

The highest pH was recorded on the forehead in the measurement after the third round of the bout, while the lowest was found for the thigh at baseline. The acidity on the arm, hand, thigh, and shin increased with each round of the bout. However, it decreased on the foot and forehead in the next two rounds (Table 6).

Table 6. Descriptive statistics for pH after WU and following successive rounds.

pH	N	Mean	Confidence: −95	Confidence: +95%	Med.	Min.	Max.	Lower Quartile	Upper Quartile	Std. Deviation
forehead (WU)	24	6.23	6.13	6.33	6.22	5.80	6.48	6.09	6.43	0.24
1	24	5.86	5.73	5.99	5.92	5.40	6.28	5.61	6.13	0.31
2	24	6.11	5.91	6.31	5.96	5.35	6.79	5.83	6.62	0.47
3	24	6.55	6.37	6.72	6.69	5.92	7.02	6.01	6.90	0.42
p				Chi^{2}Anova = 30.55 p < 0.001, η square = 0.992						
chest (WU)	24	5.81	5.74	5.88	5.87	5.51	5.97	5.68	5.96	0.17
1	24	5.65	5.43	5.86	5.83	4.91	6.30	5.10	6.11	0.51
2	24	5.90	5.64	6.16	5.92	4.93	7.01	5.38	6.04	0.62
3	24	6.20	5.97	6.44	6.21	5.31	7.16	5.76	6.52	0.57
p				Chi^{2}Anova = 36.45 p < 0.001, η square = 0.993						

Table 6. Cont.

pH	N	Mean	Confidence: −95	Confidence: +95%	Med.	Min.	Max.	Lower Quartile	Upper Quartile	Std. Deviation
arm (WU)	24	5.58	5.44	5.72	5.69	4.89	5.89	5.32	5.89	0.33
1	24	5.68	5.44	5.93	6.03	4.83	6.27	5.11	6.22	0.57
2	24	5.86	5.54	6.18	5.91	4.84	7.17	5.25	6.16	0.75
3	24	6.13	5.81	6.44	6.02	5.14	7.55	5.66	6.32	0.75
p				Chi^{2}Anova = 40.85 p < 0.001, η square = 0.994						
hand (WU)	24	5.99	5.86	6.11	6.01	5.62	6.44	5.69	6.23	0.30
1	24	6.07	5.87	6.27	6.11	5.39	6.80	5.66	6.42	0.48
2	24	6.12	5.84	6.40	6.19	5.21	7.21	5.59	6.55	0.66
3	24	6.24	6.00	6.48	6.08	5.53	7.26	5.81	6.47	0.57
p				Chi^{2}Anova = 13.85 p = 0.003, η square = 0.388						
thigh (WU)	24	5.49	5.37	5.61	5.47	5.13	5.90	5.22	5.78	0.27
1	24	5.66	5.40	5.93	5.77	4.87	6.73	5.04	5.91	0.63
2	24	5.74	5.42	6.06	5.58	4.87	7.12	5.11	6.04	0.76
3	24	5.85	5.50	6.20	5.79	4.85	7.38	5.21	6.05	0.83
p				Chi^{2}Anova = 11.25 p = 0.010, η square = 0.319						
shank (WU)	24	5.55	5.42	5.67	5.59	5.11	5.93	5.34	5.78	0.29
1	24	5.57	5.33	5.82	5.62	4.51	6.40	5.26	5.82	0.58
2	24	5.66	5.28	6.05	5.43	4.67	7.43	5.00	6.04	0.91
3	24	5.86	5.54	6.17	5.67	4.95	7.17	5.25	6.31	0.75
p				Chi^{2}Anova = 12.10 p = 0.007, η square = 0.330						
foot (WU)	24	5.91	5.71	6.12	5.68	5.52	6.87	5.62	6.20	0.48
1	24	5.66	5.41	5.90	5.54	4.99	6.83	5.28	5.72	0.58
2	24	5.74	5.50	5.99	5.47	5.07	6.82	5.29	6.03	0.58
3	24	6.11	5.78	6.44	5.92	5.25	7.63	5.57	6.36	0.78
p				Chi^{2}Anova = 38.45 p < 0.001, η square = 0.993						

p—test probability; values in bold are statistically significant.

The HR values increased in the subsequent rounds of the fight, with its peak value of 184.63 bpm (Table 7).

Table 7. Descriptive statistics for heart rate (HR) measurements following warm-up (WU) and successive rounds.

HR	N	Mean	Confidence: −95%	Confidence: +95%	Med.	Min.	Max.	Lower Quartile	Upper Quartile	Std. Deviation
WU	24	116.96	111.13	122.79	117.00	103.00	148.00	104.00	119.50	13.81
First round	24	179.50	177.03	181.97	181.00	172.00	190.00	174.00	183.00	5.85
Second round	24	183.33	181.20	185.46	185.00	175.00	190.00	179.00	187.00	5.04
Third round	24	184.63	182.03	187.22	188.00	174.00	191.00	181.00	190.00	6.13
p				Chi^{2}Anova = 59.27 p < 0.001, η square = 0.999						

p—test probability; values in bold are statistically significant.

Statistically significant correlations were demonstrated between skin temperature and pH on the chest after the first, second, and third rounds of the bout. Significant correlations were also shown after the first and second rounds on the arms. Single correlations also occurred on the shank after the second round of the bout and foot after the third round. Furthermore, numerous correlations were shown between the lower and upper limbs, chest, and arm (Table 8).

Table 8. Relationship between pH and temperature ($n = 24$).

		Temperature						
		Forehead	Chest	Arm	Hand	Thigh	Shank	Foot
pH	forehead (WU)	**−0.82**	**−0.60**	−0.24	**−0.51**	**−0.73**	−0.22	−0.16
	1	0.28	−0.45	**−0.68**	0.40	**−0.57**	−0.02	−0.31
	2	0.19	**−0.93**	**−0.73**	0.49	−0.42	−0.33	**0.53**
	3	−0.16	0.05	**−0.76**	0.24	**−0.50**	−0.18	0.21
	chest (WU)	0.39	0.14	−0.32	0.01	**0.55**	−0.22	−0.31
	1	**0.46**	−0.45	**−0.68**	0.33	**−0.57**	−0.28	−0.13
	2	0.40	**−0.97**	**−0.83**	0.39	**−0.53**	−0.39	**0.46**
	3	0.17	**−0.51**	**−0.68**	**0.45**	**−0.54**	0.05	**0.55**
	arm (WU)	**0.50**	0.22	−0.07	−0.16	0.35	**−0.41**	**−0.50**
	1	**0.54**	−0.20	−0.43	0.25	−0.42	−0.29	−0.13
	2	**0.77**	**−0.62**	−0.43	0.01	−0.34	**−0.59**	0.19
	3	**0.65**	**−0.87**	−0.16	**0.42**	−0.25	−0.24	0.18
	hand (WU)	**0.72**	**0.70**	**0.54**	0.34	**0.43**	0.29	0.07
	1	**0.64**	−0.22	**−0.57**	0.40	**−0.71**	**−0.51**	−0.35
	2	**0.62**	**−0.67**	**−0.70**	0.06	**−0.68**	**−0.68**	−0.02
	3	**0.70**	**−0.96**	−0.24	**0.53**	−0.44	**−0.48**	−0.04
	thigh (WU)	**0.92**	0.17	0.15	**0.52**	−0.02	−0.12	0.25
	1	**0.52**	−0.12	−0.25	0.07	−0.16	−0.31	0.09
	2	**0.66**	**−0.44**	−0.32	−0.09	−0.36	**−0.45**	0.04
	3	0.35	**−0.78**	−0.18	0.27	−0.33	−0.22	0.05
	shank (WU)	**0.97**	0.16	0.05	**0.65**	0.13	−0.11	0.38
	1	0.15	0.02	−0.07	0.04	**−0.45**	−0.37	−0.25
	2	**0.60**	**−0.58**	−0.43	−0.11	−0.39	**−0.43**	0.13
	3	**0.43**	**−0.83**	−0.05	0.35	−0.31	−0.27	−0.04
	foot (WU)	**0.78**	0.04	0.16	0.41	0.40	−0.36	0.16
	1	0.04	−0.32	−0.43	0.16	**−0.81**	**−0.48**	−0.40
	2	**0.58**	**−0.82**	**−0.77**	0.13	**−0.63**	**−0.51**	0.20
	3	0.31	**−0.78**	−0.41	0.32	**−0.64**	**−0.75**	**−0.41**

Values in bold are statistically significant.

There was a statistically significant correlation between the pH of the forehead skin surface and HR after the first, second, and third rounds of the bout. The relationship between HR after the third round of the bout and the pH of the chest skin surface was also significant. There was a statistically significant correlation between the thigh temperature and HR at baseline.

4. Discussion

The purpose of this study was to comprehensively determine the body composition, skin temperature, and skin pH during a real kickboxing bout in K1 style and to establish the relationships of technical and tactical skills with body composition and weight classes. The results showed significant correlations between individual body composition parameters (body mass, body fat %, muscle tissue, BMI, DCI, metabolic age, body water %) and weight class that occurred in almost measured parameters. This result showed that the lower the weight class was, the lower the muscle and body fat was in the athletes. Similarly, lighter athletes were characterized by lower BMIs and DCIs. Kickboxing is a sport characterized by weight divisions where the competitor must meet certain body mass limits [6]. A negative correlation was found between the body water percentage and the weight class, which may also explain the limits associated with a specific weight class. Athletes often aim to compete in the lowest possible weight class by reducing their body mass and often inducing dehydration [43]. The present paper determined the level of technical and tactical skills of the athletes by analyzing their kickboxing fights according to K1 rules. Technical and tactical indices are the most precise tool used to determine athletes' behavior in combat sports [4]. The statistical analysis showed a negative correlation between the weight classes and the level of technical and tactical skills of the athletes. This result can be explained by the fact that lighter competitors are characterized by greater dynamics during combat, with a greater variety and frequency of techniques used. Similar conclusions were reported by previous studies analyzing judo bouts, which highlighted technical variation in relation to specific weight classes [44,45]. Our results indicate differences in the skill used by weight category. They do not unequivocally indicate the level of these skills, but they can indicate the fact that depending on the weight category, different technical patterns dominate; lighter athletes fight faster using more techniques and heavier athletes use fewer techniques.

Our research showed that a low level of body fat and muscle tissue significantly correlates with the activeness, effectiveness, and efficiency of the attack. The body fat percentage measured among the kickboxers was estimated at a mean level of 14.09%, ranging from 5.8 to 27%. The body fat increase was connected with a heavier weight class, in which the athletes were characterized by a higher body mass and lower activeness during the fight, which translated into other performance indices (effectiveness and efficiency). Furthermore, the mean fat percentage in athletes in the present study showed an optimal range according to the accepted norms [46,47]. The body fat percentage found in the present study was similar to that reported in a previous study of boxers, where body fat ranged from 9 to 16% [48]. This may indicate a convergence in the desired low levels of body fat in representatives of both sports. A detailed analysis of the examination conducted on kickboxing athletes revealed that a low body fat percentage is a prerequisite for athletes' high sports performance [6]. Likewise, athletes' muscle tissue level in the present study was found to have an average of 65.12 kg. Muscle development is related to both genetic predisposition and the training process, which shapes mainly the leg, arm, and abdominal muscles [49]. However, scientific studies confirmed that contact sports' competition induced significant muscle fatigue and damage [50]. Therefore, optimal muscle development is essential to obtain successful performance during combat, especially for technical and tactical actions [2].

Our study showed changes in skin temperature during the fights. Regular decreases in ST were found on the chest, arm, and thigh following each round of the kickboxing fight. The decrease in skin temperature in these areas may have been related to the evaporation of excess sweat, which is an endothermic process. Hence, sweating of the skin surface is considered the most effective way for the dissipation of excess heat in the human body that appears during prolonged and/or intensive exercise [51]. A decrease in temperature can also be caused by the changed blood flow due to compensatory vasoregulation [52,53]. In this consideration, Barboza et al. [34] assessed the skin temperature of middle-distance runners during maximal exercise and showed a decrease in the upper body area's temperature, while it was increased in the upper limbs due to solicited muscles [54]. In the present study, increased skin temperature was found on the feet, which may be due to metabolic heat generation or stress [55]. During exercise, blood flow increases in order to oxygenate the tissues, and therefore, temperature may increase [56]. It should be stressed that strenuous exertion, an elevated body or ambient temperature are not the only causes of an increased rate of sweating. Strong emotions, fear, and so-called psychological stress are independent factors leading to sweating, as has been found in pianists prior and post their official performance [57].

The pH analysis of the skin showed an acidic reaction in each case. After the first round of the fight, the pH level relative to the previous measurement slightly decreased on the forehead, chest, and foot, but after the third round, it increased over the initial value. This behavior might by related to changes in chemical substances in sweat such as hydrogen ions donors, lactic acid, or their acceptors, such as ammonia [58,59]. Measurements of pH in other points of the body also showed an increase between the rounds and the resting value. Searching the other reasons for this phenomenon, it is worth emphasizing that the human body has two types of sweat glands (eccrine, apocrine), which produce sweat in different amounts, directly affecting the pH [59].

For heart rate measurements, our results showed that values increased in exercise between the baseline and the first round, which may suggest the presence of anaerobic glycolysis. Previous research reported that kickboxing fights caused substantial physiological stress [11]. Our results showed a negative correlation between skin temperature and skin pH on the chest and arm, which indicated an increase in skin temperature at lower pH values. Statistical analysis revealed a correlation between the heart rate after the first round and the pH of the skin on the forehead, which was increased. In the remaining rounds of the bout, the pH value for the forehead decreased with higher HR values, which can be explained by an anaerobic metabolism and high body acidification [11].

The increase in HR in successive rounds reflects the increase in activity of the autonomic nervous system (ANS). The same behavior of the HR was noted during the boxing fights [58]. This response of the cardiovascular system and, indirectly, the nervous system may have influenced changes in both temperature and pH in our study. The mechanism of these relationships has been discussed above.

Limitation of the Study

In the present study, heart rate was measured by wearing a measuring strap after each round. Therefore, we were not able to record the maximum heart rate during the bout. The judges did not allow the strap to be worn during the entire bout for safety reasons. An additional difficulty during the examination was the profuse perspiration, and therefore, the need to wipe the examination site. Additionally, we did not have possibility to examine athletes from all the weight categories and female athletes.

5. Conclusions

Kickboxers who compete in lower weight classes are likely to be characterized by higher technical and tactical skills. The level of body fat and muscle tissue can affect the level of technical and tactical performance. The skin temperature changed with each round of the fight, and a temperature decline was noted in the large muscle groups (chest, arm, thigh) as the fight progressed. A kickboxing fight according to K1 rules led to skin pH changes after each round of the bout in the study group.

In conclusion, it should be emphasized that the directions of pH and temperature changes observed on the skin's surface during exercise may be very different from those occurring inside the body that were well described in the literature. Advanced techniques for measuring physiological changes on the skin have only recently become available to researchers; therefore, the small number of similar experimental studies published to date do not fully explain the physiological mechanisms of the observed phenomena.

Practical Implications

In kickboxing, body composition should be constantly monitored because the measured values can affect the course of the fight and the level of technical and tactical skills. Further research should also be conducted to clarify the physiological changes of the skin's surface during combat.

Author Contributions: Conceptualization, Ł.R. and T.A.; methodology, Ł.R., T.A. and Z.O.; software, Ł.R., T.A. and W.B.; validation, Ł.R. and T.A.; formal analysis, Ł.R., T.A. and Z.O.; investigation, Ł.R. and T.A.; resources, Ł.R., T.A. and I.O.; data curation, Ł.R., T.A. and W.B.; writing—original draft preparation, Ł.R., T.A. and I.O.; writing—review and editing, Ł.R., T.A. and I.O.; visualization, Ł.R. and T.A.; supervision, Ł.R., T.A. and I.O.; project administration, Ł.R. and T.A.; funding acquisition, Ł.R. and T.A. All authors have read and agreed to the published version of the manuscript.

Funding: Open Access was financed by the program of the Minister of Science and Higher Education, entitled 'Regional Initiative for Perfection', for the years 2019–2022 (Project No. 022/RID/2018/19; a total of PLN 11,919,908).

Institutional Review Board Statement: The study was conducted according to the guidelines of the Declaration of Helsinki, and approved by the Bioethics Committee at the Regional Medical Chamber (No. 287/KBL/OIL/2020).

Informed Consent Statement: Informed consent was obtained from all subjects involved in the study.

Data Availability Statement: The data presented in this study are available on request from the corresponding author.

Conflicts of Interest: The authors declare no conflict of interest.

References

1. Di Marino, S. *A Complete Guide to Kickboxing*; Enslow Publishing: New York, NY, USA, 2018.
2. Rydzik, Ł.; Ambroży, T. Physical fitness and the level of technical and tactical training of kickboxers. *Int. J. Environ. Res. Public Health* **2021**, *18*, 3088. [CrossRef]
3. Łukasz Rydzik, P.K. *Przewodnik po Kickboxingu*; Wydawnictwo Aha: Łódź, Poland, 2018; ISBN 978-83-7299-722-8.
4. Ambroży, T.; Rydzik, Ł.; Obmiński, Z.; Klimek, A.T.; Serafin, N.; Litwiniuk, A.; Czaja, R.; Czarny, W. The Impact of Reduced Training Activity of Elite Kickboxers on Physical Fitness, Body Build, and Performance during Competitions. *Int. J. Environ. Res. Public Health* **2021**, *18*, 4342. [CrossRef]
5. Bayios, I.; Bergeles, N.K.; Apostolidis, N.G.; Noutsos, K.S.; Koskolou, M.D. Anthropometric, body composition and somatotype differences of Greek elite female basketball, volleyball and handball players. *J. Sports Med. Phys. Fitness* **2006**, *2*, 271.
6. Slimani, M.; Chaabene, H.; Miarka, B.; Franchini, E.; Chamari, K.; Cheour, F. Kickboxing review: Anthropometric, psychophysiological and activity profiles and injury epidemiology. *Biol. Sport* **2017**, *34*, 185. [CrossRef]
7. Valyakina, E. Morphological and functional features of elite male boxers and kickboxers in comparative perspective. *Mod. Univ. Sport Sci.* **2017**, 333–334.
8. Sozański, H. *Podstawy Teorii Treningu Sportowego*; Blblioteka Trenera: Warszawa, Poland, 1999; ISBN 83-86504-67-7.
9. Hall, C.J. Effects of rapid weight loss on mood and performance among amateur boxers. *Br. J. Sports Med.* **2001**, *35*, 390–395. [CrossRef] [PubMed]
10. Pettersson, S.; Berg, C.M. Hydration Status in Elite Wrestlers, Judokas, Boxers, and Taekwondo Athletes on Competition Day. *Int. J. Sport Nutr. Exerc. Metab.* **2014**, *24*, 267–275. [CrossRef]
11. Rydzik, Ł.; Maciejczyk, M.; Czarny, W.; Kędra, A.; Ambroży, T. Physiological Responses and Bout Analysis in Elite Kickboxers During International K1 Competitions. *Front. Physiol.* **2021**, *12*, 737–741. [CrossRef] [PubMed]
12. Lystad, R.P. Injuries to Professional and Amateur Kickboxing Contestants. *Orthop. J. Sport. Med.* **2015**, *3*, 232596711561241. [CrossRef]
13. Tanriverdi, F.; Unluhizarci, K.; Coksevim, B.; Selcuklu, A.; Casanueva, F.F.; Kelestimur, F. Kickboxing sport as a new cause of traumatic brain injury-mediated hypopituitarism. *Clin. Endocrinol.* **2007**, *66*, 360–366. [CrossRef]
14. Ouergui, I.; Houcine, N.; Marzouki, H.; Davis, P.; Zaouali, M.; Franchini, E.; Gmada, N.; Bouhlel, E. Development of a Noncontact Kickboxing Circuit Training Protocol That Simulates Elite Male Kickboxing Competition. *J. Strength Cond. Res.* **2015**, *29*, 3405–3411. [CrossRef]
15. Hanon, C.; Savarino, J.; Thomas, C. Blood Lactate and Acid-Base Balance of World-Class Amateur Boxers After Three 3-Minute Rounds in International Competition. *J. Strength Cond. Res.* **2015**, *29*, 942–946. [CrossRef]
16. Ouergui, I.; Davis, P.; Houcine, N.; Marzouki, H.; Zaouali, M.; Franchini, E.; Gmada, N.; Bouhlel, E. Hormonal, Physiological, and Physical Performance During Simulated Kickboxing Combat: Differences Between Winners and Losers. *Int. J. Sports Physiol. Perform.* **2016**, *11*, 425–431. [CrossRef]
17. Piil, J.F.; Kingma, B.; Morris, N.B.; Christiansen, L.; Ioannou, L.G.; Flouris, A.D.; Nybo, L. Proposed framework for forecasting heat-effects on motor-cognitive performance in the Summer Olympics. *Temperature* **2021**, *8*, 262–283. [CrossRef]
18. Benedict, F.G.; Miles, W.R.; Johnson, A. The Temperature of the Human Skin. *Proc. Natl. Acad. Sci. USA* **1919**, *5*, 218–222. [CrossRef]

19. Smith, A.D.H.; Crabtree, D.R.; Bilzon, J.L.J.; Walsh, N.P. The validity of wireless iButtons® and thermistors for human skin temperature measurement. *Physiol. Meas.* **2010**, *31*, 95–114. [CrossRef]
20. Stolwijk, J.A.J.; Hardy, J.D. Control of Body Temperature. In *Comprehensive Physiology*; Wiley: Hoboken, NJ, USA, 1977; pp. 45–68.
21. Górski, J. Fizjologia wysiłku i treningu fizycznego. *Wydaw. Lek. PZWL* **2019**, *28*, 148.
22. Tan, C.L.; Knight, Z.A. Regulation of Body Temperature by the Nervous System. *Neuron* **2018**, *98*, 31–48. [CrossRef] [PubMed]
23. Brotherhood, J.R. Heat stress and strain in exercise and sport. *J. Sci. Med. Sport* **2008**, *11*, 6–19. [CrossRef] [PubMed]
24. Schmid-Wendtner, M.-H.; Korting, H.C. The pH of the Skin Surface and Its Impact on the Barrier Function. *Skin Pharmacol. Physiol.* **2006**, *19*, 296–302. [CrossRef] [PubMed]
25. Lambers, H.; Piessens, S.; Bloem, A.; Pronk, H.; Finkel, P. Natural skin surface pH is on average below 5, which is beneficial for its resident flora. *Int. J. Cosmet. Sci.* **2006**, *28*, 359–370. [CrossRef]
26. Prakash, C.; Bhargava, P.; Tiwari, S.; Majumdar, B.; Bhargava, R.K. Skin Surface pH in Acne Vulgaris: Insights from an Observational Study and Review of the Literature. *J. Clin. Aesthet. Dermatol.* **2017**, *10*, 33–39. [CrossRef]
27. Coyle, S.; Morris, D.; Lau, K.-T.; Diamond, D.; Di Francesco, F.; Taccini, N.; Trivella, M.G.; Costanzo, D.; Salvo, P.; Porchet, J.-A.; et al. Textile sensors to measure sweat pH and sweat-rate during exercise. In Proceedings of the Proceedings of the 3d International ICST Conference on Pervasive Computing Technologies for Healthcare, London, UK, 1–3 April 2009.
28. Ma, G.; Li, C.; Luo, Y.; Mu, R.; Wang, L. High sensitive and reliable fiber Bragg grating hydrogen sensor for fault detection of power transformer. *Sens. Actuators B Chem.* **2012**, *169*, 195–198. [CrossRef]
29. Murota, H.; Matsui, S.; Ono, E.; Kijima, A.; Kikuta, J.; Ishii, M.; Katayama, I. Sweat, the driving force behind normal skin: An emerging perspective on functional biology and regulatory mechanisms. *J. Dermatol. Sci.* **2015**, *77*, 3–10. [CrossRef] [PubMed]
30. Ali, S.; Yosipovitch, G. Skin pH: From basic science to basic skin care. *Acta Derm. Venereol.* **2013**, *93*, 261–269. [CrossRef] [PubMed]
31. Cheuvront, S.N.; Carter, R.; Sawka, M.N. Fluid balance and endurance exercise performance. *Curr. Sports Med. Rep.* **2003**, *2*, 202–208. [CrossRef] [PubMed]
32. Judelson, D.A.; Maresh, C.M.; Anderson, J.M.; Armstrong, L.E.; Casa, D.J.; Kraemer, W.J.; Volek, J.S. Hydration and Muscular Performance. *Sport. Med.* **2007**, *37*, 907–921. [CrossRef]
33. Silva, A.M.; Fields, D.A.; Heymsfield, S.B.; Sardinha, L.B. Body Composition and Power Changes in Elite Judo Athletes. *Int. J. Sports Med.* **2010**, *31*, 737–741. [CrossRef]
34. Giampietro, M.; Pujia, A.; Bertini, I. Anthropometric features and body composition of young athletes practicing karate at a high and medium competitive level. *Acta Diabetol.* **2003**, *40*, s145–s148. [CrossRef]
35. Ouergui, I.; Hammouda, O.; Chtourou, H.; Zarrouk, N.; Rebai, H.; Chaouachi, A. Anaerobic upper and lower body power measurements and perception of fatigue during a kick boxing match. *J. Sports Med. Phys. Fitness* **2013**, *53*, 455–460. [PubMed]
36. Ouergui, I.; Hammouda, O.; Chtourou, H.; Gmada, N.; Franchini, E. Effects of recovery type after a kickboxing match on blood lactate and performance in anaerobic tests. *Asian J. Sports Med.* **2014**, *5*, 99–107.
37. Ouergui, I.; Benyoussef, A.; Houcine, N.; Abedelmalek, S.; Franchini, E.; Gmada, N.; Bouhlel, E.; Bouassida, A. Physiological Responses and Time-Motion Analysis of Kickboxing: Differences Between Full Contact, Light Contact, and Point Fighting Contests. *J. Strength Cond. Res.* **2019**. [CrossRef] [PubMed]
38. Ouergui, I.; Hssin, N.; Haddad, M.; Franchini, E.; Behm, D.G.; Wong, D.P.; Gmada, N.; Bouhlel, E. Time-Motion Analysis of Elite Male Kickboxing Competition. *J. Strength Cond. Res.* **2014**, *28*, 3537–3543. [CrossRef]
39. Sterkowicz-Przybycień, K. Technical diversification, body composition and somatotype of both heavy and light Polish ju-jitsukas of high level. *Sci. Sports* **2010**, *25*, 194–200. [CrossRef]
40. Burdukiewicz, A.; Pietraszewska, J.; Stachoń, A.; Andrzejewska, J. Anthropometric profile of combat athletes via multivariate analysis. *J. Sports Med. Phys. Fitness* **2018**, *58*. [CrossRef]
41. Szponar, L.; Rychlik, E.; Wolnicka, K. *Album fotografii produktów i potraw: Album of Photographs of Food Products and Dishes*; Instytut Żywności i Żywienia, 2008. Available online: http://pssebrzesko.wsse.krakow.pl/attachments/article/403/Album%20fotografii%20produktow%20i%20potraw.pdf (accessed on 1 January 2021).
42. Rydzik, Ł.; Niewczas, M.; Kędra, A.; Grymanowski, J.; Czarny, W.; Ambroży, T. Relation of indicators of technical and tactical training to demerits of kickboxers fighting in K1 formula. *Arch. Budo Sci. Martial Arts Extrem. Sport.* **2020**, *16*, 1–5.
43. Morton, J.P.; Robertson, C.; Sutton, L.; MacLaren, D.P.M. Making the Weight: A Case Study From Professional Boxing. *Int. J. Sport Nutr. Exerc. Metab.* **2010**, *20*, 80–85. [CrossRef]
44. Miarka, B.; Fukuda, H.D.; Del Vecchio, F.B.; Franchini, E. Discriminant analysis of technical-tactical actions in high-level judo athletes. *Int. J. Perform. Anal. Sport* **2016**, *16*, 30–39. [CrossRef]
45. Miarka, B.; Cury, R.; Julianetti, R.; Battazza, R.; Julio, U.F.; Calmet, M.; Franchini, E. A comparison of time-motion and technical–tactical variables between age groups of female judo matches. *J. Sports Sci.* **2014**, *32*, 1529–1538. [CrossRef] [PubMed]
46. Wald, D.; Teucher, B.; Dinkel, J.; Kaaks, R.; Delorme, S.; Boeing, H.; Seidensaal, K.; Meinzer, H.; Heimann, T. Automatic quantification of subcutaneous and visceral adipose tissue from whole-body magnetic resonance images suitable for large cohort studies. *J. Magn. Reson. Imaging* **2012**, *36*, 1421–1434. [CrossRef]
47. Leitner, B.P.; Huang, S.; Brychta, R.J.; Duckworth, C.J.; Baskin, A.S.; McGehee, S.; Tal, I.; Dieckmann, W.; Gupta, G.; Kolodny, G.M.; et al. Mapping of human brown adipose tissue in lean and obese young men. *Proc. Natl. Acad. Sci. USA* **2017**, *114*, 8649–8654. [CrossRef] [PubMed]

48. Chaabène, H.; Tabben, M.; Mkaouer, B.; Franchini, E.; Negra, Y.; Hammami, M.; Amara, S.; Chaabène, R.B.; Hachana, Y. Amateur Boxing: Physical and Physiological Attributes. *Sport. Med.* **2015**, *45*, 337–352. [CrossRef] [PubMed]
49. Bompa, T.O.; Buzzichelli, C.A. *Periodization: Theory and Methodology of Training*; Human Kinetics: Champaign, IL, USA, 2018.
50. Ghoul, N.; Tabben, M.; Miarka, B.; Tourny, C.; Chamari, K.; Coquart, J. Mixed Martial Arts Induces Significant Fatigue and Muscle Damage Up to 24 Hours Post-combat. *J. Strength Cond. Res.* **2019**, *33*, 1570–1579. [CrossRef] [PubMed]
51. Schlader, Z.J.; Simmons, S.E.; Stannard, S.R.; Mündel, T. Skin temperature as a thermal controller of exercise intensity. *Eur. J. Appl. Physiol.* **2011**, *111*, 1631–1639. [CrossRef]
52. Akimov, E.B.; Son'kin, V.D. Skin temperature and lactate threshold during muscle work in athletes. *Hum. Physiol.* **2011**, *37*, 621–628. [CrossRef]
53. Chudecka, M.; Lubkowska, A. The Use of Thermal Imaging to Evaluate Body Temperature Changes of Athletes During Training and a Study on the Impact of Physiological and Morphological Factors on Skin Temperature. *Hum. Mov.* **2012**, *13*. [CrossRef]
54. Barboza, J.A.M.; Souza, L.I.S.; Cerqueira, M.S.; de Andrade, P.R.; dos Santos, H.H.; de Almeida Ferreira, J.J. Skin temperature of middle distance runners after a maximum effort test. *Acta Sci. Health Sci.* **2020**, *42*, e48114. [CrossRef]
55. E Côrte, A.C.R.; Hernandez, A.J. Termografia Médica Infravermelha Aplicada À Medicina Do Esporte. *Rev. Bras. Med. Esporte* **2016**, *22*, 315–319. [CrossRef]
56. Sillero-Quintana, M.; Gomez-Carmona, P.M.; Fernández-Cuevas, I. Infrared Thermography as a Means of Monitoring and Preventing Sports Injuries. In *Research Anthology on Business Strategies, Health Factors, and Ethical Implications in Sports and eSports*; IGI Global: Pennsylvania, PA, USA, 2021; pp. 832–865.
57. Yoshie, M.; Kudo, K.; Ohtsuki, T. Effects of Psychological Stress on State Anxiety, Electromyographic Activity, and Arpeggio Performance in Pianists. *Med. Probl. Perform. Art.* **2008**, *23*, 120–132. [CrossRef]
58. El-Ashker, S.; Chaabene, H.; Negra, Y.; Prieske, O.; Granacher, U. Cardio-Respiratory Endurance Responses Following a Simulated 3 × 3 Minutes Amateur Boxing Contest in Elite Level Boxers. *Sports* **2018**, *6*, 119. [CrossRef]
59. Saga, K. Structure and function of human sweat glands studied with histochemistry and cytochemistry. *Prog. Histochem. Cytochem.* **2002**, *37*, 323–386. [CrossRef]

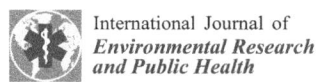

Article

Biomechanical Aspects of the Foot Arch, Body Balance and Body Weight Composition of Boys Training Football

Joanna M. Bukowska [1], Małgorzata Jekiełek [2], Dariusz Kruczkowski [3], Tadeusz Ambroży [4] and Jarosław Jaszczur-Nowicki [1,*]

[1] Department of Tourism, Recreation and Ecology, University of Warmia and Mazury, 10-719 Olsztyn, Poland; joanna.bukowska@uwm.edu.pl
[2] Department of Ergonomics and Physiological Effort, Institute of Physiotherapy, Jagiellonian University Collegium Medicum, 31-126 Krakow, Poland; malgorzata.jekielek@gmail.com
[3] Faculty of Health Sciences, Elbląg University of the Humanities and Economics, 82-300 Elbląg, Poland; dyrektor@olimpijczyk.gda.pl
[4] Institute of Sports Sciences, University of Physical Education, 31-571 Krakow, Poland; tadek@ambrozy.pl
* Correspondence: j.jaszczur-nowicki@uwm.edu.pl

Abstract: *Background:* The aim of the study is to assess the body balance and podological parameters and body composition of young footballers in the context of the control of football training. *Methods:* The study examined the distribution of the pressure of the part of the foot on the ground, the arch of the foot, and the analysis of the body composition of the boys. The pressure center for both feet and the whole body was also examined. The study involved 90 youth footballers from Olsztyn and Barczewo in three age groups: 8–10 years, 11–13 years old, and 14–16 years. The study used the Inbody 270 body composition analyzer and the EPSR1, a mat that measures the pressure distribution of the feet on the ground. *Results:* The results showed statistically significant differences in almost every case for each area of the foot between the groups of the examined boys. The most significant differences were observed for the metatarsal area and the left heel. In the case of stabilization of the whole body, statistically significant differences were noted between all study groups. In the case of the body composition parameters, in the examined boys, a coherent direction of changes was noticed for most of them. The relationships and correlations between the examined parameters were also investigated. The significance level in the study was set at $p < 0.05$. *Conclusions:* Under the training rigor, a statistically significant increase in stability was observed with age. The total length of the longitudinal arch of both feet of the examined boys showed a tendency to flatten in direct proportion to the age of the examined boys. Mean values of the body composition parameters reflect changes with the ontogenetic development, basic somatic parameters (body height and weight) and training experience, and thus with the intensity and volume of training. This indicates a correct training process that does not interfere with the proper development of the body in terms of tissue and biochemical composition.

Keywords: foot; ground pressure; body composition; body balance; football players

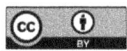

1. Introduction

The attempt to achieve the championship forced the coaches to pay more attention to training children and adolescents. This procedure seems to be fundamental, but in practice it very often causes many errors, deformations or even degenerations [1,2]. Most often, in the case of talented youth, there is a quick entry into sport for adults, often with temporary successes of young players. However, they are unprepared physically, mentally, technically and tactically. It is often accompanied by the exhaustion of a young athlete, both physically (injuries, permanent damage to the musculoskeletal system, problems in the field of motor coordination, lack of progress in the field of physical preparation) and mentally [3]. Coordination abilities can be a diagnostic tool for monitoring the dynamics of their development and on the basis of them, conclusions can be drawn about the dynamics of physical health [4]. The current knowledge and many years of training experience, not only in football, clearly show that properly selected methods and forms of training are the key to success. Perfectly matched training loads at individual stages of a player's development may bring in the future the result of an optimally prepared footballer for a world-class sport fight [3]. Football is a team game in which the players should represent a sufficiently high level of speed, strength and coordination motor skills. The level of these abilities may depend on the task performed on the pitch as well as on the sport advancement [5,6]. Coordination is one of the factors indicating a significant improvement in physical performance. This is confirmed by the directly proportional relationship between muscle strength and neuromuscular coordination [7,8]. The aim of general coordination training is to develop, improve, stabilize and restore coordination skills or performance requirements in order to be able to successfully cope with all motor tasks in sport and everyday life [9]. One of the coordination skills is balance, which is the ability to concentrate on one's own body [10]. Balance has a direct and significant influence on the ability to dribble [11]. A better balance of the body allows for better results in sports [12]. As a result of the literature review, it can be stated that people from various sports disciplines training at a higher level have better balance than people who are just starting their training [13–15]. The cause of problems and at the same time a greater risk of lower limb injuries is overweight. One of the effects of excessive fat mass in the torso reduces the degree of mobility, balance control and a decrease in postural stability [16]. The foot is an important part of the musculoskeletal system. Its function is to support the conditioning of human movement. The foot is influenced by a number of factors that have a positive effect on it or contribute to the formation of defects [17]. The use of the foot as a basic element in practicing football causes it to carry out more work than during everyday activities. Biomechanical loads that the foot is subjected to while kicking a ball, the use of special and specific footwear and the varied terrain of various sports fields (compacted earth, grass, etc.) activate a number of muscles and joints that do not function with the same intensity and mobility in everyday life [18]. Soccer players are exposed to injuries due to overload, discomfort and decreased performance due to shoe design and repetitive plantar loads [19]. The specificity of the sport discipline causes players to have different morphological profiles [17]. Laterality is also a factor that can affect foot function. Khudik, Chikurov, Voynich et al. believe that asymmetry manifests itself in the human body. Cultural factors and genetics influence the asymmetry of a given individual, and Guilherme J. et al. in their research show that training influences the functional asymmetry of the lower limbs in young football players. [20]. During the research, the following hypothesis and purpose of the research was formulated: sports activity related to football training allows for the biological development of a human being in accordance with the norms in the field of body posture and its composition. The aim of the study is to assess the physical aspects of the musculoskeletal system, related to the structure of the foot and the ability to maintain body balance, as well as to analyze the body composition of young football players in the context of football training control.

2. Materials and Methods
2.1. Participants

The study included 90 youth footballers from Olsztyn and Barczewo in three age groups: 8–10 years (mean age 9 ± 0.86 years, body weight 33.66 ± 8.51 kg, body height 136.03 ± 10.31 cm), 11–13 years (mean age 12.55 ± 0.63 years, body weight 47.83 ± 7.66 kg, height 159.79 ± 6.72 cm) and 14–16 years (mean age 14.30 ± 0.46 years, body weight 60.08 ± 10.31 kg, height 171.61 ± 6.57 cm). All boys aged 8–16, training in clubs in Olsztyn and Barczewo, who were entered into the games at the province or central level in their age categories, participated in the research. Boys under examination took part in training three times a week. Each training session consisted of a warm-up, improving football skills, shaping motor skills with or without the ball, improving individual and team behavior in specific parts of the game, playing ball, and stretching at the end of training. The research was conducted during the competition period. All respondents are players of the same league games in different age categories. The construction of the training unit between the teams was very similar and adapted to their age. All players declared their right upper and lower limbs as dominant and had no visible dysfunctions in the musculoskeletal system. Parents and trainers gave their written consent to the study. All examined boys were players of the same class of games, at different levels of classification depending on age. All coaches of the studied players have the same game goals: victory in individual matches and, as a result, obtaining the best possible place in the league. The research was conducted on the basis of the consent of the Scientific Research Ethics Committee of the University of Warmia and Mazury in Olsztyn (Decision No. 9/2018).

2.2. Instruments

The body composition analyzer Inbody 270 (Inbody Co. Ltd, Soul, Korea) was used for the research. It is a specialized medical device that uses the bioelectric impedance method to measure body composition using a quantitative method. This method is based on the ability to electrically conduct muscle tissue. Body height was measured with a Soehnle (Soehnle, Gaildorfer Straße 6, 71522 Backnang, Germany) electronic ultrasonic height measuring device. (The height measuring device performs the ultrasound measurement and the built-in tilt sensor helps to measure it precisely. The device transmits data to the computer program Lookin'Body 120 (Included in the package with the Inbody 270 device). For the measurement of foot pressure distribution and balance, the EPSR1 mat (Letsens Group, Letsens S.R.L. Via Buozzi, CastelMaggiore; Bologna, Italy) was used. The $700 \times 500 \times 5$ mm mat is equipped with 2304 pressure sensors located on the active surface. It is a diagnostic device used to evaluate the feet in static and dynamic conditions. The mat is equipped with sensors that collect the measurements for 20 seconds and transfers them to the computer using the Biomech Studio program (Biomech Studio 2.0 Manual, (Letsens Group, Letsens S.R.L. Via Buozzi, CastelMaggiore; Bologna, Italy). The following stabilometric parameters can be measured with the mat:

- COP LF—area of left foot imbalances,
- COP RF—right foot imbalances area,
- body COP—the surface of the body's center of gravity.

2.3. Procedure

The research was conducted on 5 March 2020, 11 March 2020 and 30 July 2020. The test procedure consisted of several steps. In the initial stages, consultations with trainers and parents were conducted regarding the planned study. The study schedule was also drawn up and parental consent was obtained for the study of boys. Before starting the study, a qualified person entered the data of the test person into the program, such as ID, date of birth and height. The height of the body was checked by the researcher with the help of a measuring rod, keeping an upright posture. Then, after undressing to underwear, removing jewelry and glasses, the erect participant climbed the analyzer platform so that the feet covered as much of the electrodes as possible. The device automatically started measuring the body weight. After completing the measurement, the examined person took the handles of the device in their hands with their thumb touching the upper electrode and the other fingers of the lower electrode. The subject was asked to remove the extended arms from the body so as not to touch the torso, as this could affect the reliability of the results. The feet and hands adhered to the electrodes throughout the examination, and special attention was paid to it. During the composition analysis, the boys' standards were checked by precisely referring to the body parameters generated by the program for each of them. In order to avoid errors, the tests were carried out in accordance with the procedure enclosed by the manufacturer in the device manual. The examined boys were either fasting or at least 2–3 h after a meal, and also after defecation. In order to optimize the obtained results, the test was performed in the morning, before exercise, approximately 2–3 min after changing from sitting to standing. Earlier bathing was a contraindication to the study, as it accelerates blood flow in the body, which the respondents were aware of. After the end of the test, the data were automatically sent to the Lookin'Body 120 program and the subject put down the handles of the device and left it. Then, the examined boy went to the podographic mat so that his feet were on both sides of the vertical line drawn on the mat. They were then asked to take a few steps to place their feet freely on the mat. The boy stood upright with his arms against his body, staring straight ahead. The signal remained stationary for 20 seconds. At that time, the measurements were made and transferred to a computer system using the Biomech Studio software (Biomech Studio 2.0 Manual). The diagram of the test procedure is shown in Figure 1.

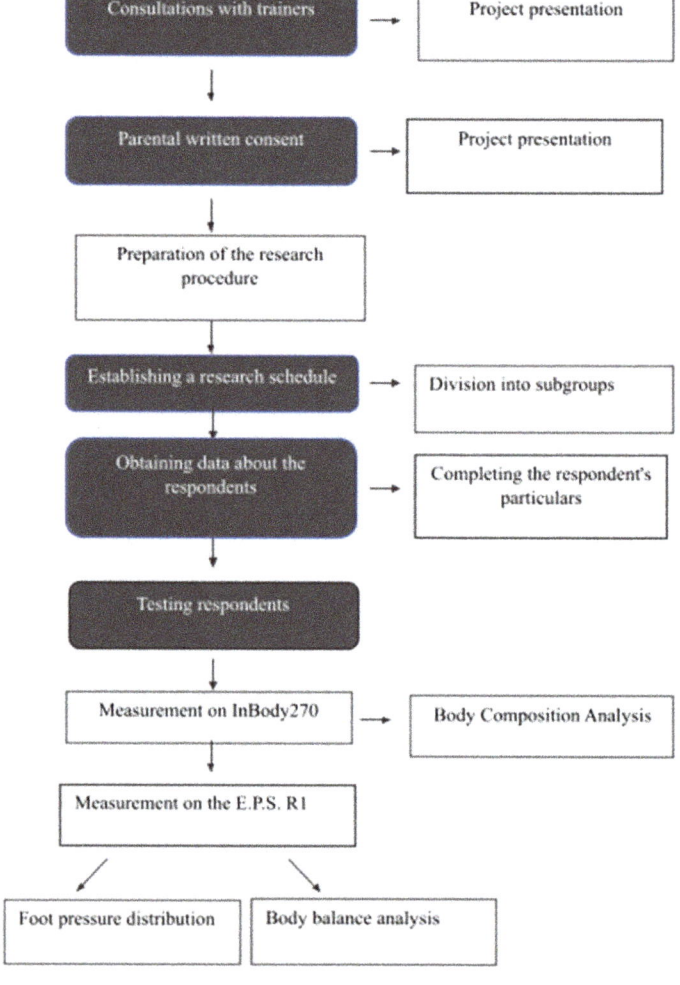

Figure 1. Scheme of the test procedure.

2.4. Statistical Analysis

The Shapiro–Wilk test was used to analyze the studied groups of boys categorized according to their age, which indicated non-compliance with the normal distribution for all measurement parameters. Therefore, in further analysis, a statistical nonparametric function was used, which is the rank test of Kruskal–Wallis. In the case of podological and stabilographic measurements, the two-tailed test with Bonferroni's correction was used due to the mean differences between the groups of boys under study. In the whole work for the characteristics of descriptive statistics, the measures of mean value, median and dispersion of quartile measurement values were used. During the statistical analysis, the Chi square test and the Spearman correlation test were also used to analyze the dependence and correlation between the obtained results. The significance level in the study was set at $p < 0.05$. Statistical analyses were performed using the Statistica program (StatSoft Polska, Kraków, Poland version 13.3).

3. Results

During the analysis, differences in the size of the foot arches were noticed for each of the studied groups of young footballers. The mean values of the pressure of the metatarsal area in the group of boys aged 8–10 years indicated significant hollowing of both feet. For the left foot, the value of the pressure area on the metatarsus was only 0.1%, and in the right foot, 0.8%. Taking into account the mean values for the group of boys aged 11–13 years, the left foot was significantly hollow (0.4%), while the right foot was in the range of the average hollow (9.8%). The results for the oldest group of boys aged 14–16 were the highest for the left foot, placing the value in the range of mean arching (12.9%) and the right foot in the range of significant arching (2.3%). The detailed results of the podiatry examination in the studied age groups are presented in Table 1.

Table 1. Characteristics of the distribution of pressure forces of the foot in the age groups of the studied boys.

	Forefoot LF (%)	Metatarsus LF (%)	Heel LF (%)	Forefoot RF (%)	Metatarsus RF (%)	Heel RF (%)
			Footballers aged 8–10 ($n = 28$)			
Me	38.40	0.10	56.70	57.30	0.80	37.95
Q_1	27.45	0.00	44.70	53.38	0.00	27.15
Q_3	49.93	2.70	71.80	65.23	6.65	43.65
			Footballers aged 11–13 ($n = 29$)			
Me	47.80	0.40	44.80	58.40	9.80	29.20
Q_1	36.50	0.00	38.10	44.50	2.30	17.60
Q_3	55.20	11.20	5510	69.40	20.50	49.50
			Footballers aged 14–16 ($n = 33$)			
Me	43.70	12.90	40.00	45.30	2.30	49.30
Q_1	39.00	7.00	37.30	37.30	0.50	43.90
Q_3	49.20	21.30	45.50	49.70	11.10	56.60

LF—left foot, RF—right foot, Me—median, Q—quartile.

Analyzing the results of the stabilographic examination, significant differences were noticed in the size of all parameters defining the field of changes in the position of the entire body, as well as the area for the left and right feet. Taking into account the total parameter of the pressure center of the whole body, the group of the youngest footballers aged 8–10 (360.62 mm^2) showed the least stability. In the following groups of boys, an increase in the stabilization of body posture was noticed, where in the group of boys aged 11–13 years, the size of the area for the whole body was 197.84 mm², while for the oldest group, aged 14–16, the mean value was 37.76 mm². The results of the stabilographic examination are presented in Table 2.

Table 2. Characteristics of the changes in the position of the center of gravity examination in the age groups.

	Body COP (mm²)	COP LF (mm²)	COP RF (mm²)
	Footballers aged 8–10 (n = 28)		
Me	360.62	40.96	73.62
Q_1	195.05	20.25	25.38
Q_3	792.63	109.44	245.89
	Footballers aged 11–13 (n = 29)		
Me	197.84	20.36	33.65
Q_1	60.96	12.25	12.54
Q_3	512.23	49.52	123.17
	Footballers aged 14–16 (n = 33)		
Me	37.76	4.33	7.30
Q_1	20.71	2.20	2.84
Q_3	72.57	9.05	14.75

COP—center of pressure, LF—left foot, RF—right foot, Me—median, Q—quartile.

The obtained results were statistically evaluated. In the podiatry study, statistically significant differences were noticed between the groups of boys, categorized in specific age groups, in almost every case for each area of the foot. The most significant differences were observed for the metatarsal area and the heel in the left foot. In the metatarsal area, significant differences were noted between all the studied groups of young footballers. Referring to the results of the evaluation of the statistical differences in the stabilographic study, significant differences were noted for all parameters. In the case of the summary parameter constituting the stabilization of the whole body, statistically significant differences were noted between all groups of the studied footballers. The results of the analysis of the statistical significance of differences in individual parameters and age groups are presented in Tables 3–5.

Table 3. Significance of differences in parameters of the distribution of pressure forces in the left foot between the studied age groups.

Variable		Forefoot LF			Metatarsus LF			Heel LF		
Kruskal–Wallis test (p)		0.100			0.000			0.001		
Age		8–10	11–13	14–16	8–10	11–13	14–16	8–10	11–13	14–16
Test post hoc with the amendment Bonferroni	8–10	X	0.100	0.546	X	1.000	0.000	X	0.122	0.001
	11–13	0.100	X	1.000	1.000	X	0.000	0.122	X	0.321
	14–16	0.546	1.000	X	0.000	0.000	X	0.001	0.321	X

LF—left foot, RF—right foot.

In the statistical analysis, differences between the groups of boys were noticed in the size of their body composition parameters. For most of them, there was a homogeneous direction of changes. A total of 80–95% of the examined boys, divided into groups, had measurement values within the normal range (TBW, proteins, FFM, WHR). In the case of the parameters related to total body water (TBW), lean body mass (FFM), skeletal muscle mass (SMM), body mass index (BMI), but also in the case of protein and mineral content in the body, the mean measurement values increased directly proportional to the age of the respondents. The differences in the mean values of the above-mentioned parameters for each group of boys were statistically significant. In the case of the percentage of adipose tissue (PBF) and the degree of obesity (obesity degree), the mean values for the subsequent study groups were inversely proportional. In their case, statistically significant differences were also noted between the boys' groups. By comparing the mean values of the parameters: total body fat mass (BFM) and the waist–hip index (WHR) and visceral fat (VFL) related to the analysis of the abdominal area, no statistically significant differences were found and the mean values for each group were almost equal. Taking into account the specificity of physical effort, football players require a high ratio of muscle mass to body fat mass, where excess fat mass leads to a significant reduction in exercise capacity. The general body mass index BMI for boys of the youngest age group remained at the lower limit of the normal range (BMI = 17.5), while in the other two groups it was at the lower limits of the normal range: BMI = 18.30 and BMI = 20.20. The gradual increase in the value of the index is closely related to the mass of skeletal muscles, where successively in the age groups of the studied footballers there is an average higher skeletal muscle mass in the body, respectively: SMM: 12.65; 20.80; 28.40. This relationship translates into mean values of lean body mass (FFM). Additionally, in the case of this parameter, the mean value increases in the subsequent age groups, respectively: FFM: 24.75; 38.40; 51.30. The analysis of body composition in terms of water content (TBW), proteins and minerals also follow the principle of a directly proportional increase in mean values in relation to the age of the studied group of boys. The mean values of the percentage of adipose tissue in the subsequent age groups of the boys under study are inversely proportional to the analyzed indicators, respectively: PBF: 22.15; 16.50; 11.30. The characteristics of body composition parameters (InBody) presented in Table 6.

Table 4. Significance of differences in parameters of the distribution of pressure forces in the right foot between the studied age groups.

Variable		Forefoot RF			Metatarsus RF			Heel RF		
Kruskal–Wallis test (p)		0.000			0.032			0.000		
Age		8–10	11–13	14–16	8–10	11–13	14–16	8–10	11–13	14–16
Test post hoc with the amendment Bonferroni	8–10	X	0.869	0.000	X	0.029	0.776	X	1.000	0.000
	11–13	0.869	X	0.003	0.029	X	0.361	1.000	X	0.000
	14–16	0.000	0.003	X	0.776	0.361	X	0.000	0.000	X

LF—left foot, RF—right foot.

Table 5. Significance of the changes in the position of the center of gravity between the studied age groups.

Variable		Body COP			LF COP			RF COP		
Kruskal–Wallis test (p)		0.000			0.000			0.000		
Age		8–10	11–13	14–16	8–10	11–13	14–16	8–10	11–13	14–16
Test post hoc with the amendment Bonferroni	8–10	X	0.013	0.000	X	0.155	0.000	X	0.012	0.000
	11–13	0.013	X	0.001	0.155	X	0.000	0.012	X	0.016
	14–16	0.000	0.001	X	0.000	0.000	X	0.000	0.000	X

COP—center of pressure, LF—left foot, RF—right foot.

During the statistical analysis, the relationships between the examined parameters were also examined. Both the relationships between the examined features and the correlation between them were analyzed. For this purpose, the Chi^2 test and the Spearman correlation test were used. In the group of the youngest boys, a statistically significant relationship and correlation between the body COP and the WHR parameter was observed. The examined boys with an increase in this parameter had a greater problem with balance while standing on both feet. However, a similar correlation was not obtained for the correlation and dependence with BMI, BFM, PBF, VFL and obesity degree. In the age group between 11 and 13 years of age, there was no correlation between body composition related to adipose tissue and body balance. In the group of the oldest boys, a statistically significant relationship and correlation between body COP and BFM was demonstrated. However, it was a negative correlation. The same relationship was noted between body COP and PBF, VFL, WHR and obesity degree. Taking into account the entire sample, there was a statistically significant correlation between body COP and BMI. With the increase in BMI, greater disturbances were noted in the examined boys. The same relationships were noted between body COP and PBF and obesity degree.

Table 6. Characteristics of selected body composition parameters (InBody) and the level of statistical significance of differences between the investigated footballers classified in age groups.

	TBW	Proteins	Minerals	BFM	FFM	SMM	BMI	PBF	WHR	VFL	Obesity Degree
				Footballers aged 8–10 ($n = 28$)							
Me	18.10	4.85	1.80	7.15	24.75	12.65	17.50	22.15	0.77	3.00	106.5
Q1	16.15	4.20	1.47	5.00	22.00	10.98	15.70	18.20	0.75	2.00	99.75
Q3	21.55	5.70	2.06	10.33	29.50	15.43	19.35	27.30	0.79	3.00	111.0
				Footballers aged 11–13 ($n = 29$)							
Me	28.20	7.50	2.74	7.60	38.40	20.80	18.30	16.50	0.77	3.00	98.00
Q1	25.90	6.90	2.52	6.10	35.40	18.80	17.10	13.00	0.76	2.00	94.00
Q3	30.80	8.20	2.92	10.50	42.00	22.70	20.10	21.50	0.79	4.00	105.00
				Footballers aged 14–16 ($n = 33$)							
Me	37.50	10.10	3.62	6.80	51.30	28.40	20.20	11.30	0.77	2.00	97.00
Q1	33.10	9.10	3.12	5.80	45.20	25.10	18.70	10.20	0.76	2.00	92.00
Q3	43.40	11.70	4.11	9.00	59.20	33.40	21.70	14.90	0.79	3.00	102.00
p	0.000	0.000	0.000	0.757	0.000	0.000	0.001	0.000	0.799	0.411	

TBW—total body water, BFM—total body fat mass, FFM—lean body mass, SMM—skeletal muscle mass, BMI—body mass index, PBF—percentage of adipose tissue, WHR—waist–hip index, VFL—visceral fat.

4. Discussion

Human biological development usually proceeds according to the norms. This enables the comparison of percentiles and the decision of whether the changes comply with the physiological norm or not. When assessing body composition, all parameters in the study group are consistent with the physiological norm. This indicates the correct selection of the examined adolescents and the proper training process, which does not disturb the proper development of the organism in terms of tissue and biochemical composition. The problem of body composition in young footballers was studied by Santos-Silva et al. The 16-week futsal training program contributed to the improvement of body composition and cardiovascular capacity in a group of boys before puberty (7–10 years). There was a significant increase in total body weight (4%), height (3%), lean body mass (8%) and a significant 6% decrease in body fat percentage [21]. The research presented in this study also shows that in older boys (14–16 years old) there was a greater percentage of boys who were below the norm than in the other groups. Similar results were obtained by Ørntoft et al. [22] found that Danish children aged 10–12 engaged in club football (FC) and other ball games

(OBGs) had more muscle mass and a lower body fat percentage than children who did not play sports in their free time (NSC). Children participating in club ball games had a higher ($p < 0.05$) lean body weight than NSC and OBG: participation in soccer classes also affects the percentage of body fat. Significant scientific reports indicate the improvement of the body's ability to maintain balance until the age of 10–12. The differences in the limits of the ability maximization are determined by the measurement method, or rather the conditions for showing the body's ability to balance. Different limits are indicated by the authors for measurements under static conditions, others under dynamic conditions. In our own study, it was observed that the body balance was better with the increasing duration of the training rigor. The oldest group of the boys under study showed the lowest balance disturbances during the stabilometric test. The research conducted by Lebiedowska M. and Syczewska M. [23] showed that despite changes in the body dimensions of children between 7 and 18 years of age in balance tests, the invariability of the swing amplitude is noticeable, which confirms the view that the same patterns of muscle activation are used in children and adolescents. Different results, but adequate to the authors of this study, were obtained by Riach C.L. and Starkes J.L. [24] who in studies of children (4–13 years old) and adults showed an age-related change in the velocity of the center of gravity and in the position of the feet. The problem of the influence of regular football training on balance was investigated by Olchowiak G. and Czwalik A. [25]. The authors carried out research on women training in football ($n = 25$) and a control group ($n = 50$). In the tests used, statistically significant differences between the groups were obtained. Women training in football showed better postural stability and balance. The study showed that regular training can improve the balance system. The authors' conclusions are consistent with the results obtained by the authors of this study, as they showed statistically significant differences between the groups in terms of body posture stability. Kumala M.S. et al. [26] also dealt with balance in athletes, comparing the balance between normal and flat feet. None of the tests performed showed statistically significant differences between the groups ($p > 0.05$) in the balance of the body. Jaszczur-Nowicki J. et al. [27–29] in their works analyze changes in the balance and distribution of pressure forces on the plantar side of the foot under the influence of various factors. In children, under the influence of an external load (backpack), the results of body balance were statistically significant. They concerned measurements of the area of the center of gravity of the body, the area of the center of gravity of the left foot and the parameter comparing the distance to area ratio. In all these parameters tested, $p < 0.05$ was obtained. The authors obtained statistically significant results in all parameters of the body balance by analyzing the influence of exercise (Harvard Step Test) on the examined parameters in students. The authors of the above studies also analyzed the distribution of pressure forces on the plantar side of the foot; in children, the results indicated that after putting on the backpack for the entire study group, statistically significant differences ($p < 0{,}05$) were found in the distribution of the foot pressure on the ground in the left foot, forefoot, and heel area. However, in the right foot, this difference was noted for the forefoot and the metatarsus. The p-value in these parameters was also below 0.05. On the other hand, among students, when comparing the mean results of measurements at rest and after exercises for the forefoot, the value of the rest vs. the post-training values for the left foot were comparable, as for the right foot. The image of the metatarsal area, being a reference to the correct longitudinal cavity of the foot. It was different for both feet when measured at rest compared to after exercise. For the heel area, the mean differences in the values between the measurements for the right and left foot was also noted. Additionally, in the author's study, differences in the pressure on the ground of individual parts of the foot between the right and left foot were noted. Systematic football training, as well as external load and physical effort, affects changes in body balance and the distribution of pressure forces on the sole of the foot. Further studies confirming the results obtained by the authors of this study are the analyses of Bibro M. et al. [29]. They took up the problem of the analysis of the arching and pressure distribution of the plantar side of the feet of young men under the influence of strength training of the lower limbs. The surveyed men were divided into two groups of 30. Group I, subjected to training, completed training in the gym including lower limb exercises within 60 minutes, and group II spent the same period of time passively, in a sitting position. In the group subjected to strength training, in the measurements before and after exercise, the lateral and medial side of the hindfoot were symmetrically loaded, while the load on the forefoot increased significantly, especially on the medial part. One hour of effort also had a slight effect on the height of the arches of both feet. Bogut I. et al. [30] conducted research on the occurrence of foot deformities in city children, as well as on possible generation and sex differences. The results of the research showed that the highest percentage of children did not have a noticeable foot deformity, so more than three-quarters of children in 2005 and 2011 had healthy feet. The only noticeable percentage of children with foot deformities relates to the first-degree flatfoot category, from 9.39% in 2005 and 14.69% in 2011. There were no significant differences in the occurrence of foot deformities between the 2005 and 2011 generations or by gender and age between and within each subgroup. The results of these studies indicate that the largest number of children aged 7–11 years did not have noticeable foot deformities, so in children studied in 2005 and 2011, so most of the children did not have deformities. The only noticeable percentage of children with foot deformity relates to the first-degree flat foot category; however, their percentage was in the range of 9–15%. The boys studied for the purposes of this study were also city dwellers. The results obtained by the authors were not compatible with the studies cited above. The author's study noted that the total length of the longitudinal arch of both feet of the examined boys showed a tendency to flatten in direct proportion to the age of the examined boys. The arches of the foot differ, however, between the right and left roof. Zdunek M.K. et al. [17] confirmed that people practicing the above disciplines have hollow long arches of the foot. Additionally, the results of the research carried out by the authors showed differences in the distribution of forces on the sole of the foot depending on the sports discipline practiced. In the throwing group, in the right and left feet, the front part of the foot was loaded more frequently, while in the jumping group, the back of the foot was more loaded in the right and left feet. The authors concluded that the observed differences probably resulted from the fact that, due to the specificity of the sports discipline, players have different morphological profiles. The authors of this study also noticed that the studied footballers were mostly characterized by a hollow longitudinal arch. Due to the specifics of their discipline, players are more likely to put stress on the rear of the left foot and the front of the right foot.

5. Conclusions

- The total length of the longitudinal arch of both feet of the examined boys showed a tendency to flatten in direct proportion to the age of the examined boys. The arches of the foot differ, however, between the right and left roof. If this tendency is maintained in the left foot, it does not take such a strong direction in the right foot.
- The youngest group of the boys under study showed the greatest deviations of the balance, while the group subjected to training for the longest time (the group of the oldest boys) had distinct smaller deviations of the pressure center.
- In the youngest group of boys, correlations between body balance deviations and waist–hip index were observed.
- The given mean values of the body composition parameters reflect changes with the ontogenetic development, basic somatic parameters (body height and weight) and training experience, and thus with the intensity and volume of training.

Some aspects require further research. The dominant side of the respondents should be taken into account, which may be the reason for the observed differences. The observed correlations may suggest a relationship between body composition parameters and the ability to maintain balance and stabilization performance.

Practical Implication

The training rigor supports the proper development of children and has a positive effect on balance and body composition. An important aspect of the training process is not to overtrain the players so that the training is beneficial and supports the natural ontogenetic development.

Author Contributions: Conceptualization, J.M.B., M.J., D.K., J.J.-N.; methodology, J.M.B., M.J., D.K., T.A., J.J.-N.; software, J.M.B., D.K., J.J.-N.; validation, J.M.B., M.J., D.K., T.A., J.J.-N.; formal analysis, J.M.B., M.J., D.K., T.A., J.J.-N.; investigation, J.M.B., M.J., D.K., J.J.-N.; resources, J.M.B., D.K., J.J.-N.; data curation, J.M.B., D.K., J.J.-N.; writing—original draft preparation, J.M.B., M.J., D.K., J.J.-N.; writing—review and editing, J.M.B., M.J., D.K., T.A., J.J.-N.; visualization, J.M.B.; supervision, J.M.B., D.K., T.A., J.J.-N.; project administration, J.M.B.; funding acquisition, J.M.B., J.J.-N. All authors have read and agreed to the published version of the manuscript.

Funding: Financing from own resources.

Institutional Review Board Statement: The study was conducted according to the guidelines of the Declaration of Helsinki. The research was conducted on the basis of the consent of the Scientific Research Ethics Committee of the University of Warmia and Mazury in Olsztyn (Decision No. 9/2018).

Informed Consent Statement: Informed consent was obtained from all subjects involved in the study.

Data Availability Statement: The data presented in this study are available on request from the corresponding author.

Conflicts of Interest: The authors declare no conflict of interest.

References

1. Jayanthi, N.; Pinkham, C.; Dugas, L.; Patrick, B.; Labella, C. Sports specialization in young athletes: Evidence-based recommendations. *Sports Health* **2013**, *5*, 251–257. [CrossRef]
2. Szwarc, A.; Jaszczur-Nowicki, J.; Aschenbrenner, P.; Zasada, M.; Padulo, J. LP Motion analysis of elite Polish soccer goalkeepers throughout a season. *Biol. Sport.* **2019**, *36*, 357–363. [CrossRef] [PubMed]
3. Egilsson, B.; Dolles, H. "From Heroes to Zeroes"-self-initiated expatriation of talented young footballers. *J. Glob. Mobil. HomeExpatr. Manag. Res.* **2017**, *5*, 174–193. [CrossRef]
4. Hirtz, P. *Koordinative Fähigkeiten im Schulsport. (Vielseiting-Variationsreichungewohnt)*; Volk und W.: Berlin, Germany, 1985.
5. Islam, M.S.; Kundu, B. Association of Dribbling with Linear and Non-linear Sprints in Young Soccer Players of Bangladesh. *Int. J. Med. Public Health* **2020**, *10*, 100–103. [CrossRef]
6. Alesi, M.; Bianco, A.; Padulo, J.; Luppina, G.; Petrucci, M.; Paoli, A.; Palma, A.; Pepi, A. Motor and cognitive growth following a Football Training Program. *Front. Psychol.* **2015**, *6*, 1627. [CrossRef] [PubMed]
7. Jaszczur-Nowicki, J.; Bukowska, J.M.; Lemanek, K.; Klimczak, J.; Kruczkowski, D. Jump height of volleyball players across the league season. *Arch Budo Sci. Martial Art Extrem. Sport* **2019**, *15*, 119–127.
8. Tieland, M.; Trouwborst, I.; Clark, B.C. Skeletal muscle performance and ageing. *J. Cachexia Sarcopenia Muscle* **2018**, *9*, 3–19. [CrossRef]
9. Golle, K.; Mechling, H.; Granacher, U. Koordinative Fähigkeiten und Koordinationstraining im Sport. In *Bewegung, Training, Leistung und Gesundheit*; Springer: Berlin/Heidelberg, Germany, 2019; pp. 1–24.
10. Ergash, N.; Kamila, K.; Kahhor, G.; Fazliddin, K. Development Of Coordination Abilities And Balance Of Primary School Age Children Gulistan State University. *Eur. J. Mol. Clin. Med.* **2020**, *7*, 5384–5389.
11. Amra, F.; Soniawan, V. The Effect of Agility, Foot-Eye Coordination, and Balance on Dribbling Ability: An Ex Post Facto Research at Balai Baru Football Academy Padang. In Proceedings of the 1st Progress in Social Science, Humanities and Education Research Symposium (PSSHERS 2019); Atlantis Press: Paris, France, 2020.
12. Mańko, G.; Kruczkowski, D.; Niźnikowski, T.; Perliński, J.; Chantsoulis, M.; Pokorska, J.; Łukaszewska, B.; Ziółkowski, A.; Graczyk, M.; Starczyńska, M.; et al. The Effect of Programed Physical Activity Measured with Levels of Body Balance Maintenance. *Med. Sci. Monit.* **2014**, *20*, 1841–1849. [CrossRef]
13. Jaszczur-Nowicki, J.; Kruczkowski, D.; Bukowska, J. Analysis of the distribution of foot force on the ground before and after a kinaesthetic stimulation. *J. Kinesiol. Exerc. Sci.* **2019**, *29*, 19–27. [CrossRef]
14. Osipov, A.; Tselovalnikova, M.; Klimas, N.; Zhavner, T.; Vapaeva, A.; Mokrous, T. Ealization of Anti Gravity fitness exercises in physical education practice of female students. *J. Phys. Educ. Sport* **2019**, *19*, 1429–1434. [CrossRef]
15. Paillard, T. Relationship Between Sport Expertise and Postural Skills. *Front. Psychol.* **2019**, *10*. [CrossRef] [PubMed]
16. Zerf, M. Body composition versus body fat percentage as predictors of posture/balance control mobility and stability among football players under 21 years. *Phys. Educ. Stud.* **2017**, *21*, 96. [CrossRef]

17. Zdunek, M.K.; Marszałek, J.; Domínguez, R. Influence of sport discipline on foot arching and load distribution: Pilot studies. *J. Phys. Educ. Sport* **2020**, *20*, 721–728. [CrossRef]
18. López, N.; Alburquerque, F.; Santos, M. SMDR Evaluation and analysis of the footprint of young individuals. A comparative study between football players and non-players. *Eur. J. Anat.* **2005**, *9*, 135–142.
19. Husain, E.; Angioi, M.; Mehta, R.; Barnett, D.N.; Okholm Kryger, K. A systematic review of plantar pressure values obtained from male and female football and the test methodologies applied. *Footwear Sci.* **2020**, *12*, 217–233. [CrossRef]
20. Guilherme, J.; Garganta, J.; Graça, A.; Seabra, A. Effects of technical training in functional asymmetry of lower limbs in young soccer players. *Rev. Bras. Cineantropometria Desempenho Humano* **2015**, *17*, 125–135. [CrossRef]
21. Santos-Silva, P.R.; Greve, J.M.D.; Novillo, H.N.E.; Haddad, S.; Santos, C.R.P.; Leme, R.B.; Franco, R.R.; Cominato, L.; Araújo, A.T.M.; Santos, F.M.; et al. Futsal improve body composition and cardiorespiratory fitness in overweight and obese children. A pilot study. *Mot. Rev. Educ. Física* **2018**, *24*. [CrossRef]
22. Ørntoft, C.; Larsen, M.N.; Madsen, M.; Sandager, L.; Lundager, I.; Møller, A.; Hansen, L.; Madsen, E.E.; Elbe, A.-M.; Ottesen, L.; et al. Physical Fitness and Body Composition in 10–12-Year-Old Danish Children in Relation to Leisure-Time Club-Based Sporting Activities. *Biomed. Res. Int.* **2018**, *2018*, 1–8. [CrossRef] [PubMed]
23. Lebiedowska, M.; Syczewska, M. Invariant sway propertis in children. *Gait Posture* **2000**, *12*, 200–204. [CrossRef]
24. Riach, C.L.; Starkes, J.L. Velocity of center of pressure excursions as an indicator of postural control system in children. *Gait Posture* **1994**, *2*, 167–172. [CrossRef]
25. Olchowik, G.; Czwalik, A. Effects of Soccer Training on Body Balance in Young Female Athletes Assessed Using Computerized Dynamic Posturography. *Appl. Sci.* **2020**, *10*, 1003. [CrossRef]
26. Kumala, M.S.; Tinduh, D.; Poerwandari, D. Comparison of Lower Extremities Physical Performance on Male Young Adult Athletes with Normal Foot and Flatfoot. *Surabaya Phys. Med. Rehabil. J.* **2019**, *1*, 6–13. [CrossRef]
27. Jaszczur-Nowicki, J.; Bukowska, J.M.; Kruczkowski, D.; Pieniążek, M.; Mańko, G.; Spieszny, M. Distribution of feet pressure on ground and maintaining body balance among 8–10-year-old children with and without external load application. *Acta Bioeng. Biomech.* **2020**, *22*. [CrossRef]
28. Jaszczur-Nowicki, J.; Bukowska, J.; Kruczkowski, D.; Spieszny, M.; Pieniążek, M.; Mańko, G. Analysis of students' foot pressure distribution on the ground, as well as their body balance before and after exercise. *Phys. Educ. Stud.* **2020**, *24*, 194–204. [CrossRef]
29. Bibro, M.; Drwal, A.; Jankowicz-Szymańska, A. Ocena wysklepienia oraz rozkładu sił nacisku podeszwowej strony stóp młodych mężczyzn pod wpływem treningu siłowego kończyn dolnych. [The assessment of the effect of strength training of lower limbs on arching and forces distribution of the sole in young. *Heal. Promot. Phys. Act.* **2018**, *3*, 7–11.
30. Bogut, I. Prevalence of Foot Deformities in Young Schoolchildren in Slavonia. *Acta Clin. Croat.* **2019**. [CrossRef]

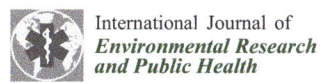

Article

Physical Fitness and the Level of Technical and Tactical Training of Kickboxers

Łukasz Rydzik * and Tadeusz Ambroży

Institute of Sports Sciences, University of Physical Education in Krakow, 31-541 Kraków, Poland; tadek@ambrozy.pl
* Correspondence: lukasz.gne@op.pl; Tel.: +48-730-696-377

Abstract: Background: Kickboxing is a dynamically progressing combat sport based on various techniques of punches and kicks. The high level of physical fitness underlies the optimal development of technique in the competitors. The objective of this study was the assessment of the level of fitness of kickboxers and the relationships between fitness and technical and tactical training. Methods: The study included 20 kickboxers aged 18–32 demonstrating the highest level of sporting performance. Their body mass ranged from 75 to 92 kg and their height from 175 to 187 cm. The selection of the group was intentional, and the criteria included training experience and the sports level assessed by the observation of the authors and opinion of the coach. The level of fitness was evaluated with the use of selected trials of International Committee on the Standardization of Physical Fitness Tests and Eurofit tests. Aerobic capacity was tested and indicators of efficiency, activeness and effectiveness of attacks were calculated. Results: A significant correlation between the indicators of technical and tactical training and results of fitness tests was shown. Conclusions: There exists a correlation between efficiency, activeness and effectiveness of attacks and the speed of upper limbs, explosive strength, static strength of a hand, agility, VO$_2$max and abdominal muscle strength.

Keywords: physical fitness; technical and tactical indicator; kickboxing

Citation: Rydzik, Ł.; Ambroży, T. Physical Fitness and the Level of Technical and Tactical Training of Kickboxers. *Int. J. Environ. Res. Public Health* **2021**, *18*, 3088. https://doi.org/10.3390/ijerph18063088

Academic Editors: Veronique Billat and Paul B. Tchounwou

Received: 7 February 2021
Accepted: 13 March 2021
Published: 17 March 2021

Publisher's Note: MDPI stays neutral with regard to jurisdictional claims in published maps and institutional affiliations.

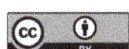

Copyright: © 2021 by the authors. Licensee MDPI, Basel, Switzerland. This article is an open access article distributed under the terms and conditions of the Creative Commons Attribution (CC BY) license (https://creativecommons.org/licenses/by/4.0/).

1. Introduction

General physical fitness is the locomotor basis on which a competitor can develop their professional techniques. There are a variety of different techniques in kickboxing which can be combined [1]. However, a proper level of technical and tactical training is the most important element of a competitor's success. Technical and tactical actions allow effective control in a bout and can almost entirely avoid a rival's attacks, simultaneously using offensive actions (counterattacks) [2]. Timing plays a key role, as it allows conducting an effective attack while simultaneously avoiding a rival's offensive actions [3]. Kickboxing is a combat sport in which competitors fight each other using kicks and punches [4]. Amateur fighters use protectors, which reduce trauma occurrence in fights [5]. There are many types of kickboxing (point fighting, light contact, kicklight, full contact, low kick) that have different rules. There are also many kickboxing organizations. The World Association of Kickboxing Organizations (WAKO) is the largest and the most significant of them [5].

Proper functioning of the cardiovascular system is the basis of the physical fitness of a kickboxer [6], which allows repeating highly intense actions during a whole fight, mainly because of the increase in the regeneration process [7]. Mean values of VO$_2$max of elite male kickboxers found in the literature range from 54 to 69 mL/kg/min [8,9].

Combat sports characterized by great intensity of actions are mostly based on anaerobic sources because decisive technical actions depend on quick and strong moves [10]. The energetic system adenosine triphosphate (ATP) and phosphocreatine (PCr) is very important for kickboxers because a proper strong blow can cause termination of a fight ahead of time (knock-out) [4,6]. A basic energetic source for this type of action includes anaerobic glycolysis; aerobic sources are important at the end of a fight (optimal aerobic and anaerobic endurance is necessary). A competitor's training should then include anaerobic power (dynamic kicks and punches) and strength and speed of upper limbs (blows and their combinations in attacks, blocks and ducks in defense) [11].

The strength of the muscles of upper and lower limbs plays an important role in winning in a kickboxing fight [12]. The results of isometric strength (e.g., the grip strength) are greatly accepted as indicators of the level of a kickboxer's strength [13,14]. The training process of kickboxers is diversified both in the context of the intensity of the training and the necessity of developing a wide range of motor skills [8,15]. Sports training in kickboxing is a subject of interest of many researchers [5,16,17]. A kickboxing fight is acyclic and its conditions change often (coordination and agility conditions). It has a holistic impact on the trainees and uses the whole organism, getting all groups of muscles active. The constantly changing situation in a bout requires good coordination and an immediate response to rival's actions. A bout duration is usually 3 × 2 min. and it characterizes many changes in effort intensity [11]. Physical effort is based on submaximal and maximal loads. The physiological profiles of competitors show that the physical training in kickboxing should be aimed at increasing both aerobic and anaerobic capacity. Due to training and starting loads (often at the level >90% VO_2max), muscle glycogen becomes the main source of energy. After terminating effort due to fatigue, glycogene is almost entirely used [18]. Using muscle glycogene in a given muscle group depends on the dynamics of movement in the ring, the frequency of changes in the intensity of the effort, methods of throwing kicks and punches and defensive reactions based mostly on anaerobic changes. Restoring glycogene takes place in after-effort restitution and its rate depends on many factors since there are moments of working on lower levels of VO_2max in competitions.

The optimal level of physical fitness of a competitor is the key element of efficiency in a sports competition. Thanks to defining the level of physical fitness, one can select training loads in the appropriate amounts of exercises with respect to both quality and quantity. Regular measurements of this level also allow the assessment of the effects of the training [19]. The strength and dynamics of upper limbs in kickboxing have been evaluated by measuring the distance in throwing a medicine ball [20,21], and the strength and the dynamics of lower limbs were evaluated by measuring the distance of a jump [8,22]. Kickboxers were observed to have high levels of strength, power, aerobic and anaerobic capacity combined with technical and tactical skills. This is the reason why physical training should be based on improving strength and capacity of the muscles in the limbs [23].

Due to detailed technical and tactical analyses it is possible to define competitors' training indicators as well as prove the existence of a relationship between the level of training and physical fitness of the participants. Technical and tactical analyses are common methods used in modifying the process of sport training in a group of martial arts and combat sports coaches and competitors. Interesting articles on this topic can be found in judo [24–26].

The results of the analysis of selected literature show that studies are concerned with success prognosis based on morpho-functional, physiological, biomechanical and psychosomatic indices [24], as well as assessment of capacity during fights [25,26]. Other studies were concerned with movement analysis [8], traumas and starting consequences [5,16]. A considerable deficit of texts regarding the level of training and the physical fitness of competitors was noted. The main objective of this paper is the assessment of the level of physical fitness of kickboxers in the highest sport level as well as finding a relationship between the fitness level and the indicators of technical and tactical training. Finding this correlation will determine whether the level of fitness influences activeness, effectiveness and efficiency of attacks and whether it allows more effective planning of sport training.

2. Materials and Methods

This study included 20 kickboxers presenting the highest level of sport. The selection of the group was intentional, and the criteria included training experience and the sports level assessed by observation of the authors and opinion of the coach. The participants were from 18 to 32 years old, their body mass ranged 75 to 92 kg and their height was between 175 and 187 cm. BMI of the participants ranged 24.13 to 28.73 kg/m^2 (Table 1).

Table 1. Anthropometric characteristic of the participants.

Variables	No	Mean	95% Confidence Interval		Median	Minimum	Maximum	1st Quartile	3rd Quartile	Standard Deviation
Body mass	20	84.90	82.59	87.21	85.50	75.00	92.00	83.00	88.50	4.93
Height	20	181.05	179.46	182.64	180.00	175.00	187.00	179.00	183.50	3.39
BMI	20	26.04	25.46	26.62	25.99	24.13	28.73	25.15	26.73	1.24

BMI-Body Mass Index.

2.1. Physical Fitness Tests

The physical fitness of the participants was assessed by selected tests taken from the tests developed by the International Committee on the Standardization of Physical Fitness Tests (ICSPFT) and European Fitness Test (EUROFIT) [27]. The entire test included the following:

1. Aerobic capacity test—VO$_2$max (description of the test below)
2. Tapping—Assessment of speed of upper hands. The subject stands in front of a table with their feet spread and puts their worst hand on a rectangular pad. Their better hand is placed on a farther disc. They should touch both discs alternatively as quick as possible. The subject makes a total of 50 moves, they touch each disc 25 times. They take two tests and the best one is noted; the time is rounded to a decimal place.
3. Standing long jump—Jumping with both feet from standing. The test measures the distance jumped in cm, which is an indicator of the possibility to quickly create strength. The subject stands with their feet lightly spread behind the start line, they bends their knees moving their arms backward, then they move their arms forward, bounce their feet from the ground and make a jump as long as possible. They land on both feet in a standing position. The test is taken twice. The longer jump is recorded, rounded to the nearest cm.
4. Grip strength using a dynamometer. Evaluating the isometric strength. The subject has their feet lightly spread, the dynamometer lies close to fingers, arm down along the body but without touching the body. Short grip on a dynamometer using maximum strength, second arm loose along the body. Best of two tests is recorded; the result is rounded to 1 kg.
5. Shuttle run (10 × 5 m). The subject runs on a signal to the second line 5 m away, crosses it with both feet and comes back. They run 10 times for a distance of 5 m, the time of the shuttle run is measured and rounded to a decimal place of a second.
6. Pull-ups—Evaluating shoulder girdle strength counting the number of repetitions. The subject catches a bar, their hands are spread in line with their shoulders and they do an overhang. On a signal they bend their arms and pull up their body so their beard should be above the bar. After a moment of rest they return to an overhang. They repeat the exercise as many times as possible. The result is the number of repetitions.
7. Sit-ups—Evaluating abdominal muscle strength. The subject lies on a mattress, their feet are 30 cm apart and their knees bent at 90 degrees, with hands on their neck. A partner holds the subject's feet so they stay on the ground. On a signal the subject performs sit-ups touching their knees with their elbows and coming back to lying down. The test lasts 30 s.
8. Flexibility test—The subject bends their torso forward when sitting down and the range of motion behind feet is measured in cm. The sitting subject moves a ruler with their hands on a box with a scale. The best of two tests is recorded.
9. Cooper's test—Running endurance—12-min run, distance is measured.

The tests were done by the authors, with tests 1–4 on the first day, and tests 5–9 on the second. The volume of training was reduced to 30–40% two days before the tests.

2.2. Measuring the Indicators of Technical and Tactical Training

The analysis of a sports bout was done based on digital recording of a fight. Then, the indicators of technical and tactical training were computed using the following formulas [5].

Efficiency of the attack (S_a)

$$Sa = \frac{n}{N}$$

n—Number of attacks awarded 1 pt.*
* In K1 formula each fair hit is awarded 1 pt.
N—Number of bouts.
Effectiveness of the attack (E_a)

$$Ea = \frac{number\ of\ efective\ attacks}{number\ of\ all\ attacks} \times 100$$

* An effective attack is a technical action awarded a point.
* Number of all attacks is the number of all offensive actions.
Activeness of the attack (A_a)

$$Aa = \frac{number\ of\ all\ registered\ offensive\ actions\ of\ a\ kickboxer}{number\ of\ bouts\ fought\ by\ a\ kickboxer}$$

2.3. VO$_2$max Measurement

The test of maximal oxygen intake (VO$_2$max) was done with the use of the Margaria test. The participants climbed a step 40 cm tall. In the first 6-minute period the frequency of climbing was 15/min, in the second was 25/min. During both parts, heart rate was measured with sportster (Polar). The maximal oxygen intake was computed based on the formula in [28].

$$VO_2max = \frac{HRmax(VO2II - VO2I) + HRII * VO2I * VO2II}{HRII - HRI}$$

where:
HRmax—max heart rate [beats/min.]
*HRmax computed according to Tanaka 2001 (208 − 0.7*age) [29]
HRI—heart rate during I part [beats/min.]
HRII—heart rate during II part [beats/min.]
VO2I—estimated oxygen intake during I part [mL/O /kg/min],
that requires ca. 22.0 [mL/O /kg/min]
VO2II—estimated oxygen intake during II part [mL/O /kg/min],
that requires ca. 23.4 [mL/O /kg/min]

2.4. Bioethical Committee

Prior to participation in the tests, the competitors were informed about the research procedures, which were in accordance with the ethical principles of the Declaration of Helsinki WMADH (2000). Obtaining the competitors' written consent was the condition for their participation in the project. The research was approved by the Bioethics Committee at the Regional Medical Chamber (No. 287/KBL/OIL/2020).

2.5. Statistical Analysis

Statistical analysis of the data was done with the use of Statistica 13.1 by StatSoft. Parametric tests were used due to meeting the basic assumptions concerning the consistency of studied distributions to a normal distribution and the homogeneity of the variance. The consistency of the distributions to a normal distribution was evaluated with the use of a Shapiro–Wilk test, and the homogeneity of variance was evaluated with the use of a Levene test. All descriptive statistics (mean, median, minimum, maximum, 95% confidence intervals, 1st and 3rd quartile and standard deviation) were computed for all variables. The correlation of two variables of a normal distribution was evaluated with the use of a Pearson's linear correlation coefficient. The level of statistical significance was set to $p < 0.05$.

3. Results

The results of the fitness tests of the participants are shown in Table 2.

Table 2. The rezults of fitness test.

Variables	Number	Mean	95% Confidence Interval		Median	Minimum	Maximum	1st Quartile	3rd Quartile	Standard Dev.
Plate tapping [s]	20	7.64	7.17	8.10	7.25	6.46	9.43	6.89	8.18	1.00
Standing long jump [cm]	20	205.25	198.14	212.36	210.00	167.00	225.00	198.00	216.50	15.19
Cooper's test [m]	20	3086.20	2928.53	3243.87	3003.50	2656.00	3920.00	2837.00	3327.50	336.88
Static strength of a right hand [kg]	20	55.96	55.06	56.85	56.16	51.22	58.65	55.06	57.13	1.91
Static strength of a left hand [kg]	20	54.70	53.67	55.73	55.12	50.26	58.30	53.22	56.44	2.20
Pull-ups on a bar [n]	20	18.05	16.21	19.89	17.00	10.00	26.00	15.50	21.50	3.94
Shuttle run [s]	20	11.02	10.62	11.42	10.93	10.01	13.45	10.36	11.38	0.85
Flexibility [cm]	20	15.98	15.67	16.29	15.90	15.00	18.00	15.65	16.30	0.65
Sit-ups [n]	20	30.35	28.03	32.67	31.50	23.00	39.00	25.50	34.50	4.97

The mean level of aerobic capacity was 47.65 mL/kg/min and the results ranged from 41 to 56 (Table 3).

Table 3. VO2max.

Variables	Number	Mean	95% Confidence Interval		Median	Minimum	Maximum	1st Quartile	3rd Quartile	Standard Dev.
VO$_2$max [mL/kg/min]	20	47.65	45.59	49.71	49.00	41.00	56.00	43.00	51.00	4.39

Activeness of the attack was 96.8 on average and it ranged from 64 to 133. Effectiveness of the attack was 47.85 on average and it ranged from 40.6 to 56.32. Efficiency of the attack was 50.45 on average and it ranged from 45 to 56 (Tables 3 and 4).

Table 4. Activeness, effectiveness and efficiency of attacks.

Variables	Number	Mean	95% Confidence Interval		Median	Minimum	Maximum	1st Quartile	3rd Quartile	Standard Dev.
Activeness	20	96.80	89.46	104.14	92.00	64.00	133.00	89.00	102.50	15.69
Effectiveness	20	47.84	45.00	50.69	45.29	40.60	56.32	42.44	53.79	6.08
Efficiency	20	50.45	48.83	52.07	50.50	45.00	56.00	48.00	53.00	3.47

A strong negative correlation between aerobic capacity and the speed of upper limb and between aerobic capacity and shuttle run was shown as well as a strong positive correlation between aerobic capacity and standing long jump and between aerobic capacity and endurance. There was also a strong correlation between VO$_2$max and static strength of both hands and between VO$_2$max and abdominal muscle strength. It was also proven that body mass was strongly positively correlated with the speed of upper limbs and shuttle run as well as being negatively correlated with standing long jump and endurance. Participants who were quicker and more agile also had higher levels of the indicators of activeness, effectiveness and efficiency of attacks (strong negative correlation of the indicators with speed and shuttle run and strong positive correlation with standing long jump and endurance). Participants who had higher results of standing long jump or Cooper's test also had higher levels of the indicators. The efficiency of attacks was correlated with abdominal muscle strength (Table 5).

Table 5. The influence of selected variables on the results of fitness tests.

Pearson's Linear Correlation Coefficient r Level of Significance p	VO_2max	Body Mass	Height	BMI	Activeness	Effectiveness	Efficiency
Plate tapping [s]	−0.89 0.001	0.80 0.001	0.52 0.020	0.55 0.013	−0.55 0.013	−0.79 0.001	−0.82 0.001
Standing long jump [cm]	0.85 0.001	−0.72 0.001	−0.57 0.009	−0.40 0.077	0.52 0.019	0.74 0.001	0.85 0.001
Cooper's test [m]	0.87 0.001	−0.87 0.001	−0.59 0.007	−0.50 0.026	0.80 0.001	0.67 0.001	0.70 0.001
Static strength of a right hand [kg]	0.74 0.001	−0.60 0.005	−0.61 0.004	−0.22 0.350	0.50 0.026	0.51 0.021	0.77 0.001
Static strength of a left hand [kg]	0.67 0.001	−0.55 0.012	−0.42 0.065	−0.54 0.015	0.34 0.143	0.65 0.002	0.73 0.001
Pull-ups on a bar [n]	−0.22 0.349	0.28 0.238	0.44 0.052	−0.07 0.766	−0.19 0.430	−0.19 0.415	−0.22 0.349
Shuttle run [s]	−0.85 0.001	0.82 0.001	0.71 0.001	0.33 0.155	−0.63 0.003	−0.70 0.001	−0.85 0.001
Flexibility [cm]	−0.14 0.550	−0.01 0.970	0.14 0.561	−0.03 0.903	−0.06 0.805	−0.06 0.817	−0.10 0.666
Sit-ups [n]	0.52 0.019	−0.26 0.263	−0.28 0.234	−0.13 0.587	0.13 0.587	0.42 0.068	0.49 0.027

Participants who had higher levels of VO_2max also had higher levels of indicators of activeness, effectiveness and efficiency of attacks. All correlations were strong and statistically significant. Moreover, lighter and shorter participants also had higher levels of the indicators. Correlations between body mass and the levels of indicators of activeness, effectiveness and efficiency of attacks were strong and the correlations between the height and the levels of indicators of activeness, effectiveness and efficiency of attacks were medium; all correlations were significant. Effectiveness of the attack was significantly negatively correlated to the BMI of the participants. The correlation had a medium strength (Table 6).

Table 6. The influence of selected variables on the activeness, the effectiveness and the efficiency of attacks.

Pearson's Linear Correlation Coefficient (r) Level of Significance p	VO_2max	Body Mass	Height	BMI
Activeness	0.72 0.001	−0.82 0.001	−0.58 0.007	−0.35 0.131
Effectiveness	0.70 0.001	−0.74 0.001	−0.58 0.007	−0.51 0.021
Efficiency	0.88 0.001	−0.71 0.001	−0.69 0.001	−0.32 0.175

4. Discussion

A kickboxing bout in a K1 rules competition is dynamic as well as comprehensive in the technical and tactical aspects [4]. Contenders who fight in the highest level competitions must have proper aerobic capacity. In this study, the mean result of the participants' level of VO_2max was 47.65 mL/kg/min, which can be interpreted as a high level of aerobic capacity [16,17]. In other combat sports the mean level of competitors' VO_2max was as follows: 40.8 mL/kg/min (judokas), 50.3 mL/kg/min (boxers), 58.4 mL/kg/min (MMA fighters) [30–32]. The participants of this study had better VO_2max level than judokas, but were worse than MMA fighters and comparable to boxers. Statistical analysis showed a strong and significant correlation between the level of VO_2max and the activeness, the effectiveness and the efficiency of the participants. This can show that the level of indicators of technical and tactical training depends on aerobic capacity and they can be related to general endurance of the organism (VO_2max underlies the endurance) that is considered as the basis of physical possibilities of a competitor [33]. Statistical analysis also showed significant negative correlations between the speed of upper limbs and the indicators of technical and tactical training. The correlations were strong (with the efficiency of the attack) and medium (with other indices). Similarly, there were strong (with the efficiency) and medium (with other indices) correlations between shuttle run and the indicators. Thus it follows that the competitors whose results in speed and agility test were worse, were more active and had greater effectiveness and efficiency of their attacks than the participants with better results in those tests. The higher the speed of the upper limbs, the higher the number of competitor's actions involving hand techniques in a round. Good upper limb speed also corresponds to better defensive actions. Due to great similarity in the actions involving upper limbs in both boxers and kickboxers, the analysis of the results of this study could be also done in the study of boxers and the results would be similar [34,35]. Competitors who had quicker upper limbs were able to use more techniques which resulted in increasing their activeness, effectiveness and efficiency indicators. Similar results were reached in assessing agility (as speed and coordination) which is characteristic and significant in kickboxing competitions. Thanks to a high level of agility it is possible to move more smoothly in a ring, which makes attacks more effective (one can surprise a rival with feints, change of pace and anticipating the attack) and improves defensive actions (dodging, ducks, turns). Speed and coordination are basic elements of a kickboxing fight and they underlie proper timing, which means using a technique in the right moment [8,15,23].

There were strong positive correlations between the results of most of the fitness tests and the levels of the indicators of technical and tactical training. It was shown that a high level of maximum anaerobic power was assessed with the use of the standing long jump test. It is worth noticing that Ambroży et al. proved that a high round kick was the most effective lower limb technique, and could often end a fight with a knock-out [4]. Dynamic strength determines the efficiency of doing kicks and it could also improve the indicators of technical and tactical training [36]. Static strength is an important element of the motor preparation of a competitor. Its high level gives the possibility of increasing the technical potential of a kickboxer [37]. In this study we showed the existence of medium strength significant correlations between the technical and tactical training indicators and the static strength of a hand. The analysis of the results shows that there is a medium strength relationship between the abdominal muscle strength and the effectiveness of a competitor in a kickboxing fight. The training process in kickboxing is based on comprehensive development of abdominal muscles, which guarantees an effective defense, protecting a fighter's torso. This is the reason why this relationship can be a direct effect of the training methods used.

This study showed a negative correlation between body mass and height vs. the level of indicators of technical and tactical training. The strength of the correlations was usually medium, and only in the case of the relationship between body mass and activeness of the attack was the correlation strong. Participants competing in lower weight categories can punch and kick faster but at the cost of the strength of a blow [38]. That could be a reason why lighter and shorter participants had better results of activeness, but also effectiveness and efficiency of attacks in comparison to heavier and taller kickboxers. Tests conducted in this study did not prove the existence of significant relationships between shoulder girdle strength (pull-ups) and the level of the indicators of technical and tactical training. Thus it follows that shoulder girdle strength is not a significant element of a kickboxing competition according to K1 rules. Similarly, there was no significant relationship between the level of agility and the level of the indicators of technical and tactical training. Competitors fighting according to K1 rules use mostly low kicks on the thigh or high round kicks that do not require an above average developed agility level.

This way of fighting could point, for example, to the lack of agility predispositions in some competitors, which, as can be seen, is not an element that could decide the win in a kickboxing fight.

5. Conclusions

Activeness, effectiveness and efficiency of the competitors expressed by the indicators of technical and tactical training show a strong correlation to the level of maximum oxygen intake VO_2max. It follows that kickboxers should work out the optimal level of aerobic capacity in a preparation term and then maintain this during the competitions. It should impact their starting possibilities.

The level of the speed of upper limbs and agility influence the starting possibilities measured with the use of the indicators of technical and tactical preparations. This is closely connected to efficiency of a kickboxing fight.

Efficiency, effectiveness and activeness of an attack depend on the level of muscle strength of upper, middle and lower parts of the body.

Somatic features of the competitors influence activeness, effectiveness and efficiency of attacks. The relationships show the necessity of controlling body mass before the start of a competition and keeping it at the optimum level in the aspect of weight categories.

Practical Implication

The training process of kickboxers fighting according to K1 rules should be based on the comprehensive development of a competitor in the aspects of strength, speed and endurance, while keeping the optimal body weight should underlie the training process.

Author Contributions: Conceptualization, Ł.R.; methodology, Ł.R.; validation, Ł.R.; formal analysis, Ł.R., T.A.; resources, Ł.R.; data curation, Ł.R.; writing—original draft preparation, Ł.R., T.A.; writing—review and editing, Ł.R., T.A.; supervision, T.A.; project administration, Ł.R.; funding acquisition, T.A. All authors have read and agreed to the published version of the manuscript. Please turn to the CRediT taxonomy for the term explanation. Authorship must be limited to those who have contributed substantially to the work reported.

Funding: This research received no external funding.

Institutional Review Board Statement: The research was approved by the Bioethics Committee at the Regional Medical Chamber (No. 287/KBL/OIL/2020)

Informed Consent Statement: Informed consent was obtained from all subjects involved in the study.

Data Availability Statement: The data presented in this study are available on request from the corresponding author.

Conflicts of Interest: The authors declare no conflict of interest.

References

1. Di Marino, S. *A Complete Guide to Kickboxing*; Enslow Publishing: New York, NY, USA, 2018.
2. Adam, M.; Sterkowicz-Przybycień, K. The efficiency of tactical and technical actions of the national teams of Japan and Russia at the World Championships in Judo (2013, 2014 and 2015). *Biomed. Hum. Kinet.* **2018**, *10*, 45–52. [CrossRef]
3. Malkov, O.B.; Romashov, A.A. Key differences in combat tactics, action triggers and self-commands in taekwondo and boxing. *Theory Pract. Phys. Cult.* **2018**, *7*, 21.
4. Ambroży, T.; Rydzik, Ł.; Kędra, A.; Ambroży, D.; Niewczas, M.; Sobiło, E.; Czarny, W. The effectiveness of kickboxing techniques and its relation to fights won by knockout. *Arch. Budo* **2020**, *16*, 11–17.
5. Rydzik, Ł.; Niewczas, M.; Kędra, A.; Grymanowski, J.; Czarny, W.; Ambroży, T. Relation of indicators of technical and tactical training to demerits of kickboxers fighting in K1 formula. *Arch. Budo Sci. Martial Arts Extrem. Sport.* **2020**, *16*, 1–5.

6. Buse, G.J. Kickboxing. In *Combat Sports Medicine. London*; Springer: London, UK, 2009; pp. 331–351.
7. Crisafulli, A.; Vitelli, S.; Cappai, I.; Milia, R.; Tocco, F.; Melis, F.; Concu, A. Physiological responses and energy cost during a simulation of a Muay Thai boxing match. *Appl. Physiol. Nutr. Metab.* **2009**, *34*, 143–150. [CrossRef] [PubMed]
8. Ouergui, I.; Hssin, N.; Haddad, M.; Padulo, J.; Franchini, E.; Gmada, N.; Bouhlel, E. The effects of five weeks of kickboxing training on physical fitness. *Muscles Ligaments Tendons J.* **2014**, *4*, 106–113. [CrossRef] [PubMed]
9. Ouergui, I.; Davis, P.; Houcine, N.; Marzouki, H.; Zaouali, M.; Franchini, E.; Gmada, N.; Bouhlel, E. Hormonal, Physiological, and Physical Performance During Simulated Kickboxing Combat: Differences Between Winners and Losers. *Int. J. Sports Physiol. Perform.* **2016**, *11*, 425–431. [CrossRef] [PubMed]
10. Chaabène, H.; Tabben, M.; Mkaouer, B.; Franchini, E.; Negra, Y.; Hammami, M.; Amara, S.; Chaabène, R.B.; Hachana, Y. Amateur Boxing: Physical and Physiological Attributes. *Sport. Med.* **2015**, *45*, 337–352. [CrossRef] [PubMed]
11. Łukasz Rydzik, P.K. *Przewodnik po Kickboxingu*; Wydawnictwo Aha: Łódź, Poland, 2018; ISBN 978-83-7299-722-8.
12. Zabukovec, R.; Tiidus, P.M. Physiological and anthropometric profile of elite kickboxers. *J. Strength Cond. Res.* **1995**, *9*, 240–242.
13. Salci, Y. The metabolic demands and ability to sustain work outputs during kickboxing competitions. *Int. J. Perform. Anal. Sport* **2015**, *15*, 39–52. [CrossRef]
14. Machado, S.; Souza, R.A.; Simão, A.; Jerônimo, D.; Silva, N.; Osorio, R.; Magini, M. Comparative study of isokinetic variables of the knee in taekwondo and kickboxing athletes. *Fit. Perform. J.* **2009**, *8*, 407–411. [CrossRef]
15. Buse, G.J.; Santana, J.C. Conditioning Strategies for Competitive Kickboxing. *Strength Cond. J.* **2008**, *30*, 42–48. [CrossRef]
16. Myers, J.; Kaminsky, L.A.; Lima, R.; Christle, J.W.; Ashley, E.; Arena, R. A Reference Equation for Normal Standards for VO2 Max: Analysis from the Fitness Registry and the Importance of Exercise National Database (FRIEND Registry). *Prog. Cardiovasc. Dis.* **2017**, *60*, 21–29. [CrossRef] [PubMed]
17. Silva, G.; Oliveira, N.L.; Aires, L.; Mota, J.; José Oliveira, J.C.R. Calculation and validation of models for estimating VO2 max from the 20-m shuttle run test in children and adolescents. *Arch. Exerc. Heal. Diseose* **2012**, *3*, 145–152. [CrossRef]
18. Górski, J. *Fizjologia Wysiłku i Treningu Fizycznego*; PZWL Wydawnictwo Lekarskie: Warszawa, Poland, 2019; ISBN 978-83-200-5676-1.
19. Mancha-Triguero, D.; García-Rubio, J.; Calleja-González, J.; Ibáñez, S.J. Physical fitness in basketball players: A systematic review. *J. Sports Med. Phys. Fit.* **2019**, *59*. [CrossRef] [PubMed]
20. Slimani, M.; Miarka, B.; Briki, W.; Cheour, F. Comparison of Mental Toughness and Power Test Performances in High-Level Kickboxers by Competitive Success. *Asian J. Sports Med.* **2016**, *7*, e30840. [CrossRef] [PubMed]
21. Ouergui, I.; Hammouda, O.; Chtourou, H.; Zarrouk, N.; Rebai, H.; Chaouachi, A. Anaerobic upper and lower body power measurements and perception of fatigue during a kick boxing match. *J. Sports Med. Phys. Fit.* **2013**, *53*, 455–460.
22. Nikolaïdis, P.; Fragkiadiakis, G.; Papadopoulos, V.; Karydis, N. Differences in Force-Velocity Characteristics of Upper and Lower Limbs of Male Kickboxers. *Balt. J. Health Phys. Act.* **2011**, *3*. [CrossRef]
23. Slimani, M.; Chaabene, H.; Miarka, B.; Franchini, E.; Chamari, K.; Cheour, F. Kickboxing review: Anthropometric, psychophysiological and activity profiles and injury epidemiology. *Biol. Sport* **2017**, *34*, 185–196. [CrossRef]
24. Kłys, A.; Sterkowicz-Przybycień, K.; Marek Adam, C.C. Performance analysis considering the technical-tactical variables in female judo athletes at different sport skill levels: Optimization of predictors. *J. Phys. Educ. Sport* **2020**, *20*, 1775–1782. [CrossRef]
25. Coswig, V.S.; Gentil, P.; Bueno, J.C.A.; Follmer, B.; Marques, V.A.; Del Vecchio, F.B. Physical fitness predicts technical-tactical and time-motion profile in simulated Judo and Brazilian Jiu-Jitsu matches. *PeerJ* **2018**, *6*, e4851. [CrossRef]
26. Miarka, B.; Pérez, D.I.V.; Aedo-Muñoz, E.; da Costa, L.O.F.; Brito, C.J. Technical-Tactical Behaviors Analysis of Male and Female Judo Cadets' Combats. *Front. Psychol.* **2020**, *11*. [CrossRef]
27. Talaga, J. *Sprawność Fizyczna Ogólna-Testy*; Zysk i S-ka: Poznań, Poland, 2004.
28. Halicka-Ambroziak, H.D.; Jusiak, R.; Martyn, A.; Opaszowski, B.H.; Szarska-Martyn, I.; Tyszkiewicz, M.; Wit, B. *Wskazówki do Ćwiczeń z Fizjologii dla Studentów Wychowania Fizycznego*; AWF Warszawa: Warszawa, Poland, 2004.
29. Tanaka, H.; Monahan, K.D.; Seals, D.R. Age-predicted maximal heart rate revisited. *J. Am. Coll. Cardiol.* **2001**, *37*, 153–156. [CrossRef]
30. Pałka, T.; Lech, G.; Tyka, A.; Tyka, A.; Sterkowicz-Przybycień, K.; Sterkowicz, S.; Cebula, A.; Stawiarska, A. Differences in the level of anaerobic and aerobic components of physical capacity in judoists at different age. *Arch. Budo* **2013**, *9*, 195–203.
31. Ambroży, T.; Snopkowski, P.; Mucha, D.; Tota, Ł. Observation and analysis of a boxing fight. *Secur. Econ. Law* **2015**, *4*, 58–71.
32. Tota, Ł.; Drwal, T.; Maciejczyk, M.; Szyguła, Z.; Pilch, W.; Pałka, T.; Lech, G. Effects of original physical training program on changes in body composition, upper limb peak power and aerobic performance of a mixed martial arts fighter. *Med. Sport* **2014**, *18*, 78–83. [CrossRef]
33. Boehncke, S.; Poettgen, K.; Maser-Gluth, C.; Reusch, J.; Boehncke, W.-H.; Badenhoop, K. Endurance capabilities of triathlon competitors with type 1 diabetes mellitus. *Dtsch. Med. Wochenschr.* **2009**, *134*, 677–682. [CrossRef] [PubMed]
34. Kimm, D.; Thiel, D.V. Hand Speed Measurements in Boxing. *Procedia Eng.* **2015**, *112*, 502–506. [CrossRef]
35. Sanchez Rodríguez, D.A.; Bohórquez Aldana, A.F. Análisis de la velocidad y la aceleración entre un golpe de boxeo y uno de taekwondo. *Rev. U.D.C.A Actual. Divulg. Científica* **2020**, *23*. [CrossRef]
36. Jalilov, A.A.; Balashova, V.F.; Podlubnaya, A.A. Elementary kicking leg movement biomechanics for body kicks in kickboxing. *Theory Pract. Phys. Cult.* **2019**, *1*, 90–93.

37. Suchomel, T.J.; Nimphius, S.; Bellon, C.R.; Stone, M.H. The Importance of Muscular Strength: Training Considerations. *Sport. Med.* **2018**, *48*, 765–785. [CrossRef] [PubMed]
38. Syrlybayev, S.; Iskakov, T.; Baltina, A. Study the impact force in boxing. *J. Phys. Educ. Sport* **2019**, *19*, 1720–1727. [CrossRef]

MDPI
St. Alban-Anlage 66
4052 Basel
Switzerland
Tel. +41 61 683 77 34
Fax +41 61 302 89 18
www.mdpi.com

International Journal of Environmental Research and Public Health Editorial Office
E-mail: ijerph@mdpi.com
www.mdpi.com/journal/ijerph

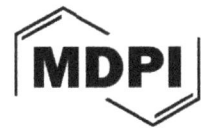

www.ingramcontent.com/pod-product-compliance
Lightning Source LLC
LaVergne TN
LVHW070426100526
838202LV00014B/1537